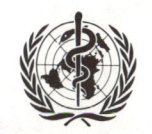

WORLD HEALTH ORGANIZATION

INTERNATIONAL AGENCY FOR RESEARCH ON CANCER

IARC MONOGRAPHS
ON THE
EVALUATION OF CARCINOGENIC RISKS TO HUMANS

Hepatitis Viruses

VOLUME 59

This publication represents the views and expert opinions
of an IARC Working Group on the
Evaluation of Carcinogenic Risks to Humans,
which met in Lyon,

8–15 June 1993

1994

IARC MONOGRAPHS

In 1969, the International Agency for Research on Cancer (IARC) initiated a programme on the evaluation of the carcinogenic risk of chemicals to humans involving the production of critically evaluated monographs on individual chemicals. In 1980 and 1986, the programme was expanded to include evaluations of carcinogenic risks associated with exposures to complex mixtures and other agents.

The objective of the programme is to elaborate and publish in the form of monographs critical reviews of data on carcinogenicity for agents to which humans are known to be exposed and on specific exposure situations; to evaluate these data in terms of human risk with the help of international working groups of experts in chemical carcinogenesis and related fields; and to indicate where additional research efforts are needed.

This project is supported by PHS Grant No. 5-UO1 CA33193-12 awarded by the US National Cancer Institute, Department of Health and Human Services. Additional support has been provided since 1986 by the Commission of the European Communities.

©International Agency for Research on Cancer 1994

ISBN 92 832 1259 2

ISSN 0250-9555

Publications of the World Health Organization enjoy copyright protection in accordance with the provisions of Protocol 2 of the Universal Copyright Convention.

All rights reserved. Application for rights of reproduction or translation, in part or *in toto*, should be made to the International Agency for Research on Cancer.

Distributed for the International Agency for Research on Cancer
by the Secretariat of the World Health Organization, Geneva

PRINTED IN THE UNITED KINGDOM

CONTENTS

NOTE TO THE READER 9

LIST OF PARTICIPANTS 11

PREAMBLE 17
    Background 17
    Objective and Scope 17
    Selection of Topics for Monographs 18
    Data for Monographs 19
    The Working Group 19
    Working Procedures 19
    Exposure Data 20
    Studies of Cancer in Humans 21
    Studies of Cancer in Experimental Animals 25
    Other Relevant Data 27
    Summary of Data Reported 28
    Evaluation 30
    References 34

GENERAL REMARKS 39

THE MONOGRAPHS

Hepatitis B virus 45
    1. Exposure data 45
        1.1 Structure and biology of hepatitis B virus (HBV) 45
            1.1.1 Structure of the virus 45
            1.1.2 Structure of HBV genome and gene products 45
            1.1.3 Replication of HBV 47
            1.1.4 HBV and related animal viruses 48
            1.1.5 HBV mutants 48
            1.1.6 Host range and target cells of HBV infection 50
        1.2 Methods of detection 50
            1.2.1 In serum and plasma 50
            1.2.2 In liver tissues 52

CONTENTS

    1.2.3 Interpretation of serological markers of HBV infection 53
  1.3 Epidemiology of infection 54
    1.3.1 Transmission 54
    1.3.2 Determinants of chronic infection 55
    1.3.3 Global patterns of chronic infection 55
  1.4 Clinical diseases (other than cancer) 57
    1.4.1 Acute infection 59
    1.4.2 Chronic infection 59
    1.4.3 Extrahepatic manifestations 61
  1.5 Therapy and immunoprophylaxis 62
    1.5.1 Therapy 62
    1.5.2 Immunoprophylaxis 63
2. Studies of cancer in humans 66
  2.1 Case series and case reports 66
    2.1.1 Hepatocellular carcinoma 66
    2.1.2 Other cancers 67
  2.2 Descriptive studies 67
  2.3 Cohort studies 67
    2.3.1 Prospective studies of general population groups 67
    2.3.2 Prospective studies of blood donors 70
    2.3.3 Prospective studies of populations with pre-existing disease 71
  2.4 Case–control studies 72
    2.4.1 Hepatocellular carcinoma 72
    2.4.2 Cholangiocarcinoma 97
    2.4.3 Other cancers 97
3. Studies of cancer in experimental animals 97
  3.1 Primates 97
    3.1.1 Infection with HBV 97
    3.1.2 Infection with HBV with concomitant administration of chemical
       carcinogens 99
  3.2 Transgenic mice 100
    3.2.1 With no concomitant administration of chemical carcinogens . . . 100
    3.2.2 With concomitant administration of known chemical
       carcinogens 100
  3.3 Woodchucks (*Marmota monax*) 103
    3.3.1 Hepatocellular carcinoma in woodchucks naturally infected with
       woodchuck hepatitis virus 103
    3.3.2 Hepatocellular carcinoma in woodchucks experimentally infected
       with woodchuck hepatitis virus 105
    3.3.3 Hepatocellular carcinoma in woodchucks experimentally infected
       with ground squirrel hepatitis virus 106

CONTENTS

  3.4 Ground squirrels, ducks and other species 106
    3.4.1 Beechey ground squirrels 106
    3.4.2 Richardson ground squirrels 108
    3.4.3 Ducks 109
    3.4.4 Other species 113
4. Other relevant data 113
  4.1 Pathology 113
    4.1.1 Acute hepatitis 113
    4.1.2 Chronic hepatitis 114
    4.1.3 Cirrhosis 114
    4.1.4 Evolution of hepatocellular carcinoma from cirrhosis 115
    4.1.5 Hepatocellular carcinoma 116
  4.2 Molecular biology 116
    4.2.1 Integration of HBV DNA 117
    4.2.2 Expression and potential oncogenic properties of HBV gene products 120
    4.2.3 Genetic alterations in hepatocellular carcinoma 123
  4.3 Other observations relevant to possible mechanisms of action of HBV in carcinogenesis 125
    4.3.1 Cell division and tissue regeneration in response to HBV infection 125
    4.3.2 Immune response 125
    4.3.3 Hepatocellular carcinoma-associated tumour markers 126
    4.3.4 Role of aflatoxins and possible modification of the effect of HBV 126
5. Summary of data reported and evaluation 126
  5.1 Exposure data 126
  5.2 Human carcinogenicity data 127
  5.3 Animal carcinogenicity data 128
  5.4 Other relevant data 128
  5.5 Evaluation 129
6. References 129

Hepatitis C virus 165

1. Exposure data 165
  1.1 Structure and biology of hepatitis C virus (HCV) 165
    1.1.1 Structure of the virus 165
    1.1.2 Structure of HCV genome and gene products 165
    1.1.3 Replication and gene expression of HCV 165
    1.1.4 HCV animal models 167
    1.1.5 Genotypes of HCV 167

CONTENTS

        1.1.6   Host range and target cells of HCV infection 167
   1.2   Methods of detection 168
        1.2.1   In serum and plasma 168
        1.2.2   In liver tissues 170
        1.2.3   Interpretation of serological markers of HCV infection 170
   1.3   Epidemiology of infection 171
        1.3.1   Parenteral exposure 173
        1.3.2   Non-parenteral exposure 175
   1.4   Clinical diseases (other than cancer) 179
        1.4.1   Acute infection 179
        1.4.2   Chronic infection 179
        1.4.3   Extrahepatic manifestations 180
   1.5   Therapy 181
        1.5.1   Acute and fulminant HCV infection 181
        1.5.2   Chronic HCV infection 181
2.   Studies of cancer in humans 182
   2.1   Case series 182
   2.2   Cohort studies 182
   2.3   Case–control studies 186
        2.3.1   First-generation assays 186
        2.3.2   Second-generation assays 190
   2.4   Modifying effects of seropositivity for hepatitis B surface antigen 195
3.   Studies of cancer in experimental animals 195
4.   Other relevant data 198
   4.1   Pathology 198
        4.1.1   Acute infection 198
        4.1.2   Chronic infection 199
        4.1.3   Cirrhosis and hepatocellular carcinoma 199
   4.2   Molecular biology 199
   4.3   Other observations relevant to possible mechanisms of action of HCV
        in carcinogenesis 200
5.   Summary of data reported and evaluation 200
   5.1   Exposure data 200
   5.2   Human carcinogenicity data 201
   5.3   Animal carcinogenicity data 202
   5.4   Other relevant data 202
   5.5   Evaluation 202
6.   References 202

CONTENTS

Hepatitis D virus 223
1. Exposure data 223
   1.1 Structure and biology of hepatitis D virus (HDV) 223
      1.1.1 Structure of the virus 223
      1.1.2 Structure of HDV genome and gene products 223
      1.1.3 Replication of HDV 225
      1.1.4 HDV-related animal models 225
      1.1.5 HDV mutants 225
      1.1.6 HDV-HBV interaction 226
      1.1.7 Host range and target cells of HDV infection 226
   1.2 Methods of detection 227
      1.2.1 In serum and plasma 227
      1.2.2 In liver tissues 227
      1.2.3 Serological markers of HDV infection 228
   1.3 Epidemiology of infection 229
      1.3.1 Prevalence 229
      1.3.2 Transmission 232
   1.4 Clinical diseases (other than cancer) 233
      1.4.1 Acute infection 233
      1.4.2 Chronic infection 234
   1.5 Therapy and immunoprophylaxis 235
      1.5.1 Therapy 235
      1.5.2 Immunoprophylaxis 235
2. Studies of cancer in humans 236
   2.1 Case series 236
   2.2 Case-control studies 236
3. Studies of cancer in experimental animals 239
4. Other relevant data 239
   4.1 Pathology 239
      4.1.1 Acute infection 239
      4.1.2 Chronic infection 240
      4.1.3 Cirrhosis 240
   4.2 Other observations relevant to possible mechanisms of action of HDV in carcinogenesis 240
5. Summary of data reported and evaluation 241
   5.1 Exposure data 241
   5.2 Human carcinogenicity data 242
   5.3 Animal carcinogenicity data 242
   5.4 Other relevant data 242
   5.5 Evaluation 242

CONTENTS

6. References 242
SUMMARY OF FINAL EVALUATIONS 255
SUPPLEMENTARY CORRIGENDA TO VOLUMES 1–58 257
CUMULATIVE INDEX TO THE *MONOGRAPHS* SERIES 259

NOTE TO THE READER

The term 'carcinogenic risk' in the *IARC Monographs* series is taken to mean the probability that exposure to an agent will lead to cancer in humans.

Inclusion of an agent in the *Monographs* does not imply that it is a carcinogen, only that the published data have been examined. Equally, the fact that an agent has not yet been evaluated in a monograph does not mean that it is not carcinogenic.

The evaluations of carcinogenic risk are made by international working groups of independent scientists and are qualitative in nature. No recommendation is given for regulation or legislation.

Anyone who is aware of published data that may alter the evaluation of the carcinogenic risk of an agent to humans is encouraged to make this information available to the Unit of Carcinogen Identification and Evaluation, International Agency for Research on Cancer, 150 cours Albert Thomas, 69372 Lyon Cedex 08, France, in order that the agent may be considered for re-evaluation by a future Working Group.

Although every effort is made to prepare the monographs as accurately as possible, mistakes may occur. Readers are requested to communicate any errors to the Unit of Carcinogen Identification and Evaluation, so that corrections can be reported in future volumes.

This volume is dedicated to Dr Lorenzo Tomatis, who initiated the *IARC Monographs* series in 1971 and retired in December 1993 after 12 years as Director of the Agency. The unflagging integrity and wisdom of Lorenzo Tomatis are the foundations for the respect that the *Monographs* command internationally.

IARC WORKING GROUP ON THE EVALUATION OF CARCINOGENIC RISKS TO HUMANS: HEPATITIS VIRUSES

Lyon, 8–15 June 1993

LIST OF PARTICIPANTS

Members[1]

V. Beral, Cancer Epidemiology Unit, Gibson Building, The Radcliffe Infirmary, Oxford OX2 6HE, United Kingdom

H. Blum, Department of Internal Medicine, Medical Clinic B, Rämistrasse 100, 8091 Zurich, Switzerland (*Vice-Chairman*)

M.-A. Buendia, Retroviruses Building, Pasteur Institute, 28 rue du Docteur Roux, 75724 Paris Cédex 15, France

J.R. Craig, St Jude Medical Center, 101 E. Valencia Mesa Drive, Fullerton, CA 92634, USA

T.A. Dragani, Division of Experimental Oncology A, National Institute for the Study and Treatment of Tumours, via Venezian 1, 20133 Milano, Italy

Y.T. Gao, Department of Epidemiology, Shanghai Cancer Institute, Shanghai, China

J.W. Grisham, The University of North Carolina at Chapel Hill, The School of Medicine, Department of Pathology, CB 7525, Brinkhous-Bullitt Building, Chapel Hill, NC 27599–7525, USA

A.J. Hall, Communicable Diseases Epidemiology Unit, London School of Hygiene and Tropical Medicine, Keppel Street, London WC1E 7HT, United Kingdom

J. Kaldor, National Centre in HIV Epidemiology and Clinical Research, St Vincent's Medical Centre, 2nd floor, 376 Victoria Street, Sydney, NSW 2010, Australia

M.C. Kew, Department of Medicine, University of Witwatersrand Medical School, 7 York Road, Parktown, 2193 Johannesburg, South Africa

---

[1]Unable to attend: C. Bréchot, INSERM U 75, Necker–Enfants Malades, 156 rue de Vaugirard, 75742 Paris Cédex 15, France; M. Colombo, Institute of Internal Medicine, via Pace 9, 20122 Milan, Italy; J.L. Gerin, Department of Microbiology, Georgetown University School of Medicine—School of Dentistry, 5640 Fishers Lane, Rockville, MD 20852, USA

G.M. Kirby, Lady Davis Research Institute, Jewish General Hospital, 3755 Cote St Catherine Road, Montréal, Québec, Canada H3T 1E2

W.T. London, Fox Chase Cancer Center, Liver Cancer Prevention Center, 7701 Burholme Avenue, Philadelphia, PA 19111, USA

P.L. Marion, Department of Medicine, Division of Infectious Diseases, Stanford University School of Medicine, Stanford, CA 94305, USA

A.B. Miller, Department of Preventive Medicine and Biostatistics, Faculty of Medicine, McMurrich Building, University of Toronto, Toronto, Ontario, Canada M5S 1A8 (*Chairman*)

J. Monjardino, Department of Medicine, St Mary's Hospital Medical School, London W2 1PG, United Kingdom

N. Müller, Department of Epidemiology, Harvard School of Public Health, 677 Huntington Avenue, Boston, MA 02115, USA

K. Nishioka, Japanese Red Cross Central Blood Center, 1–31 Hiroo 4-Chome, Shibuya-ku, Tokyo 150, Japan

M. Ozturk, Léon Bérard Centre, 28 rue Laënnec, 69373 Lyon Cédex 08, France

D. Trichopoulos, Department of Epidemiology, Harvard School of Public Health, 677 Huntington Avenue, Boston, MA 02115, USA

IARC Secretariat

B. Armstrong, Deputy Director[1]
P. Boffetta, Unit of Analytical Epidemiology
F.X. Bosch, Unit of Field and Intervention Studies[2]
E. Cardis, Unit of Analytical Epidemiology
M.-J. Ghess, Unit of Carcinogen Identification and Evaluation
E. Heseltine, 24290 St Léon-sur-Vézère, France
M.A. Kane, Microbiology and Immunology Support Services, World Health Organization, 1211 Geneva 27, Switzerland
V. Krutovskikh, Unit of Multistage Carcinogenesis
D. McGregor, Unit of Carcinogen Identification and Evaluation
D. Mietton, Unit of Carcinogen Identification and Evaluation
H. Møller, Unit of Carcinogen Identification and Evaluation
R. Montesano, Unit of Mechanisms of Carcinogenesis
N. Muñoz, Unit of Field and Intervention Studies
C. Partensky, Unit of Carcinogen Identification and Evaluation
I. Peterschmitt, Unit of Carcinogen Identification and Evaluation, Geneva, Switzerland
L. Tomatis, Director
H. Vainio, Unit of Carcinogen Identification and Evaluation

---

[1]Present adress: Australian Institute of Health and Welfare, GPO Box 570, Canberra ACT 2601, Australia
[2]Present address: Institut d'Oncologia, Unitat d'Epidemiologia, Hospital Duran i Reynals, Autovia Castelldefels K. 2,7, E-08907 Hospitalet del Llobregat (Barcelona), Spain

J. Wilbourn, Unit of Carcinogen Identification and Evaluation
C. Wild, Unit of Mechanisms of Carcinogenesis

Secretarial assistance

M. Lézère
J. Mitchell
S. Reynaud

PREAMBLE

IARC MONOGRAPHS PROGRAMME ON THE EVALUATION OF CARCINOGENIC RISKS TO HUMANS[1]

PREAMBLE

1. BACKGROUND

In 1969, the International Agency for Research on Cancer (IARC) initiated a programme to evaluate the carcinogenic risk of chemicals to humans and to produce monographs on individual chemicals. The *Monographs* programme has since been expanded to include consideration of exposures to complex mixtures of chemicals (which occur, for example, in some occupations and as a result of human habits) and of exposures to other agents, such as radiation and viruses. With Supplement 6 (IARC, 1987a), the title of the series was modified from *IARC Monographs on the Evaluation of the Carcinogenic Risk of Chemicals to Humans* to *IARC Monographs on the Evaluation of Carcinogenic Risks to Humans*, in order to reflect the widened scope of the programme.

The criteria established in 1971 to evaluate carcinogenic risk to humans were adopted by the working groups whose deliberations resulted in the first 16 volumes of the *IARC Monographs* series. Those criteria were subsequently updated by further ad-hoc working groups (IARC, 1977, 1978, 1979, 1982, 1983, 1987b, 1988, 1991a; Vainio *et al.*, 1992).

2. OBJECTIVE AND SCOPE

The objective of the programme is to prepare, with the help of international working groups of experts, and to publish in the form of monographs, critical reviews and evaluations of evidence on the carcinogenicity of a wide range of human exposures. The *Monographs* may also indicate where additional research efforts are needed.

The *Monographs* represent the first step in carcinogenic risk assessment, which involves examination of all relevant information in order to assess the strength of the available evidence that certain exposures could alter the incidence of cancer in humans. The second step is quantitative risk estimation. Detailed, quantitative evaluations of epidemiological data may be made in the *Monographs*, but without extrapolation beyond the range of the data

---

[1]This project is supported by PHS Grant No. 5-UO1 CA33193-12 awarded by the US National Cancer Institute, Department of Health and Human Services. Since 1986, the programme has also been supported by the Commission of the European Communities.

available. Quantitative extrapolation from experimental data to the human situation is not undertaken.

The term 'carcinogen' is used in these monographs to denote an exposure that is capable of increasing the incidence of malignant neoplasms; the induction of benign neoplasms may in some circumstances (see p. 26) contribute to the judgement that the exposure is carcinogenic. The terms 'neoplasm' and 'tumour' are used interchangeably.

Some epidemiological and experimental studies indicate that different agents may act at different stages in the carcinogenic process, and several different mechanisms may be involved. The aim of the *Monographs* has been, from their inception, to evaluate evidence of carcinogenicity at any stage in the carcinogenesis process, independently of the underlying mechanisms. Information on mechanisms may, however, be used in making the overall evaluation (IARC, 1991a; Vainio *et al.*, 1992; see also pp. 32–34).

The *Monographs* may assist national and international authorities in making risk assessments and in formulating decisions concerning any necessary preventive measures. The evaluations of IARC working groups are scientific, qualitative judgements about the evidence for or against carcinogenicity provided by the available data. These evaluations represent only one part of the body of information on which regulatory measures may be based. Other components of regulatory decisions may vary from one situation to another and from country to country, responding to different socioeconomic and national priorities. **Therefore, no recommendation is given with regard to regulation or legislation, which are the responsibility of individual governments and/or other international organizations.**

The *IARC Monographs* are recognized as an authoritative source of information on the carcinogenicity of a wide range of human exposures. A users' survey, made in 1988, indicated that the *Monographs* are consulted by various agencies in 57 countries. Each volume is generally printed in 4000 copies for distribution to governments, regulatory bodies and interested scientists. The *Monographs* are also available *via* the Distribution and Sales Service of the World Health Organization.

3. SELECTION OF TOPICS FOR MONOGRAPHS

Topics are selected on the basis of two main criteria: (a) there is evidence of human exposure, and (b) there is some evidence or suspicion of carcinogenicity. The term 'agent' is used to include individual chemical compounds, groups of related chemical compounds, physical agents (such as radiation) and biological factors (such as viruses). Exposures to mixtures of agents may occur in occupational exposures and as a result of personal and cultural habits (like smoking and dietary practices). Chemical analogues and compounds with biological or physical characteristics similar to those of suspected carcinogens may also be considered, even in the absence of data on a possible carcinogenic effect in humans or experimental animals.

The scientific literature is surveyed for published data relevant to an assessment of carcinogenicity. The IARC surveys of chemicals being tested for carcinogenicity (IARC, 1973–1992) and directories of on-going research in cancer epidemiology (IARC, 1976–1992) often indicate those exposures that may be scheduled for future meetings. Ad-hoc working groups convened by IARC in 1984, 1989 and 1991 gave recommendations as to which agents should be evaluated in the *IARC Monographs* series (IARC, 1984, 1989, 1991b).

As significant new data on subjects on which monographs have already been prepared become available, re-evaluations are made at subsequent meetings, and revised monographs are published.

4. DATA FOR MONOGRAPHS

The *Monographs* do not necessarily cite all the literature concerning the subject of an evaluation. Only those data considered by the Working Group to be relevant to making the evaluation are included.

With regard to biological and epidemiological data, only reports that have been published or accepted for publication in the openly available scientific literature are reviewed by the working groups. In certain instances, government agency reports that have undergone peer review and are widely available are considered. Exceptions may be made on an ad-hoc basis to include unpublished reports that are in their final form and publicly available, if their inclusion is considered pertinent to making a final evaluation (see pp. 30 *et seq.*). In the sections on chemical and physical properties, on analysis, on production and use and on occurrence, unpublished sources of information may be used.

5. THE WORKING GROUP

Reviews and evaluations are formulated by a working group of experts. The tasks of the group are: (i) to ascertain that all appropriate data have been collected; (ii) to select the data relevant for the evaluation on the basis of scientific merit; (iii) to prepare accurate summaries of the data to enable the reader to follow the reasoning of the Working Group; (iv) to evaluate the results of epidemiological and experimental studies on cancer; (v) to evaluate data relevant to the understanding of mechanism of action; and (vi) to make an overall evaluation of the carcinogenicity of the exposure to humans.

Working Group participants who contributed to the considerations and evaluations within a particular volume are listed, with their addresses, at the beginning of each publication. Each participant who is a member of a working group serves as an individual scientist and not as a representative of any organization, government or industry. In addition, nominees of national and international agencies and industrial associations may be invited as observers.

6. WORKING PROCEDURES

Approximately one year in advance of a meeting of a working group, the topics of the monographs are announced and participants are selected by IARC staff in consultation with other experts. Subsequently, relevant biological and epidemiological data are collected by IARC from recognized sources of information on carcinogenesis, including data storage and retrieval systems such as BIOSIS, Chemical Abstracts, CANCERLIT, MEDLINE and TOXLINE—including EMIC and ETIC for data on genetic and related effects and reproductive and developmental effects, respectively.

For chemicals and some complex mixtures, the major collection of data and the preparation of first drafts of the sections on chemical and physical properties, on analysis, on production and use and on occurrence are carried out under a separate contract funded by the US National Cancer Institute. Representatives from industrial associations may assist in the preparation of sections on production and use. Information on production and trade is obtained from governmental and trade publications and, in some cases, by direct contact with industries. Separate production data on some agents may not be available because their publication could disclose confidential information. Information on uses may be obtained from published sources but is often complemented by direct contact with manufacturers. Efforts are made to supplement this information with data from other national and international sources.

Six months before the meeting, the material obtained is sent to meeting participants, or is used by IARC staff, to prepare sections for the first drafts of monographs. The first drafts are compiled by IARC staff and sent, prior to the meeting, to all participants of the Working Group for review.

The Working Group meets in Lyon for seven to eight days to discuss and finalize the texts of the monographs and to formulate the evaluations. After the meeting, the master copy of each monograph is verified by consulting the original literature, edited and prepared for publication. The aim is to publish monographs within nine months of the Working Group meeting.

The available studies are summarized by the Working Group, with particular regard to the qualitative aspects discussed below. In general, numerical findings are indicated as they appear in the original report; units are converted when necessary for easier comparison. The Working Group may conduct additional analyses of the published data and use them in their assessment of the evidence; the results of such supplementary analyses are given in square brackets. When an important aspect of a study, directly impinging on its interpretation, should be brought to the attention of the reader, a comment is given in square brackets.

7. EXPOSURE DATA

Sections that indicate the extent of past and present human exposure, the sources of exposure, the people most likely to be exposed and the factors that contribute to the exposure are included at the beginning of each monograph.

Most monographs on individual chemicals, groups of chemicals or complex mixtures include sections on chemical and physical data, on analysis, on production and use and on occurrence. In monographs on, for example, physical agents, occupational exposures and cultural habits, other sections may be included, such as: historical perspectives, description of an industry or habit, chemistry of the complex mixture or taxonomy. Monographs on biological agents have sections on structure and biology, methods of detection, epidemiology of infection and clinical disease other than cancer.

For chemical exposures, the Chemical Abstracts Services Registry Number, the latest Chemical Abstracts Primary Name and the IUPAC Systematic Name are recorded; other synonyms are given, but the list is not necessarily comprehensive. For biological agents, taxonomy and structure are described, and the degree of variability is given, when applicable.

Information on chemical and physical properties and, in particular, data relevant to identification, occurrence and biological activity are included. For biological agents, mode of replication, life cycle, target cells, persistence and latency and host response are given. A description of technical products of chemicals includes trades names, relevant specifications and available information on composition and impurities. Some of the trade names given may be those of mixtures in which the agent being evaluated is only one of the ingredients.

The purpose of the section on analysis or detection is to give the reader an overview of current methods, with emphasis on those widely used for regulatory purposes. Methods for monitoring human exposure are also given, when available. No critical evaluation or recommendation of any of the methods is meant or implied. The IARC publishes a series of volumes, *Environmental Carcinogens: Methods of Analysis and Exposure Measurement* (IARC, 1978–93), that describe validated methods for analysing a wide variety of chemicals and mixtures. For biological agents, methods of detection and exposure assessment are described, including their sensitivity, specificity and reproducibility.

The dates of first synthesis and of first commercial production of a chemical or mixture are provided; for agents which do not occur naturally, this information may allow a reasonable estimate to be made of the date before which no human exposure to the agent could have occurred. The dates of first reported occurrence of an exposure are also provided. In addition, methods of synthesis used in past and present commercial production and different methods of production which may give rise to different impurities are described.

Data on production, international trade and uses are obtained for representative regions, which usually include Europe, Japan and the USA. It should not, however, be inferred that those areas or nations are necessarily the sole or major sources or users of the agent. Some identified uses may not be current or major applications, and the coverage is not necessarily comprehensive. In the case of drugs, mention of their therapeutic uses does not necessarily represent current practice nor does it imply judgement as to their therapeutic efficacy.

Information on the occurrence of an agent or mixture in the environment is obtained from data derived from the monitoring and surveillance of levels in occupational environments, air, water, soil, foods and animal and human tissues. When available, data on the generation, persistence and bioaccumulation of the agent are also included. In the case of mixtures, industries, occupations or processes, information is given about all agents present. For processes, industries and occupations, a historical description is also given, noting variations in chemical composition, physical properties and levels of occupational exposure with time and place. For biological agents, the epidemiology of infection is described.

Statements concerning regulations and guidelines (e.g., pesticide registrations, maximal levels permitted in foods, occupational exposure limits) are included for some countries as indications of potential exposures, but they may not reflect the most recent situation, since such limits are continuously reviewed and modified. The absence of information on regulatory status for a country should not be taken to imply that that country does not have regulations with regard to the exposure. For biological agents, legislation and control, including vaccines and therapy, are described.

8. STUDIES OF CANCER IN HUMANS

(a) *Types of studies considered*

Three types of epidemiological studies of cancer contribute to the assessment of carcinogenicity in humans—cohort studies, case–control studies and correlation (or ecological) studies. Rarely, results from randomized trials may be available. Case reports of cancer in humans may also be reviewed.

Cohort and case–control studies relate individual exposures under study to the occurrence of cancer in individuals and provide an estimate of relative risk (ratio of incidence in those exposed to incidence in those not exposed) as the main measure of association.

In correlation studies, the units of investigation are usually whole populations (e.g., in particular geographical areas or at particular times), and cancer frequency is related to a summary measure of the exposure of the population to the agent, mixture or exposure circumstance under study. Because individual exposure is not documented, however, a causal relationship is less easy to infer from correlation studies than from cohort and case–control studies. Case reports generally arise from a suspicion, based on clinical experience, that the concurrence of two events—that is, a particular exposure and occurrence of a cancer—has happened rather more frequently than would be expected by chance. Case reports usually lack complete ascertainment of cases in any population, definition or enumeration of the population at risk and estimation of the expected number of cases in the absence of exposure. The uncertainties surrounding interpretation of case reports and correlation studies make them inadequate, except in rare instances, to form the sole basis for inferring a causal relationship. When taken together with case–control and cohort studies, however, relevant case reports or correlation studies may add materially to the judgement that a causal relationship is present.

Epidemiological studies of benign neoplasms, presumed preneoplastic lesions and other end-points thought to be relevant to cancer are also reviewed by working groups. They may, in some instances, strengthen inferences drawn from studies of cancer itself.

(b) Quality of studies considered

The *Monographs* are not intended to summarize all published studies. Those that are judged to be inadequate or irrelevant to the evaluation are generally omitted. They may be mentioned briefly, particularly when the information is considered to be a useful supplement to that in other reports or when they provide the only data available. Their inclusion does not imply acceptance of the adequacy of the study design or of the analysis and interpretation of the results, and limitations are clearly outlined in square brackets at the end of the study description.

It is necessary to take into account the possible roles of bias, confounding and chance in the interpretation of epidemiological studies. By 'bias' is meant the operation of factors in study design or execution that lead erroneously to a stronger or weaker association than in fact exists between disease and an agent, mixture or exposure circumstance. By 'confounding' is meant a situation in which the relationship with disease is made to appear stronger or to appear weaker than it truly is as a result of an association between the apparent causal factor and another factor that is associated with either an increase or decrease in the incidence of the disease. In evaluating the extent to which these factors have been minimized in an individual study, working groups consider a number of aspects of design and analysis as described in the report of the study. Most of these considerations apply equally to case–control, cohort and correlation studies. Lack of clarity of any of these aspects in the reporting of a study can decrease its credibility and the weight given to it in the final evaluation of the exposure.

Firstly, the study population, disease (or diseases) and exposure should have been well defined by the authors. Cases of disease in the study population should have been identified in a way that was independent of the exposure of interest, and exposure should have been assessed in a way that was not related to disease status.

Secondly, the authors should have taken account in the study design and analysis of other variables that can influence the risk of disease and may have been related to the exposure of interest. Potential confounding by such variables should have been dealt with either in the design of the study, such as by matching, or in the analysis, by statistical adjustment. In cohort studies, comparisons with local rates of disease may be more appropriate than those with national rates. Internal comparisons of disease frequency among individuals at different levels of exposure should also have been made in the study.

Thirdly, the authors should have reported the basic data on which the conclusions are founded, even if sophisticated statistical analyses were employed. At the very least, they should have given the numbers of exposed and unexposed cases and controls in a case–control study and the numbers of cases observed and expected in a cohort study. Further tabulations by time since exposure began and other temporal factors are also important. In a cohort study, data on all cancer sites and all causes of death should have been given, to reveal the possibility of reporting bias. In a case–control study, the effects of investigated factors other than the exposure of interest should have been reported.

Finally, the statistical methods used to obtain estimates of relative risk, absolute rates of cancer, confidence intervals and significance tests, and to adjust for confounding should have been clearly stated by the authors. The methods used should preferably have been the generally accepted techniques that have been refined since the mid-1970s. These methods have been reviewed for case–control studies (Breslow & Day, 1980) and for cohort studies (Breslow & Day, 1987).

(c) *Inferences about mechanism of action*

Detailed analyses of both relative and absolute risks in relation to temporal variables, such as age at first exposure, time since first exposure, duration of exposure, cumulative exposure and time since exposure ceased, are reviewed and summarized when available. The analysis of temporal relationships can be useful in formulating models of carcinogenesis. In particular, such analyses may suggest whether a carcinogen acts early or late in the process of carcinogenesis, although at best they allow only indirect inferences about the mechanism of action. Special attention is given to measurements of biological markers of carcinogen exposure or action, such as DNA or protein adducts, as well as markers of early steps in the carcinogenic process, such as proto-oncogene mutation, when these are incorporated into epidemiological studies focused on cancer incidence or mortality. Such measurements may allow inferences to be made about putative mechanisms of action (IARC, 1991a; Vainio *et al.*, 1992).

(d) *Criteria for causality*

After the quality of individual epidemiological studies of cancer has been summarized and assessed, a judgement is made concerning the strength of evidence that the agent, mixture or exposure circumstance in question is carcinogenic for humans. In making their judgement, the Working Group considers several criteria for causality. A strong association (i.e., a large relative risk) is more likely to indicate causality than a weak association, although it is recognized that relative risks of small magnitude do not imply lack of causality and may be important if the disease is common. Associations that are replicated in several studies of the same design or using different epidemiological approaches or under different circumstances of exposure are more likely to represent a causal relationship than isolated observations from single studies. If there are inconsistent results among investigations, possible reasons are sought (such as differences in amount of exposure), and results of studies judged to be of high quality are given more weight than those from studies judged to be methodologically less sound. When suspicion of carcinogenicity arises largely from a single study, these data are not combined with those from later studies in any subsequent reassessment of the strength of the evidence.

If the risk of the disease in question increases with the amount of exposure, this is considered to be a strong indication of causality, although absence of a graded response is not necessarily evidence against a causal relationship. Demonstration of a decline in risk after cessation of or reduction in exposure in individuals or in whole populations also supports a causal interpretation of the findings.

Although a carcinogen may act upon more than one target, the specificity of an association (i.e., an increased occurrence of cancer at one anatomical site or of one morphological type) adds plausibility to a causal relationship, particularly when excess cancer occurrence is limited to one morphological type within the same organ.

Although rarely available, results from randomized trials showing different rates among exposed and unexposed individuals provide particularly strong evidence for causality.

When several epidemiological studies show little or no indication of an association between an exposure and cancer, the judgement may be made that, in the aggregate, they show evidence of lack of carcinogenicity. Such a judgement requires first of all that the studies giving rise to it meet, to a sufficient degree, the standards of design and analysis described above. Specifically, the possibility that bias, confounding or misclassification of exposure or outcome could explain the observed results should be considered and excluded with reasonable certainty. In addition, all studies that are judged to be methodologically sound should be consistent with a relative risk of unity for any observed level of exposure and, when considered together, should provide a pooled estimate of relative risk which is at or near unity and has a narrow confidence interval, due to sufficient population size. Moreover, no individual study nor the pooled results of all the studies should show any consistent tendency for relative risk of cancer to increase with increasing level of exposure. It is important to note that evidence of lack of carcinogenicity obtained in this way from several epidemiological studies can apply only to the type(s) of cancer studied and to dose levels and intervals between first exposure and observation of disease that are the same as or less than those observed in all the studies. Experience with human cancer indicates that, in some cases, the period from first exposure to the development of clinical cancer is seldom less than 20 years; latent periods substantially shorter than 30 years cannot provide evidence for lack of carcinogenicity.

9. STUDIES OF CANCER IN EXPERIMENTAL ANIMALS

All known human carcinogens that have been studied adequately in experimental animals have produced positive results in one or more animal species (Wilbourn *et al.*, 1986; Tomatis *et al.*, 1989). For several agents (aflatoxins, 4-aminobiphenyl, azathioprine, betel quid with tobacco, BCME and CMME (technical grade), chlorambucil, chlornaphazine, ciclosporin, coal-tar pitches, coal-tars, combined oral contraceptives, cyclophosphamide, diethylstilboestrol, melphalan, 8-methoxypsoralen plus UVA, mustard gas, myleran, 2-naphthylamine, nonsteroidal oestrogens, oestrogen replacement therapy/steroidal oestrogens, solar radiation, thiotepa and vinyl chloride), carcinogenicity in experimental animals was established or highly suspected before epidemiological studies confirmed the carcinogenicity in humans (Vainio *et al.*, 1994). Although this association cannot establish that all agents and mixtures that cause cancer in experimental animals also cause cancer in humans, nevertheless, **in the absence of adequate data on humans, it is biologically plausible and prudent to regard agents and mixtures for which there is sufficient evidence (see p. 31) of carcinogenicity in experimental animals as if they presented a carcinogenic risk to humans.** The possibility that a given agent may cause cancer through a species-specific mechanism which does not operate in humans (see p. 32) should also be taken into consideration.

The nature and extent of impurities or contaminants present in the chemical or mixture being evaluated are given when available. Animal strain, sex, numbers per group, age at start of treatment and survival are reported.

Other types of studies summarized include: experiments in which the agent or mixture was administered in conjunction with known carcinogens or factors that modify carcinogenic effects; studies in which the end-point was not cancer but a defined precancerous lesion; and experiments on the carcinogenicity of known metabolites and derivatives.

For experimental studies of mixtures, consideration is given to the possibility of changes in the physicochemical properties of the test substance during collection, storage, extraction, concentration and delivery. Chemical and toxicological interactions of the components of mixtures may result in nonlinear dose–response relationships.

An assessment is made as to the relevance to human exposure of samples tested in experimental animals, which may involve consideration of: (i) physical and chemical characteristics, (ii) constituent substances that indicate the presence of a class of substances, (iii) the results of tests for genetic and related effects, including genetic activity profiles, DNA adduct profiles, proto-oncogene mutation and expression and suppressor gene inactivation. The relevance of results obtained, for example, with animal viruses analogous to the virus being evaluated in the monograph must also be considered. They may provide biological and mechanistic information relevant to the understanding of the process of carcinogenesis in humans and may strengthen the plausibility of a conclusion that the biological agent that is being evaluated is carcinogenic in humans.

(a) Qualitative aspects

An assessment of carcinogenicity involves several considerations of qualitative importance, including (i) the experimental conditions under which the test was performed, including route and schedule of exposure, species, strain, sex, age, duration of follow-up; (ii) the consistency of the results, for example, across species and target organ(s); (iii) the spectrum of neoplastic response, from preneoplastic lesions and benign tumours to malignant neoplasms; and (iv) the possible role of modifying factors.

As mentioned earlier (p. 19), the *Monographs* are not intended to summarize all published studies. Those studies in experimental animals that are inadequate (e.g., too short a duration, too few animals, poor survival; see below) or are judged irrelevant to the evaluation are generally omitted. Guidelines for conducting adequate long-term carcinogenicity experiments have been outlined (e.g., Montesano *et al.*, 1986).

Considerations of importance to the Working Group in the interpretation and evaluation of a particular study include: (i) how clearly the agent was defined and, in the case of mixtures, how adequately the sample characterization was reported; (ii) whether the dose was adequately monitored, particularly in inhalation experiments; (iii) whether the doses and duration of treatment were appropriate and whether the survival of treated animals was similar to that of controls; (iv) whether there were adequate numbers of animals per group; (v) whether animals of both sexes were used; (vi) whether animals were allocated randomly to groups; (vii) whether the duration of observation was adequate; and (viii) whether the data were adequately reported. If available, recent data on the incidence of specific tumours in historical controls, as well as in concurrent controls, should be taken into account in the evaluation of tumour response.

When benign tumours occur together with and originate from the same cell type in an organ or tissue as malignant tumours in a particular study and appear to represent a stage in the progression to malignancy, it may be valid to combine them in assessing tumour incidence (Huff *et al.*, 1989). The occurrence of lesions presumed to be preneoplastic may in certain instances aid in assessing the biological plausibility of any neoplastic response observed. If an agent or mixture induces only benign neoplasms that appear to be end-points that do not readily undergo transition to malignancy, it should nevertheless be suspected of being a carcinogen and it requires further investigation.

(b) Quantitative aspects

The probability that tumours will occur may depend on the species, sex, strain and age of the animal, the dose of the carcinogen and the route and length of exposure. Evidence of an increased incidence of neoplasms with increased level of exposure strengthens the inference of a causal association between the exposure and the development of neoplasms.

The form of the dose–response relationship can vary widely, depending on the particular agent under study and the target organ. Both DNA damage and increased cell division are important aspects of carcinogenesis, and cell proliferation is a strong determinant of dose–response relationships for some carcinogens (Cohen & Ellwein, 1990). Since many chemicals require metabolic activation before being converted into their reactive intermediates, both metabolic and pharmacokinetic aspects are important in determining the dose–response pattern. Saturation of steps such as absorption, activation, inactivation and elimination may produce nonlinearity in the dose–response relationship, as could saturation of processes such as DNA repair (Hoel *et al.*, 1983; Gart *et al.*, 1986).

(c) Statistical analysis of long-term experiments in animals

Factors considered by the Working Group include the adequacy of the information given for each treatment group: (i) the number of animals studied and the number examined histologically, (ii) the number of animals with a given tumour type and (iii) length of survival. The statistical methods used should be clearly stated and should be the generally accepted techniques refined for this purpose (Peto *et al.*, 1980; Gart *et al.*, 1986). When there is no difference in survival between control and treatment groups, the Working Group usually compares the proportions of animals developing each tumour type in each of the groups. Otherwise, consideration is given as to whether or not appropriate adjustments have been made for differences in survival. These adjustments can include: comparisons of the proportions of tumour-bearing animals among the effective number of animals (alive at the time the first tumour is discovered), in the case where most differences in survival occur before tumours appear; life-table methods, when tumours are visible or when they may be considered 'fatal' because mortality rapidly follows tumour development; and the Mantel-Haenszel test or logistic regression, when occult tumours do not affect the animals' risk of dying but are 'incidental' findings at autopsy.

In practice, classifying tumours as fatal or incidental may be difficult. Several survival-adjusted methods have been developed that do not require this distinction (Gart *et al.*, 1986), although they have not been fully evaluated.

10. OTHER RELEVANT DATA

In coming to an overall evaluation of carcinogenicity in humans (see p. 32), the Working Group also considers related data. The nature of the information selected for summary depends on the agent being considered.

For chemicals and complex mixtures of chemicals such as those in some occupational situations and in cultural habits (e.g., tobacco smoking), the other data considered to be relevant are divided into those on absorption, distribution, metabolism and excretion; those on toxic effects; reproductive and developmental effects; and genetic and related effects.

Concise information is given on absorption, distribution (including placental transfer) and excretion in both humans and experimental animals. Kinetic factors that may affect the dose–response relationship, such as saturation of uptake, protein binding, metabolic activation, detoxification and DNA repair processes, are mentioned. Studies that indicate the metabolic fate of the agent in humans and in experimental animals are summarized briefly, and comparisons of data from humans and animals are made when possible. Comparative information on the relationship between exposure and the dose that reaches the target site may be of particular importance for extrapolation between species. Data are given on acute and chronic toxic effects (other than cancer), such as organ toxicity, increased cell proliferation, immunotoxicity and endocrine effects. The presence and toxicological significance of cellular receptors is described. Effects on reproduction, teratogenicity, fetotoxicity and embryotoxicity are also summarized briefly.

Tests of genetic and related effects are described in view of the relevance of gene mutation and chromosomal damage to carcinogenesis (Vainio *et al.*, 1992). The adequacy of the reporting of sample characterization is considered and, where necessary, commented upon; with regard to complex mixtures, such comments are similar to those described for animal carcinogenicity tests on p. 25. The available data are interpreted critically by phylogenetic group according to the end-points detected, which may include DNA damage, gene mutation, sister chromatid exchange, micronucleus formation, chromosomal aberrations, aneuploidy and cell transformation. The concentrations employed are given, and mention is made of whether use of an exogenous metabolic system *in vitro* affected the test result. These data are given as listings of test systems, data and references; bar graphs (activity profiles) and corresponding summary tables with detailed information on the preparation of the profiles (Waters *et al.*, 1987) are given in appendices.

Positive results in tests using prokaryotes, lower eukaryotes, plants, insects and cultured mammalian cells suggest that genetic and related effects could occur in mammals. Results from such tests may also give information about the types of genetic effect produced and about the involvement of metabolic activation. Some end-points described are clearly genetic in nature (e.g., gene mutations and chromosomal aberrations), while others are to a greater or lesser degree associated with genetic effects (e.g., unscheduled DNA synthesis). In-vitro tests for tumour-promoting activity and for cell transformation may be sensitive to changes that are not necessarily the result of genetic alterations but that may have specific relevance to the process of carcinogenesis. A critical appraisal of these tests has been published (Montesano *et al.*, 1986).

Genetic or other activity manifest in experimental mammals and humans is regarded as being of greater relevance than that in other organisms. The demonstration that an agent or mixture can induce gene and chromosomal mutations in whole mammals indicates that it may have carcinogenic activity, although this activity may not be detectably expressed in any or all species. Relative potency in tests for mutagenicity and related effects is not a reliable indicator of carcinogenic potency. Negative results in tests for mutagenicity in selected tissues from animals treated *in vivo* provide less weight, partly because they do not exclude the possibility of an effect in tissues other than those examined. Moreover, negative results in short-term tests with genetic end-points cannot be considered to provide evidence to rule out carcinogenicity of agents or mixtures that act through other mechanisms (e.g., receptor-mediated effects, cellular toxicity with regenerative proliferation, peroxisome proliferation) (Vainio *et al.*, 1992). Factors that may lead to misleading results in short-term tests have been discussed in detail elsewhere (Montesano *et al.*, 1986).

When available, data relevant to mechanisms of carcinogenesis that do not involve structural changes at the level of the gene are also described.

The adequacy of epidemiological studies of reproductive outcome and genetic and related effects in humans is evaluated by the same criteria as are applied to epidemiological studies of cancer.

Structure–activity relationships that may be relevant to an evaluation of the carcinogenicity of an agent are also described.

For biological agents—viruses, bacteria and parasites—other data relevant to carcinogenicity include descriptions of the pathology of infection, molecular biology (integration and expression of viruses, and any genetic alterations seen in human tumours) and other observations, which might include cellular and tissue responses to infection, immune response and the presence of tumour markers.

11. SUMMARY OF DATA REPORTED

In this section, the relevant epidemiological and experimental data are summarized. Only reports, other than in abstract form, that meet the criteria outlined on p. 19 are considered for evaluating carcinogenicity. Inadequate studies are generally not summarized: such studies are usually identified by a square-bracketed comment in the preceding text.

(a) Exposures

Human exposure to chemicals and complex mixtures is summarized on the basis of elements such as production, use, occurrence in the environment and determinations in human tissues and body fluids. Quantitative data are given when available. Exposure to biological agents is described in terms of transmission, and prevalence of infection.

(b) Carcinogenicity in humans

Results of epidemiological studies that are considered to be pertinent to an assessment of human carcinogenicity are summarized. When relevant, case reports and correlation studies are also summarized.

(c) Carcinogenicity in experimental animals

Data relevant to an evaluation of carcinogenicity in animals are summarized. For each animal species and route of administration, it is stated whether an increased incidence of neoplasms or preneoplastic lesions was observed, and the tumour sites are indicated. If the agent or mixture produced tumours after prenatal exposure or in single-dose experiments, this is also indicated. Negative findings are also summarized. Dose–response and other quantitative data may be given when available.

(d) Other data relevant to an evaluation of carcinogenicity and its mechanisms

Data on biological effects in humans that are of particular relevance are summarized. These may include toxicological, kinetic and metabolic considerations and evidence of DNA binding, persistence of DNA lesions or genetic damage in exposed humans. Toxicological information, such as that on cytotoxicity and regeneration, receptor binding and hormonal and immunological effects, and data on kinetics and metabolism in experimental animals are given when considered relevant to the possible mechanism of the carcinogenic action of the agent. The results of tests for genetic and related effects are summarized for whole mammals, cultured mammalian cells and nonmammalian systems.

When available, comparisons of such data for humans and for animals, and particularly animals that have developed cancer, are described.

Structure–activity relationships are mentioned when relevant.

For the agent, mixture or exposure circumstance being evaluated, the available data on end-points or other phenomena relevant to mechanisms of carcinogenesis from studies in humans, experimental animals and tissue and cell test systems are summarized within one or more of the following descriptive dimensions:

(i) Evidence of genotoxicity (i.e., structural changes at the level of the gene): for example, structure–activity considerations, adduct formation, mutagenicity (effect on specific genes), chromosomal mutation/aneuploidy

(ii) Evidence of effects on the expression of relevant genes (i.e., functional changes at the intracellular level): for example, alterations to the structure or quantity of the product of a proto-oncogene or tumour suppressor gene, alterations to metabolic activation/-inactivation/DNA repair

(iii) Evidence of relevant effects on cell behaviour (i.e., morphological or behavioural changes at the cellular or tissue level): for example, induction of mitogenesis, compensatory cell proliferation, preneoplasia and hyperplasia, survival of premalignant or malignant cells (immortalization, immunosuppression), effects on metastatic potential

(iv) Evidence from dose and time relationships of carcinogenic effects and interactions between agents: for example, early/late stage, as inferred from epidemiological studies; initiation/promotion/progression/malignant conversion, as defined in animal carcinogenicity experiments; toxicokinetics

These dimensions are not mutually exclusive, and an agent may fall within more than one of them. Thus, for example, the action of an agent on the expression of relevant genes could be summarized under both the first and second dimension, even if it were known with reasonable certainty that those effects resulted from genotoxicity.

12. EVALUATION

Evaluations of the strength of the evidence for carcinogenicity arising from human and experimental animal data are made, using standard terms.

It is recognized that the criteria for these evaluations, described below, cannot encompass all of the factors that may be relevant to an evaluation of carcinogenicity. In considering all of the relevant data, the Working Group may assign the agent, mixture or exposure circumstance to a higher or lower category than a strict interpretation of these criteria would indicate.

(a) Degrees of evidence for carcinogenicity in humans and in experimental animals and supporting evidence

These categories refer only to the strength of the evidence that an exposure is carcinogenic and not to the extent of its carcinogenic activity (potency) nor to the mechanisms involved. A classification may change as new information becomes available.

An evaluation of degree of evidence, whether for a single agent or a mixture, is limited to the materials tested, as defined physically, chemically or biologically. When the agents evaluated are considered by the Working Group to be sufficiently closely related, they may be grouped together for the purpose of a single evaluation of degree of evidence.

(i) *Carcinogenicity in humans*

The applicability of an evaluation of the carcinogenicity of a mixture, process, occupation or industry on the basis of evidence from epidemiological studies depends on the variability over time and place of the mixtures, processes, occupations and industries. The Working Group seeks to identify the specific exposure, process or activity which is considered most likely to be responsible for any excess risk. The evaluation is focused as narrowly as the available data on exposure and other aspects permit.

The evidence relevant to carcinogenicity from studies in humans is classified into one of the following categories:

Sufficient evidence of carcinogenicity: The Working Group considers that a causal relationship has been established between exposure to the agent, mixture or exposure circumstance and human cancer. That is, a positive relationship has been observed between the exposure and cancer in studies in which chance, bias and confounding could be ruled out with reasonable confidence.

Limited evidence of carcinogenicity: A positive association has been observed between exposure to the agent, mixture or exposure circumstance and cancer for which a causal interpretation is considered by the Working Group to be credible, but chance, bias or confounding could not be ruled out with reasonable confidence.

Inadequate evidence of carcinogenicity: The available studies are of insufficient quality, consistency or statistical power to permit a conclusion regarding the presence or absence of a causal association, or no data on cancer in humans are available.

Evidence suggesting lack of carcinogenicity: There are several adequate studies covering the full range of levels of exposure that human beings are known to encounter, which are mutually consistent in not showing a positive association between exposure to the agent, mixture or exposure circumstance and any studied cancer at any observed level of exposure. A conclusion of 'evidence suggesting lack of carcinogenicity' is inevitably limited to the cancer sites, conditions and levels of exposure and length of observation covered by the available studies. In addition, the possibility of a very small risk at the levels of exposure studied can never be excluded.

In some instances, the above categories may be used to classify the degree of evidence related to carcinogenicity in specific organs or tissues.

(ii) *Carcinogenicity in experimental animals*

The evidence relevant to carcinogenicity in experimental animals is classified into one of the following categories:

Sufficient evidence of carcinogenicity: The Working Group considers that a causal relationship has been established between the agent or mixture and an increased incidence of malignant neoplasms or of an appropriate combination of benign and malignant neoplasms in (a) two or more species of animals or (b) in two or more independent studies in one species carried out at different times or in different laboratories or under different protocols.

Exceptionally, a single study in one species might be considered to provide sufficient evidence of carcinogenicity when malignant neoplasms occur to an unusual degree with regard to incidence, site, type of tumour or age at onset.

Limited evidence of carcinogenicity: The data suggest a carcinogenic effect but are limited for making a definitive evaluation because, e.g., (a) the evidence of carcinogenicity is restricted to a single experiment; or (b) there are unresolved questions regarding the adequacy of the design, conduct or interpretation of the study; or (c) the agent or mixture increases the incidence only of benign neoplasms or lesions of uncertain neoplastic potential, or of certain neoplasms which may occur spontaneously in high incidences in certain strains.

Inadequate evidence of carcinogenicity: The studies cannot be interpreted as showing either the presence or absence of a carcinogenic effect because of major qualitative or quantitative limitations, or no data on cancer in experimental animals are available.

Evidence suggesting lack of carcinogenicity: Adequate studies involving at least two species are available which show that, within the limits of the tests used, the agent or mixture is not carcinogenic. A conclusion of evidence suggesting lack of carcinogenicity is inevitably limited to the species, tumour sites and levels of exposure studied.

(b) *Other data relevant to the evaluation of carcinogenicity*

Other evidence judged to be relevant to an evaluation of carcinogenicity and of sufficient importance to affect the overall evaluation is then described. This may include data on preneoplastic lesions, tumour pathology, genetic and related effects, structure–activity relationships, metabolism and pharmacokinetics, physicochemical parameters and analogous biological agents.

Data relevant to mechanisms of the carcinogenic action are also evaluated. The strength of the evidence that any carcinogenic effect observed is due to a particular mechanism is assessed, using terms such as weak, moderate or strong. Then, the Working Group assesses if that particular mechanism is likely to be operative in humans. The strongest indications that a particular mechanism operates in humans come from data on humans or biological specimens obtained from exposed humans. The data may be considered to be especially relevant if they show that the agent in question has caused changes in exposed humans that are on the causal pathway to carcinogenesis. Such data may, however, never become available, because it is at least conceivable that certain compounds may be kept from human use solely on the basis of evidence of their toxicity and/or carcinogenicity in experimental systems.

For complex exposures, including occupational and industrial exposures, chemical composition and the potential contribution of carcinogens known to be present are considered by the Working Group in its overall evaluation of human carcinogenicity. The Working Group also determines the extent to which the materials tested in experimental systems are related to those to which humans are exposed.

(c) *Overall evaluation*

Finally, the body of evidence is considered as a whole, in order to reach an overall evaluation of the carcinogenicity to humans of an agent, mixture or circumstance of exposure.

An evaluation may be made for a group of chemical compounds that have been evaluated by the Working Group. In addition, when supporting data indicate that other, related compounds for which there is no direct evidence of capacity to induce cancer in humans or in animals may also be carcinogenic, a statement describing the rationale for this conclusion is added to the evaluation narrative; an additional evaluation may be made for this broader group of compounds if the strength of the evidence warrants it.

The agent, mixture or exposure circumstance is described according to the wording of one of the following categories, and the designated group is given. The categorization of an agent, mixture or exposure circumstance is a matter of scientific judgement, reflecting the strength of the evidence derived from studies in humans and in experimental animals and from other relevant data.

Group 1—The agent (mixture) is carcinogenic to humans.
The exposure circumstance entails exposures that are carcinogenic to humans.

This category is used when there is *sufficient evidence* of carcinogenicity in humans. Exceptionally, an agent (mixture) may be placed in this category when evidence in humans is less than sufficient but there is *sufficient evidence* of carcinogenicity in experimental animals and strong evidence in exposed humans that the agent (mixture) acts through a relevant mechanism of carcinogenicity.

Group 2

This category includes agents, mixtures and exposure circumstances for which, at one extreme, the degree of evidence of carcinogenicity in humans is almost sufficient, as well as those for which, at the other extreme, there are no human data but for which there is evidence of carcinogenicity in experimental animals. Agents, mixtures and exposure circumstances are assigned to either group 2A (probably carcinogenic to humans) or group 2B (possibly carcinogenic to humans) on the basis of epidemiological and experimental evidence of carcinogenicity and other relevant data.

Group 2A—The agent (mixture) is probably carcinogenic to humans.
The exposure circumstance entails exposures that are probably carcinogenic to humans.

This category is used when there is *limited evidence* of carcinogenicity in humans and *sufficient evidence* of carcinogenicity in experimental animals. In some cases, an agent (mixture) may be classified in this category when there is *inadequate evidence* of carcinogenicity in humans and *sufficient evidence* of carcinogenicity in experimental animals and strong evidence that the carcinogenesis is mediated by a mechanism that also operates in humans. Exceptionally, an agent, mixture or exposure circumstance may be classified in this category solely on the basis of *limited evidence* of carcinogenicity in humans.

Group 2B—The agent (mixture) is possibly carcinogenic to humans.
The exposure circumstance entails exposures that are possibly carcinogenic to humans.

This category is used for agents, mixtures and exposure circumstances for which there is *limited evidence* of carcinogenicity in humans and less than *sufficient evidence* of carcinogenicity in experimental animals. It may also be used when there is *inadequate evidence* of carcinogenicity in humans but there is *sufficient evidence* of carcinogenicity in experimental animals. In some instances, an agent, mixture or exposure circumstance for which there is *inadequate evidence* of carcinogenicity in humans but *limited evidence* of carcinogenicity in experimental animals together with supporting evidence from other relevant data may be placed in this group.

Group 3—The agent (mixture or exposure circumstance) is not classifiable as to its carcinogenicity to humans.

This category is used most commonly for agents, mixtures and exposure circumstances for which the evidence of carcinogenicity is inadequate in humans and inadequate or limited in experimental animals.

Exceptionally, agents (mixtures) for which the evidence of carcinogenicity is inadequate in humans but sufficient in experimental animals may be placed in this category when there is strong evidence that the mechanism of carcinogenicity in experimental animals does not operate in humans.

Agents, mixtures and exposure circumstances that do not fall into any other group are also placed in this category.

Group 4—The agent (mixture) is probably not carcinogenic to humans.

This category is used for agents or mixtures for which there is *evidence suggesting lack of carcinogenicity* in humans and in experimental animals. In some instances, agents or mixtures for which there is *inadequate evidence* of carcinogenicity in humans but *evidence suggesting lack of carcinogenicity* in experimental animals, consistently and strongly supported by a broad range of other relevant data, may be classified in this group.

References

Breslow, N.E. & Day, N.E. (1980) *Statistical Methods in Cancer Research*, Vol. 1, *The Analysis of Case-control Studies* (IARC Scientific Publications No. 32), Lyon, IARC

Breslow, N.E. & Day, N.E. (1987) *Statistical Methods in Cancer Research*, Vol. 2, *The Design and Analysis of Cohort Studies* (IARC Scientific Publications No. 82), Lyon, IARC

Cohen, S.M. & Ellwein, L.B. (1990) Cell proliferation in carcinogenesis. *Science*, 249, 1007–1011

Gart, J.J., Krewski, D., Lee, P.N., Tarone, R.E. & Wahrendorf, J. (1986) *Statistical Methods in Cancer Research*, Vol. 3, *The Design and Analysis of Long-term Animal Experiments* (IARC Scientific Publications No. 79), Lyon, IARC

Hoel, D.G., Kaplan, N.L. & Anderson, M.W. (1983) Implication of nonlinear kinetics on risk estimation in carcinogenesis. *Science*, 219, 1032–1037

Huff, J.E., Eustis, S.L. & Haseman, J.K. (1989) Occurrence and relevance of chemically induced benign neoplasms in long-term carcinogenicity studies. *Cancer Metastasis Rev.*, 8, 1–21

IARC (1973–1992) *Information Bulletin on the Survey of Chemicals Being Tested for Carcinogenicity/Directory of Agents Being Tested for Carcinogenicity*, Numbers 1–15, Lyon

> Number 1 (1973)   52 pages
> Number 2 (1973)   77 pages
> Number 3 (1974)   67 pages
> Number 4 (1974)   97 pages
> Number 5 (1975)   88 pages
> Number 6 (1976)   360 pages
> Number 7 (1978)   460 pages
> Number 8 (1979)   604 pages
> Number 9 (1981)   294 pages
> Number 10 (1983) 326 pages
> Number 11 (1984) 370 pages
> Number 12 (1986) 385 pages
> Number 13 (1988) 404 pages
> Number 14 (1990) 369 pages
> Number 15 (1992) 317 pages

IARC (1976–1992)

> *Directory of On-going Research in Cancer Epidemiology 1976*. Edited by C.S. Muir & G. Wagner, Lyon

Directory of On-going Research in Cancer Epidemiology 1977 (IARC Scientific Publications No. 17). Edited by C.S. Muir & G. Wagner, Lyon

Directory of On-going Research in Cancer Epidemiology 1978 (IARC Scientific Publications No. 26). Edited by C.S. Muir & G. Wagner, Lyon

Directory of On-going Research in Cancer Epidemiology 1979 (IARC Scientific Publications No. 28). Edited by C.S. Muir & G. Wagner, Lyon

Directory of On-going Research in Cancer Epidemiology 1980 (IARC Scientific Publications No. 35). Edited by C.S. Muir & G. Wagner, Lyon

Directory of On-going Research in Cancer Epidemiology 1981 (IARC Scientific Publications No. 38). Edited by C.S. Muir & G. Wagner, Lyon

Directory of On-going Research in Cancer Epidemiology 1982 (IARC Scientific Publications No. 46). Edited by C.S. Muir & G. Wagner, Lyon

Directory of On-going Research in Cancer Epidemiology 1983 (IARC Scientific Publications No. 50). Edited by C.S. Muir & G. Wagner, Lyon

Directory of On-going Research in Cancer Epidemiology 1984 (IARC Scientific Publications No. 62). Edited by C.S. Muir & G. Wagner, Lyon

Directory of On-going Research in Cancer Epidemiology 1985 (IARC Scientific Publications No. 69). Edited by C.S. Muir & G. Wagner, Lyon

Directory of On-going Research in Cancer Epidemiology 1986 (IARC Scientific Publications No. 80). Edited by C.S. Muir & G. Wagner, Lyon

Directory of On-going Research in Cancer Epidemiology 1987 (IARC Scientific Publications No. 86). Edited by D.M. Parkin & J. Wahrendorf, Lyon

Directory of On-going Research in Cancer Epidemiology 1988 (IARC Scientific Publications No. 93). Edited by M. Coleman & J. Wahrendorf, Lyon

Directory of On-going Research in Cancer Epidemiology 1989/90 (IARC Scientific Publications No. 101). Edited by M. Coleman & J. Wahrendorf, Lyon

Directory of On-going Research in Cancer Epidemiology 1991 (IARC Scientific Publications No. 110). Edited by M. Coleman & J. Wahrendorf, Lyon

Directory of On-going Research in Cancer Epidemiology 1992 (IARC Scientific Publications No. 117). Edited by M. Coleman, J. Wahrendorf & E. Demaret, Lyon

IARC (1977) *IARC Monographs Programme on the Evaluation of the Carcinogenic Risk of Chemicals to Humans. Preamble* (IARC intern. tech. Rep. No. 77/002), Lyon

IARC (1978) *Chemicals with* Sufficient Evidence *of Carcinogenicity in Experimental Animals*—IARC Monographs *Volumes 1–17* (IARC intern. tech. Rep. No. 78/003), Lyon

IARC (1978–1993) *Environmental Carcinogens. Methods of Analysis and Exposure Measurement*:

    Vol. 1. *Analysis of Volatile Nitrosamines in Food* (IARC Scientific Publications No. 18). Edited by R. Preussmann, M. Castegnaro, E.A. Walker & A.E. Wasserman (1978)

    Vol. 2. *Methods for the Measurement of Vinyl Chloride in Poly(vinyl chloride), Air, Water and Foodstuffs* (IARC Scientific Publications No. 22). Edited by D.C.M. Squirrell & W. Thain (1978)

    Vol. 3. *Analysis of Polycyclic Aromatic Hydrocarbons in Environmental Samples* (IARC Scientific Publications No. 29). Edited by M. Castegnaro, P. Bogovski, H. Kunte & E.A. Walker (1979)

    Vol. 4. *Some Aromatic Amines and Azo Dyes in the General and Industrial Environment* (IARC Scientific Publications No. 40). Edited by L. Fishbein, M. Castegnaro, I.K. O'Neill & H. Bartsch (1981)

Vol. 5. *Some Mycotoxins* (IARC Scientific Publications No. 44). Edited by L. Stoloff, M. Castegnaro, P. Scott, I.K. O'Neill & H. Bartsch (1983)

Vol. 6. N-*Nitroso Compounds* (IARC Scientific Publications No. 45). Edited by R. Preussmann, I.K. O'Neill, G. Eisenbrand, B. Spiegelhalder & H. Bartsch (1983)

Vol. 7. *Some Volatile Halogenated Hydrocarbons* (IARC Scientific Publications No. 68). Edited by L. Fishbein & I.K. O'Neill (1985)

Vol. 8. *Some Metals: As, Be, Cd, Cr, Ni, Pb, Se, Zn* (IARC Scientific Publications No. 71). Edited by I.K. O'Neill, P. Schuller & L. Fishbein (1986)

Vol. 9. *Passive Smoking* (IARC Scientific Publications No. 81). Edited by I.K. O'Neill, K.D. Brunnemann, B. Dodet & D. Hoffmann (1987)

Vol. 10. *Benzene and Alkylated Benzenes* (IARC Scientific Publications No. 85). Edited by L. Fishbein & I.K. O'Neill (1988)

Vol. 11. *Polychlorinated Dioxins and Dibenzofurans* (IARC Scientific Publications No. 108). Edited by C. Rappe, H.R. Buser, B. Dodet & I.K. O'Neill (1991)

Vol. 12. *Indoor Air* (IARC Scientific Publications No. 109). Edited by B. Seifert, H. van de Wiel, B. Dodet & I.K. O'Neill (1993)

IARC (1979) *Criteria to Select Chemicals for* IARC Monographs (IARC intern. tech. Rep. No. 79/003), Lyon

IARC (1982) *IARC Monographs on the Evaluation of the Carcinogenic Risk of Chemicals to Humans, Supplement 4, Chemicals, Industrial Processes and Industries Associated with Cancer in Humans (IARC Monographs, Volumes 1 to 29)*, Lyon

IARC (1983) *Approaches to Classifying Chemical Carcinogens According to Mechanism of Action* (IARC intern. tech. Rep. No. 83/001), Lyon

IARC (1984) *Chemicals and Exposures to Complex Mixtures Recommended for Evaluation in* IARC Monographs *and Chemicals and Complex Mixtures Recommended for Long-term Carcinogenicity Testing* (IARC intern. tech. Rep. No. 84/002), Lyon

IARC (1987a) *IARC Monographs on the Evaluation of Carcinogenic Risks to Humans*, Supplement 6, *Genetic and Related Effects: An Updating of Selected* IARC Monographs *from Volumes 1 to 42*, Lyon

IARC (1987b) *IARC Monographs on the Evaluation of Carcinogenic Risks to Humans*, Supplement 7, *Overall Evaluations of Carcinogenicity: An Updating of* IARC Monographs *Volumes 1 to 42*, Lyon

IARC (1988) *Report of an IARC Working Group to Review the Approaches and Processes Used to Evaluate the Carcinogenicity of Mixtures and Groups of Chemicals* (IARC intern. tech. Rep. No. 88/002), Lyon

IARC (1989) *Chemicals, Groups of Chemicals, Mixtures and Exposure Circumstances to be Evaluated in Future IARC Monographs, Report of an ad hoc Working Group* (IARC intern. tech. Rep. No. 89/004), Lyon

IARC (1991a) *A Consensus Report of an* IARC Monographs *Working Group on the Use of Mechanims of Carcinogenesis in Risk Identification* (IARC intern. tech. Rep. No. 91/002), Lyon

IARC (1991b) *Report of an Ad-hoc* IARC Monographs *Advisory Group on Viruses and Other Biological Agents Such as Parasites* (IARC intern. tech. Rep. No. 91/001), Lyon

Montesano, R., Bartsch, H., Vainio, H., Wilbourn, J. & Yamasaki, H., eds (1986) *Long-term and Short-term Assays for Carcinogenesis—A Critical Appraisal* (IARC Scientific Publications No. 83), Lyon, IARC

Peto, R., Pike, M.C., Day, N.E., Gray, R.G., Lee, P.N., Parish, S., Peto, J., Richards, S. & Wahrendorf, J. (1980) Guidelines for simple, sensitive significance tests for carcinogenic effects in long-term animal experiments. In: *IARC Monographs on the Evaluation of the Carcinogenic Risk of Chemicals to Humans*, Supplement 2, *Long-term and Short-term Screening Assays for Carcinogens: A Critical Appraisal*, Lyon, pp. 311–426

Tomatis, L., Aitio, A., Wilbourn, J. & Shuker, L. (1989) Human carcinogens so far identified. *Jpn. J. Cancer Res.*, *80*, 795–807

Vainio, H., Magee, P., McGregor, D. & McMichael, A., eds (1992) *Mechanisms of Carcinogenesis in Risk Identification* (IARC Scientific Publications No. 116), Lyon, IARC

Vainio, H., Wilbourn, J. & Tomatis, L. (1994) Identification of environmental carcinogens: the first step in risk assessment. In: Mehlman, M.A. & Upton, A., eds, *The Identification and Control of Environmental and Occupational Diseases*, Princeton, Princeton Scientific Publishing Company (in press)

Waters, M.D., Stack, H.F., Brady, A.L., Lohman, P.H.M., Haroun, L. & Vainio, H. (1987) Appendix 1. Activity profiles for genetic and related tests. In: *IARC Monographs on the Evaluation of Carcinogenic Risks to Humans*, Suppl. 6, *Genetic and Related Effects: An Updating of Selected IARC Monographs from Volumes 1 to 42*, Lyon, IARC, pp. 687–696

Wilbourn, J., Haroun, L., Heseltine, E., Kaldor, J., Partensky, C. & Vainio, H. (1986) Response of experimental animals to human carcinogens: an analysis based upon the IARC Monographs Programme. *Carcinogenesis*, *7*, 1853–1863

GENERAL REMARKS ON THE AGENTS CONSIDERED

This fifty-ninth volume of *IARC Monographs on the Evaluation of Carcinogenic Risks to Humans* contains monographs on three human hepatotropic viruses—hepatitis B virus (HBV), hepatitis C virus (HCV) and hepatitis D virus (HDV, also known as the delta agent). Until now, the subjects of *IARC Monographs* have been mainly single chemical compounds and, to a lesser extent, groups of chemicals, complex mixtures, cultural habits, occupational exposure circumstances and physical agents. The inclusion of biological agents in the programme was considered by an advisory group which met in 1991 (IARC, 1991). The report of that group recommended inclusion of biological agents, and the human hepatotropic viruses were given high priority for evaluation.

At least five viruses (hepatitis A virus, HBV, HCV, HDV and hepatitis E virus) cause a similar acute illness in humans and are known as hepatitis viruses. They are, however, very different in structure and biology. Serological testing is necessary for accurate diagnosis. A few other viruses, such as yellow fever virus, Epstein-Barr virus and cytomegalovirus, may also induce acute viral hepatitis.

The three viruses considered in this volume have as a common feature that the liver disease they cause can have a chronic course. Hepatitis A and E viruses induce an acute clinical illness similar to that caused by HBV and HCV, but they do not appear to induce chronic liver infection. The few studies that have been done found no association between infection with hepatitis A virus and hepatocellular carcinoma (Drucker *et al.*, 1979; Tabor *et al.*, 1980), and no studies of hepatitis E virus have been reported in this connection. Infection with these two viruses was therefore not evaluated in this volume.

Chronic infection with HBV is highly prevalent in many human populations, particularly in developing countries. Over 300 million people are estimated to be chronically infected worldwide (IARC, undated), and between 250 000 and 1 million people die annually from HBV-associated disease, including fulminant liver failure, cirrhosis and hepatocellular carcinoma. The worldwide prevalence of HCV infection is less variable than that of HBV. About 50% of those infected with HCV develop chronic disease. HDV occurs only in the presence of HBV infection; however, there is marked variability in the prevalence of HDV infection among HBV carriers.

The worldwide incidence of primary cancer of the liver (ICD 155) was estimated at some 300 000 cases in 1985, the sex ratio varying from 1.3 to 3.7 in different parts of the world (Parkin *et al.*, 1993). An overview of studies in which the presence of hepatitis B surface antigen was used as a marker of chronic infection suggests that the proportion of hepatocellular carcinomas that is attributable to chronic infection with HBV ranges from a few percent in industrialized countries to more than 50% in some populations in Africa and Asia (Tomatis *et al.*, 1990). Estimates of the burden of cancer associated with HCV infection are not yet available.

In the evaluation of the three viral agents considered in this volume, the same principles were used as in previous monographs (see Preamble). Exposure to the viruses, however, was evaluated in epidemiological investigations on the basis of viral markers in sera and other tissues of study subjects; in other monographs, exposure assessment was based on measurements in the environment of subjects, on data from records or on information reported by the subjects themselves. The biological markers used to determine exposure in the studies reported in the present monographs are thus more direct than the methods used in monographs on non-biological agents.

Of relevance to the assessment that chronic HBV infection introduces a risk for developing hepatocellular carcinoma in humans is identification of species-specific, HBV-related viruses in the woodchuck (woodchuck hepatitis virus) and the Beechey ground squirrel (ground squirrel hepatitis virus), which are associated with the development of hepatocellular carcinomas in those animals. The Working Group did not formally evaluate those viruses but considered that the studies provide biological and mechanistic information relevant to the understanding of the process of carcinogenesis of HBV in humans. The interpretation of studies in experimental animals in evaluating the carcinogenic risk of viral infection in humans poses further complications not ordinarily encountered with chemicals or physical factors: Each hepadnavirus infects only a limited host range; for example, convincing evidence that HBV infects species other than chimpanzees and man is lacking. It is therefore impossible to assess directly the carcinogenicity of HBV in two or more species of animal, as is done with chemicals and physical factors. Somewhat similar considerations apply to experimental studies of HCV and HDV.

Hepatocellular carcinomas can develop in transgenic mice genetically engineered to express selected portions of the HBV genome. A high rate of expression of some, but not all, HBV genes in hepatocytes of transgenic mice is correlated with the development of neoplasia in these animals. Nevertheless, it does not appear possible at this time to apply these observations directly to evaluation of the carcinogenic risk of HBV.

Evaluation of the carcinogenicity of HDV represents a special situation: HDV infection appears to occur only in people who are also infected with HBV. HDV is not, therefore, biologically active in the absence of HBV. In order to evaluate whether or not HDV is a cause of cancer, cancer incidence must be compared in people with both HBV and HDV infection and in people with HBV only; HDV infection may be considered to be a cause of cancer if the lifetime cumulative incidence of cancer in people with both infections is higher than in those with HBV alone, or if cancers occur earlier in those with both infections than in those with HBV infection alone.

References

Drucker, J.A., Coursaget, P., Maupas, P., Goudeau, A., Gerety, R.J., Chiron, J.P., Denis, F. & Diop Mar, I. (1979) Hepatitis A infection and primary hepatocellular carcinoma. *Biomedicine*, **31**, 23–25

IARC (1991) *Report of an Ad-hoc IARC Monographs Advisory Group on Viruses and Other Biological Agents such as Parasites* (IARC int. tech. Rep. No. 91/001), Lyon

IARC (undated) *Hepatitis B and Liver Cancer. The Gambia Hepatitis Intervention Study*, Lyon

Parkin, D.M., Pisani, P. & Ferlay, J. (1993) Estimates of the worldwide incidence of eighteen major cancers in 1985. *Int. J. Cancer*, **54**, 594–606

Tabor, E., Trichopoulos, D., Manousos, O., Zavitsanos, X., Drucker, J.A. & Gerety, R.J. (1980) Absence of an association between past infection with hepatitis A virus and primary hepatocellular carcinoma. *Int. J. Epidemiol.*, **9**, 221–223

Tomatis, L., Aitio, A., Day, N.E., Heseltine, E., Kaldor, J., Miller, A.B., Parkin, D.M. & Riboli, E., eds (1990) *Cancer: Causes, Occurrence and Control* (IARC Scientific Publications No. 100), Lyon, IARC, pp. 184–186

THE MONOGRAPHS

HEPATITIS B VIRUS

1. Exposure Data

1.1 Structure and biology of hepatitis B virus (HBV)

1.1.1 *Structure of the virus*

The structure of hepatitis B virus (HBV) has been characterized in great detail (Tiollais & Buendia, 1991). HBV belongs to a group of hepatotropic DNA viruses (hepadnaviruses) that includes the hepatitis viruses of the woodchuck (Summers *et al.*, 1978), ground squirrel (Marion *et al.*, 1980), Pekin duck (Mason *et al.*, 1980) and heron (Sprengel *et al.*, 1988).

HBV is a small virus, about 42 nm in diameter ('Dane particle'), composed of a lipid-bilayer envelope containing hepatitis B surface antigen (HBsAg) and an internal nucleo-capsid structure (core). The nucleocapsid consists of the core protein and the viral DNA genome, which is about 3200 base pairs (about 2100 kDa) in length, with an associated DNA polymerase/reverse transcriptase (Tiollais *et al.*, 1985; Blum *et al.*, 1989a).

1.1.2 *Structure of HBV genome and gene products*

The viral genome is a partially double-stranded, circular DNA molecule. The genome has four open reading frames, three of which encode for viral proteins whose structures and functions have been well characterized (Fig. 1) (Blum *et al.*, 1989a).

(*a*) *HBsAg*

Hepatitis B surface antigen, formerly termed 'Australia antigen' (Le Bouvier, 1971), serum hepatitis antigen, hepatitis antigen and hepatitis associated antigen, is encoded by the pre-surface and surface genes; with lipid, it makes up the envelope of the virus. Excess HBsAg occurs abundantly in serum as small (22 nm) spherical or filamentous, non-infectious particles. In natural infection, the ratio of non-infectious HBsAg particles to virions is about 1000 to 1. Three different HBsAgs are synthesized: the large HBsAg (encoded by pre-S1, pre-S2 and S genes), the middle HBsAg (encoded by pre-S2 and S genes) and the major HBsAg (encoded by the S gene) (Tiollais *et al.*, 1985; Blum *et al.*, 1989a). The large HBsAg presumably mediates binding of the virus to the cell (Neurath *et al.*, 1986, 1990). The function of the middle HBsAg is unknown. The major HBsAg represents the predominant structural protein of the viral envelope (Tiollais *et al.*, 1985) (Fig. 2).

Fig. 1. The hepatitis B viral DNA genome consists of a complete minus strand and an incomplete plus strand, with a cohesive overlap of their 5' regions. In the cohesive region, there are two direct repeat sequences (DR1 and DR2), which are important in viral replication. The four open reading frames are indicated as arrows.

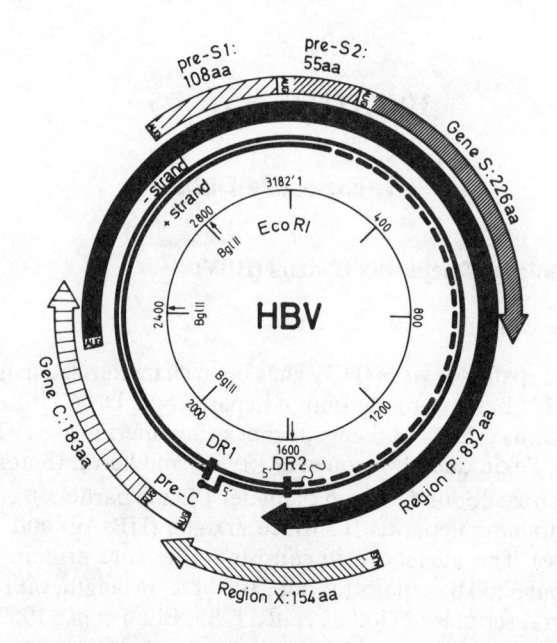

Adapted from Tiollais *et al.* (1985); Blum *et al.* (1989a)

Fig. 2. Structure of hepatitis B virus, showing surface (HBsAgs) and core (HBcAg) antigens

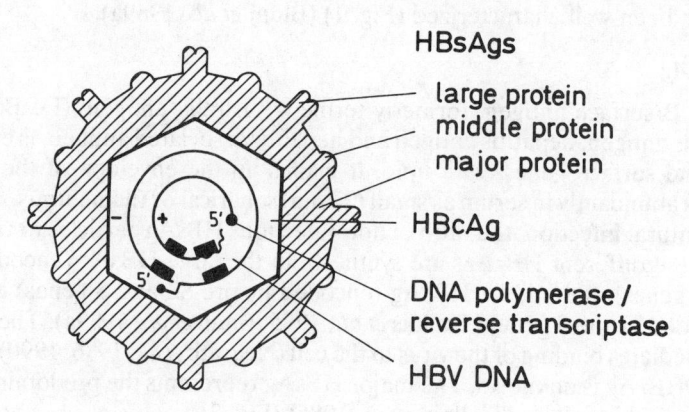

From Blum *et al.* (1989a)

HBsAg carries a group-specific determinant, *a*, common to all subtypes of this antigen, and two additional subtypic determinants, *d* or *y* and *w* or *r*. As a result, four major subtypes of HBsAg exist: adw, adr, ayw and ayr (Le Bouvier, 1971; Bancroft et al., 1972). They have distinct distributions worldwide and may therefore be useful for tracing the source of infection, e.g. *w* is commoner than *r* in the USA, but *r* is commonest in Thailand (Bancroft et al., 1972).

The group-specific determinant *a* is encoded by the S genic region, encompassing roughly codons 124 to 147. This epitope is highly immunogenic, resulting in an anti-HBs response after natural infection (Carman et al., 1993) or vaccination (Halliday et al., 1992).

(b) *HBsAg and HBeAg*

The hepatitis B core antigen (HBcAg) and its antigenically distinct processed product, hepatitis B envelope antigen (HBeAg), are encoded by the pre-core/core (HBe-C/C) gene. The core (C) gene is transcribed into a core protein which packages the pre-genomic RNA to yield 'core particles'. The pre-C/C gene is transcribed into a pre-C/C fusion protein (Blum et al., 1989a). The core antigen represents the major structural component of the nuclear capsid (Fig. 2). After truncation at its amino and carboxy termini, this protein is detectable in serum as HBeAg, usually indicating a high level of viral replication in the liver.

(c) *Viral DNA polymerase/reverse transcriptase*

The hepadnaviral polymerase gene encodes for a protein with a calculated molecular weight of 93.2 kDa. Genetic analysis has demonstrated that the enzyme consists of several functional domains arranged in order from the amino to the carboxy terminus: (i) terminal protein, which presumably serves as a protein primer for reverse transcription of the RNA pre-genome into minus-strand DNA; (ii) a spacer region, which can be deleted without loss of enzyme activity; (iii) DNA polymerase/reverse transcriptase activity; and (iv) RNase H activity. HBV and duck hepatitis B virus polymerases have been expressed *in vitro* (Bartenschlager et al., 1992; Howe et al., 1992; Wang & Seeger, 1992).

(d) *HBxAg*

The fourth open reading frame, which is conserved in all mammalian but not avian hepadnaviruses, encodes for a small protein, X. The biological functions of this protein for the viral life cycle and for the pathobiology of HBV have not been firmly established. The X gene product (HBxAg) has been shown to activate transcription of HBV, other viral sequences and a variety of cellular genes (Kekulé et al., 1993). HBxAg does not seem to be required for HBV replication or gene expression *in vitro* (Blum et al., 1992). Data in the woodchuck model suggest, however, that a woodchuck hepatitis virus X-minus mutant is not infectious *in vivo* (Chen et al., 1993).

1.1.3 *Replication of HBV*

The hepadnaviral genomes are of similar size and structure and replicate asymmetrically via reverse transcription of an RNA intermediate (Summers & Mason, 1982). The replication strategy of HBV has been analysed in great detail both biochemically and genetically (Seeger et al., 1986; Will et al., 1987). Although hepadnaviruses are similar to retroviruses, their mode of replication is unique (Miller & Robinson, 1986), with homologies only to the cauliflower mosaic DNA virus (Toh et al., 1983).

1.1.4 HBV and related animal viruses

Similarities and differences between HBV and the related mammalian viruses of the woodchuck (WHV) and ground squirrel (GSHV) and the related avian viruses of Pekin duck (DHBV) and heron (HHBV) have been reviewed (Wain-Hobson, 1984; Mason & Taylor, 1989; Schödel et al., 1989, 1991). All hepadnaviruses have a similar sized, partially double-stranded genome of about 3000 base pairs, which replicates asymmetrically by reverse transcription of an intermediate RNA template, the pre-genome (Ganem & Varmus, 1987; Feitelson, 1992). Further, the genetic organization of these genomes is identical, except that the avian viruses (DHBV and HHBV) lack the X open reading frame. While hepadnaviruses have a high species specificity of infection, the DNA sequences of HBV and WHV are highly homologous, which results in cross-reactivity between HBsAg and WHsAg (Wain-Hobson, 1984). Further, GSHV has been shown to infect woodchucks (Seeger et al., 1991). Avian hepadnaviruses are more divergent in genomic structure and sequence. Calculations show DNA homologies of about 82% between GSHV and WHV and about 55% between GSHV and HBV, while only scattered homologies were apparent between DHBV and the other hepadnaviruses (reviewed by Sherker & Marion, 1991).

1.1.5 HBV mutants

The existence of HBV mutants was suspected for many years on the basis of the finding of HBV DNA in liver and serum from HBsAg-seronegative patients with or without antibodies to HBV. Conventional cloning techniques or polymerase chain reaction (PCR) amplification were used to clone and sequence viral DNA from sera and liver biopsy specimens, and naturally occurring mutations were identified in all viral genes. PCR allows amplification and detection of viral DNA at a sensitivity equal to that of tests of transmission in chimpanzees in vivo (Ulrich et al., 1989). The PCR product can be sequenced directly or after cloning into an appropriate vector.

In the woodchuck model, the mutation rate has been estimated to be less than or equal to 2×10^{-4} base substitutions per genome and year of replication (Girones & Miller, 1989). The hepadnaviral genome therefore appears to be relatively stable during replication in its natural host. The mutation rate of hepadnaviruses is 100–1000 times lower than that of RNA viruses but about 100 times higher than that of other DNA viruses. Since HBV infection frequently persists in humans for many years or decades, base changes can accumulate over time and may eventually result in a significant number of mutations. In addition, defective viral genomes containing major deletions occur frequently in individuals chronically infected with HBV (Takeda et al., 1990). These defective viruses probably arise during active viral replication, but their contribution to the pathogenesis of HBV-related liver disease remains unclear.

(a) *Pre-S and S gene mutants* (Carman et al., 1993)

While various naturally occurring mutations in the pre-S and S genes have been described, including deletions and point mutations leading to subtypic changes (Le Bouvier,

1971; Okamoto *et al.*, 1987; Lai *et al.*, 1991), a potentially important naturally occurring mutation affects the group-specific determinant *a*. A child from southern Italy, for example, who was infected by HBV despite passive–active immunization at birth and development of an anti-HBs response was found to carry a virus with a mutation in codon 145 of the S gene, resulting in a glycine to arginine substitution. This substitution results in loss of the *a* determinant against which the vaccine-induced anti-HBs response is mainly directed (Carman *et al.*, 1990; Harrison *et al.*, 1991; Waters *et al.*, 1992). Similar findings have been reported from Japan (Fujii *et al.*, 1992; Okamoto *et al.*, 1992), where not only the mutation in codon 145 but a further mutation in codon 126 of the S gene was detected (an asparagine to threonine or isoleucine substitution), which also resulted in loss of the *a* determinant (Okamoto *et al.*, 1992). In liver transplant recipients with chronic hepatitis B treated with a human monoclonal anti-HBs antibody, mutations similar to those described above have been identified in the S gene (McMahon, G. *et al.*, 1992). The transmission efficiency of these mutants has not been established.

Other mutations in pre-S and S genes may affect the sensitivity of antigen–antibody tests routinely used to detect HBsAg in serum. This may be especially relevant for assays based on antigen capture or detection using monoclonal anti-HBs antibodies that may not bind to the mutant HBsAg.

(b)   Pre-C and C gene mutants

Attention has recently focused on mutations identified in the pre-core (pre-C) or core (C) gene region of the viral genome in patients who seroconverted from HBeAg to anti-HBe without loss of viral replication. The mutations in the pre-C gene identified to date most frequently induce a stop codon at the end of the pre-C region (Carman *et al.*, 1989; Akahane *et al.*, 1990; Brunetto *et al.*, 1990; Santantonio *et al.*, 1991a), resulting in an inability to produce HBeAg. While a pre-C stop codon mutation does not interfere with viral replication (Tong *et al.*, 1990), these mutations were found in clinically asymptomatic individuals, in patients with severe and active liver disease (Carman *et al.*, 1989; Akahane *et al.*, 1990; Brunetto *et al.*, 1990; Tong *et al.*, 1990; Naoumov *et al.*, 1992) and in patients with a fulminant course of HBV infection (Terazawa *et al.*, 1990; Carman *et al.*, 1991a,b; Hasegawa *et al.*, 1991; Kojima *et al.*, 1991; Kosaka *et al.*, 1991; Liang *et al.*, 1991a). Given the different clinical presentations of patients with pre-C stop codon mutants and the fact that in any patient with chronic HBV infection many mutants may coexist ('quasispecies') and multiple mutations may be found in a single viral genome, the causal relationship between the pre-C stop codon mutation and a particular course of the disease is unclear. A study in the woodchuck model suggests, however, that the pre-C stop codon may prevent persistence of WHV infection without affecting acute pathogenicity (Chen, H.-S. *et al.*, 1992).

Relatively few mutations have so far been identified in the C gene. In a patient seropositive for human immunodeficiency virus, cytomegalovirus, HBsAg and HBeAg and seronegative for anti-HBc, Bhat *et al.* (1990) identified a viral mutant with two point mutations in the pre-C and C genes as well as an in-frame 36-base pair insertion in the pre-C region. In contrast, in a study of children with HBV infection seronegative for anti-HBc who were undergoing chemotherapy for malignancies, no pre-C or C mutation was found (Melegari *et al.*, 1991). Recent evidence suggests, however, that mutations in the core gene (codons

84–101) are correlated with the severity of liver disease, possibly by altering recognition of infected cells by cytotoxic T cells (Ehata *et al.*, 1992).

(c) *X gene mutants*

Three naturally occurring mutations in the X gene have been described: a replication-competent HBV genome with a pre-X open reading frame (Loncarevic *et al.*, 1990); an HBV variant with an 8-base pair deletion at the 3′ end of the X gene (Repp *et al.*, 1992); and a replication-competent HBV variant with a fused X–C reading frame, resulting from a single nucleotide insertion in the X–C overlapping region (Kim *et al.*, 1992). The functional significance of X gene mutations is unclear.

(d) *Polymerase gene mutants*

In a patient serologically immune to HBV infection, a viral genome was identified with a point mutation in the protein region of the polymerase gene which terminated HBV replication through loss of RNA encapsidation function; this defect could be transcomplemented by a normal polymerase (Blum *et al.*, 1991). A further naturally occurring polymerase-defective variant was detected in the DHBV system, as a point mutation in the region of the gene that encodes for RNase H activity (Chen, Y. *et al.*, 1992). The functional significance of this mutation is unclear.

1.1.6 *Host range and target cells of HBV infection*

The host range of HBV and the related viruses in woodchuck, ground squirrel, Pekin duck and heron is very narrow. HBV, for example, infects only humans and chimpanzees. This narrow host range is believed to reflect the specificity of the liver-cell receptor for HBV, which interacts with an epitope in the pre-S1 region, 21–47, and which is also found on cells of extrahepatic origin (Neurath *et al.*, 1986, 1990).

In permissive hosts, viral antigens and nucleic acids are found primarily in liver cells. By use of molecular techniques, hepadnaviruses have also been detected in cells other than hepatocytes (Blum *et al.*, 1989b), e.g. bile-duct epithelial cells, endothelial cells in liver (Blum *et al.*, 1983), pancreas, adrenal cortex, kidney, skin, spleen and bone-marrow cells (Halpern *et al.*, 1983, 1984; Tagawa *et al.*, 1985; Tiollais *et al.*, 1985; Freiman *et al.*, 1988; Yoffe *et al.*, 1990; Mason *et al.*, 1992) and various peripheral white blood cells. The biological significance of HBV in cells other than hepatocytes remains largely undefined (Omata, 1990). Activation of HBV has been observed in peripheral blood mononuclear cells (Bouffard *et al.*, 1992), and persistent HBV infection of mononuclear blood cells without concomitant liver infection has been demonstrated (Féray *et al.*, 1990).

1.2 Methods of detection

Infection is detected on the basis of assays for viral antigens, antibodies and nucleic acids.

1.2.1 *In serum and plasma*

(a) *HBsAg and anti-HBs*

Tests for HBsAg developed in 1965 (Sherker & Marion, 1991) have since been improved significantly with regard to sensitivity and specificity. The early, less sensitive methods identified only patients with high titres of surface antigen. More recent methods, such as reverse passive haemagglutination and enzyme immunoassay/radioimmunoassay (EIA/RIA), are highly sensitive and specific and allow detection of HbsAg at 100–200 pg/ml serum, that is, about 3×10^7 HBsAg particles/ml (Dusheiko et al., 1992), and these are the assays used most commonly for HBsAg in serum. In reverse passive haemagglutination, fixed erythrocytes coated with anti-HBs are added to test samples, and haemagglutination patterns are read. In EIA/RIA, a sandwich method, with anti-HBs as both absorbed reagent and label or conjugate, has been employed. Anti-HBs is measured by passive haemagglutination of fixed erythrocytes coated with HBsAg or by an EIA/RIA sandwich method with HBsAg as the adsorbed reagent and label or conjugate.

(b) Pre-S antigens and antibodies

Pre-S antigens and antibodies are measured by research procedures (Itoh et al., 1986; Coursaget et al., 1990). The significance of these markers in natural infection or protection is not known.

(c) HBcAg and anti-HBc

HBcAg is not routinely detected in serum; in contrast, anti-HBc is a useful serological marker for current or past HBV infection. Total anti-HBc is measured by the haemagglutination inhibition method (Iizuka et al., 1992) or by competitive binding EIA/RIA. Anti-HBc tests have limited specificity, especially at low titres. Commercial tests for both immunoglobulin (Ig) M and total anti-HBc are available; high titres of IgM class anti-HBc are typically present in acute HBV infection. As IgG class anti-HBc appears and is predominant in the course of chronic infection, IgM-anti-HBc may be a useful marker to differentiate between acute and chronic infection.

(d) HBeAg and anti-HBe

HBeAg can be measured by sandwich EIA/RIA using anti-HBe as the capture antibody. Early tests for HBeAg, such as gel diffusion, had little sensitivity, and the results of studies based on such tests must be interpreted with caution. Anti-HBe can be measured by competitive binding.

(e) HBxAg and anti-HBx

HBxAg and anti-HBx are determined by an enzyme-linked immunoabsorbent assay (ELISA) (Horiike et al., 1991), which is not available commercially.

(f) HBV DNA

HBV DNA in serum can be detected by hybridization analysis (filter hybridization or liquid-phase hybridization) or PCR amplification followed by hybridization.

Hybridization assays: In filter hybridization, a test sample is denatured by the addition of sodium hydroxide and filtered through a nitrocellulose membrane to bind DNA. The membrane is then incubated with cloned labelled HBV DNA. If the test sample contains HBV DNA, the labelled probe is annealed to the membrane-bound viral DNA and can be detected by autoradiography. The sensitivity of this assay is 0.1–1 pg HBV DNA, or about

10^3–10^5 virions. In liquid-phase hybridization, HBV DNA exposed by virion lysis is mixed with a labelled HBV probe. This test system is available commercially, is better standardized than filter hybridization and has the same sensitivity; it is, however, costly and time-consuming (Dusheiko et al., 1992).

Polymerase chain reaction (PCR): The amplification of HBV DNA by PCR is an extremely sensitive test: theoretically, one genome equivalent per sample, at least 10 000 times more sensitive than dot–blot hybridization or RIA of HBsAg; it also facilitates analysis of the sequence of the amplified genomes. Contamination remains the major difficulty of this method, and extreme care must be taken at each step to avoid it. Negative and positive control samples, including reaction mixtures without DNA, should be analysed in each test (Dusheiko et al., 1992; Seelig et al., 1992). PCR followed by sequencing has also been used for subtyping HBV and for characterizing and identifying HBV mutants.

Table 1 gives information on the relative sensitivities and specificities of the tests for HBV markers.

Table 1. Relative sensitivities and specificities of tests for hepatitis B viral markers in serum

Marker[a]	Test	Relative sensitivity	Relative specificity
HBsAg	Immunodiffusion	Low	High
	Counterimmunoelectrophoresis	Low	High
	Complement fixation	Medium	High
	Immune adherence	Medium	High
	Reverse passive haemagglutination	Medium	High
	Radioimmunoassay	High	High
	Enzyme immunoassay	High	High
Anti-HBs	Passive haemagglutination	Medium	High
	Radioimmunoassay/enzyme immunoassay	High	High
Anti-HBc	Haemagglutination inhibition	Medium	Medium
	Radioimmunoassay/enzyme immunoassay	High	Medium
HBeAg/anti-HBe	Immunodiffusion	Low	High
	Radioimmunoassay/enzyme immunoassay	High	High
HBV DNA	Hybridization analysis	Medium	High
	Polymerase chain reaction	High	High

[a]HBsAg, hepatitis B surface antigen; anti-HBs, antibody to hepatitis B surface antigen; anti-HBc, antibody to hepatitis B core antigen; HBeAg, hepatitis B envelope antigen; anti-HBe, antibody to hepatitis B envelope antigen; HBV DNA, hepatitis B viral DNA

1.2.2 *In liver tissues*

(a) *HBsAg and HBcAg*

Both HBsAg and HBcAg can be detected by a direct immunofluorescence method in formalin-fixed, paraffin-embedded liver specimens (Yoshizawa et al., 1977). [The sensitivity is limited, however, as shown by the fact that 35–40% of individuals seropositive for HBV markers have no detectable level of antigen in tissues.] HBsAg can also be detected in infected liver cells by histochemical staining, such as with orcein and other reagents for staining elastic fibres (Shikata et al., 1974). These methods were used to locate HBsAg and HBcAg in liver cells.

(b) HBV DNA

HBV DNA can be detected in liver tissue by Southern blot hybridization of extracted DNA or by in-situ hybridization. The major contribution of Southern blot analysis is physical characterization of HBV DNA and especially the distinction between extrachromosomal viral replication and integration of viral sequences into the cellular genome (Tiollais et al., 1985). HBV-specific antigen and DNA can be detected simultaneously in paraffin-embedded liver tissue by immunohistochemistry and in-situ hybridization using a digoxigenin-label probe, without significant reduction in the sensitivity of either assay (Han et al., 1992). HBV DNA can also be detected at high sensitivity in formalin-fixed, paraffin-embedded liver tissue by PCR, at a level correlated with serological and immunohistochemical markers (Lampertico et al., 1990; Diamantis et al., 1992).

1.2.3 Interpretation of serological markers of HBV infection

Typical patterns of serological markers in HBV infection are summarized in Table 2. Further information and correlations with the clinical course of disease are given in section 1.4.

Table 2. Typical serological patterns in HBV infection

Infection status	HBsAg	Anti–HBc IgM	Anti–HBc Total	HBeAg	Anti–HBe	Anti–HBs
Acute infection[a]	+	+	+	+	–	–
Chronic infection with high levels of viral replication	+	–	+	+	–	–
Chronic infection with low levels of viral replication[b]	+	–	+	–	+	–
Recovery from acute infection before development of anti-HBs	–	+	+	–	+	–
Low titre; possible false positive	–	–	+	–	–	–
High titre; possible 'low level carrier'	–	–	+	–	+	–
Recovery from acute infection, indicating immunity	–	–	+	–	+	+
Vaccine response[c]	–	–	–	–	–	+
Susceptible to HBV infection	–	–	–	–	–	–

For abbreviations, see footnote to Table 1.
[a]Reactivated chronic disease may have this pattern with sensitive anti-HBc IgM assays.
[b]Some patients may be seronegative for HBeAg and anti-HBe.
[c]In unvaccinated individuals, a high titre may represent immunity or be nonspecific; low titres are often nonspecific.

1.3 Epidemiology of infection

1.3.1 Transmission

Hepatitis B virus is transmitted from a person who has circulating virus and is HBsAg seropositive. The person may have an acute infection or be a carrier, a carrier being defined as a person who is seropositive for HBsAg on at least two occasions six months apart. Individuals who are HBeAg seropositive are particularly infectious, since the presence of this antigen is correlated with the level of serum HBV DNA.

The mode of transmission of virus to a susceptible individual varies with age. Transmission occurs at three important times of life: at birth (Mitsuda et al., 1989), in early childhood and in adult life. Neonates born to HBeAg-seropositive carriers have an approximately 85% chance of becoming infected, whereas children of HBeAg-seronegative carriers have only a 31% probability of infection (Beasley et al., 1977). The precise mode of perinatal transmission is unclear.

Infection in childhood is associated with living in households in which there is one or more infected sibling; the risk of infection increases with their number (Whittle et al., 1990). The mode of transmission in childhood is unclear. Traditional practices, such as scarification, ear piercing, circumcision and tatooing, have been proposed (Struve, 1992), but controlled studies have failed to confirm them as risk factors (Fox et al., 1988). HBV transmission through the use of contaminated needles, syringes and acupuncture equipment has been well documented (Kent et al., 1988). Skin lesions, in particular tropical ulcers, have been proposed as a source of infection (Foster et al., 1984), but, again, the evidence is not strong. Arthropods have been suggested as a means of transmission on the basis of studies of mosquitoes (Prince et al., 1972), bedbugs (Wills et al., 1977) and tampans (Joubert et al., 1985). One study found a significant association between infection of HBeAg-seropositive people and infestation of beds with bugs (Vall Mayans et al., 1990). Actual arthropod transmission has not been confirmed.

In adult life, parenteral and sexual transmission are the most important routes. The use of contaminated needles by intravenous drug users[1] is a very well documented form of transmission. For example, in a study of drug users in Sweden, 74% of men and 80% of women had markers of past infection, whereas only 1% and 5%, respectively, in the general population did so (Struve, 1992). In surveillance programmes, it was estimated that 27% of patients with acute hepatitis B in the USA in 1988 (Alter et al., 1990) and 24% in the United Kingdom in 1985-88 (Polakoff, 1990) were intravenous drug users. Blood transfusion and administration of blood products for bleeding disorders were important sources of parenteral exposure, but the risk has now been virtually eliminated by screening blood sources and by treatment of blood products.

Szmuness et al. (1975a) indicated the importance of sexual intercourse in transmission of HBV. They compared the prevalence of past infection in spouses of 280 people with and 238 without persistent infection and the cumulative prevalence in women, homosexual men and

---

[1]The term 'intravenous drug use' refers to the practice of self-injecting drugs for recreational purposes. It is assumed to cover intravenous injection as well as intramuscular and other forms of injection.

attendees at sexually transmitted disease clinics. The results clearly showed that the virus could be transmitted sexually. The prevalence of past infection was 10% in spouses of non-carriers and 27% in spouses of carriers. Homosexual men had a prevalence of 48%, but no increase was seen in homosexual women. Subsequent studies of sexual activity showed that the number of sexual partners, duration of sexual activity and a history of sexually transmitted disease were all risk factors for HBV infection (Alter *et al.*, 1989; Rosenblum *et al.*, 1992; Osmond *et al.*, 1993). In surveillance studies of patients with acute hepatitis B, a history of multiple sexual partners was also found to be an important risk factor; 7% of all such patients in the USA and the United Kingdom had a history of homosexuality (Alter *et al.*, 1990; Kingsley *et al.*, 1990; Polakoff, 1990), and 26% in the USA were heterosexual (Alter *et al.*, 1990). The largest proportion of patients in these surveillance studies reported no known risk factor. Some infection may be intra-familial (Szmuness *et al.*, 1975b), from a household carrier. This form of transmission was associated with skin lesions in one case–control study (Bernier *et al.*, 1982). In both developed (Szmuness *et al.*, 1978a) and developing (Toukan, 1987) countries, infection is associated with low socio-economic status.

1.3.2 Determinants of chronic infection

Age at infection is the major determinant of whether a person becomes a carrier. Perinatal transmission confers the highest probability of becoming a carrier, with 80 to about 100% of infected children becoming carriers (Beasley *et al.*, 1977; Wong *et al.*, 1984). In children aged 1–10, the risk is 20–40% and appears to decline across this interval (McMahon *et al.*, 1985; Coursaget *et al.*, 1987). In adolescence and adult life, the probability of chronic infection following infection is in the range 0–10% (Nielsen *et al.*, 1971; McMahon *et al.*, 1985). The relationship has been reviewed recently (Edmunds *et al.*, 1993), and there is no evidence of geographical heterogeneity.

This profile of risk for chronic infection contrasts with the risk for acute clinical hepatitis. Symptomatic infection is unusual in childhood but affects 30–60% of individuals in adolescence and adult life (McMahon *et al.*, 1985).

The risk of becoming a carrier after infection is greater in males than in females in a ratio of about 1.6:1 (London, 1979). The sex ratio of prevalent carriers in the population increases with age because of longer chronic infection in males (Coursaget *et al.*, 1987).

People whose immune system is suppressed, for example by cytotoxic drugs or the human immunodeficiency virus, appear to have a higher risk of chronic infection. They may also convert from apparent immunity to active infection.

1.3.3 Global patterns of chronic infection

WHO classifies hepatitis B endemicity by the proportion of the adult population who are hepatitis B carriers. Populations with 0–2% carriers are regarded as having low endemicity, 2–7% as intermediate and 8% or greater as high endemicity (Fig. 3).

The prevalence of infection is low in North America, western Europe, Australia and South America, with the exception of the Amazon basin. In these populations, a steady increase in prevalence of viral markers is seen with age. In the USA, blacks have a higher prevalence of infection than whites, particularly at older ages (McQuillan *et al.*, 1989).

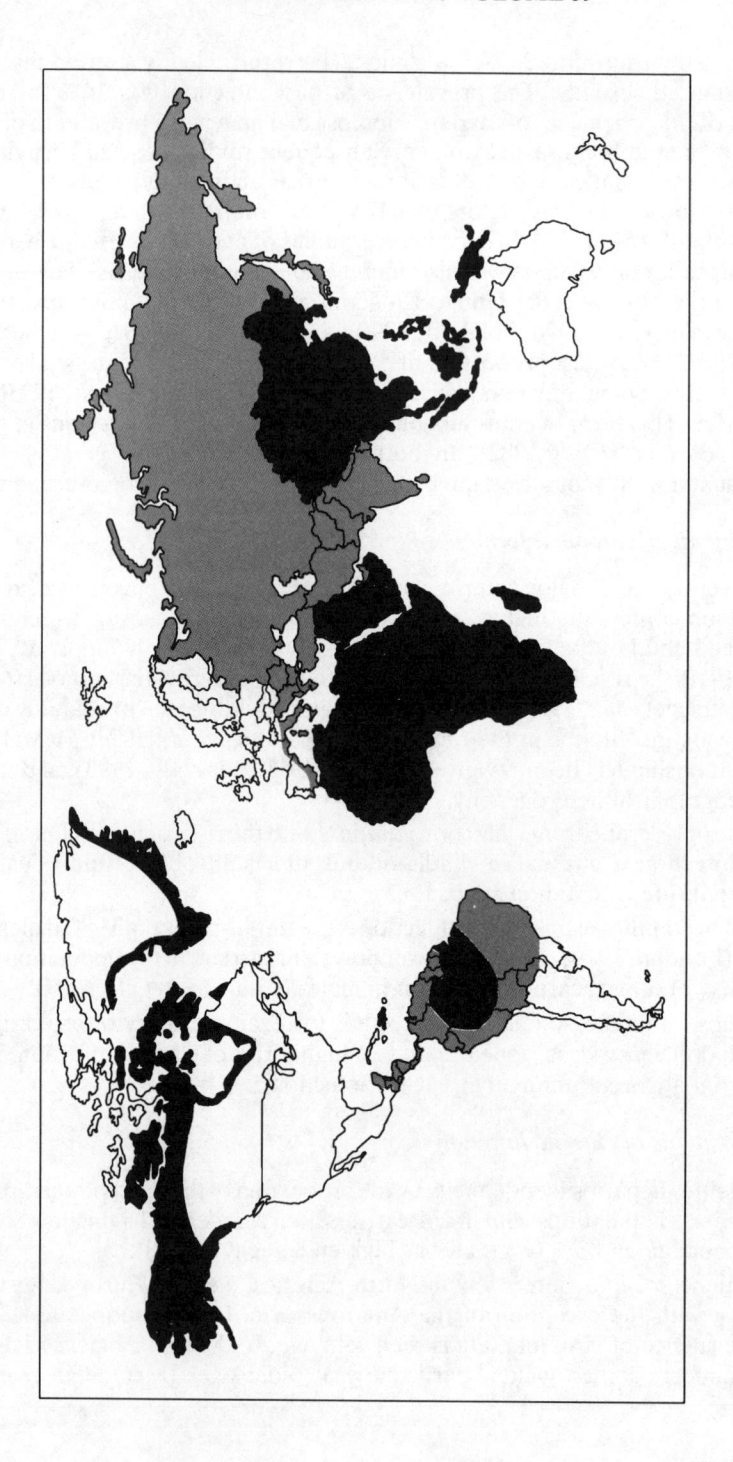

Fig. 3. Geographic pattern of the prevalence of hepatitis B

Black: ≥ 8% – high; grey: 2-7.9% – intermediate; white: < 2% – low
From WHO (undated)

Intermediate levels of prevalence are found in eastern and southern Europe, in the Middle East, Japan and South Asia; high prevalences are found in China, Southeast Asia and sub-Saharan Africa (Prince, 1970; Szmuness, 1975).

High endemicity is associated with infection in childhood, as shown by the results of population-based surveys of hepatitis B markers before vaccination became widespread (Table 3). In Asia, perinatal transmission plays an important role in childhood infection: 30–40% of carriers are infected around the time of birth; in contrast, only 5–10% of carriers in Africa had perinatal infection. The proportion of mothers who are carriers is similar in Asia and sub-Saharan Africa (15–20%); however, 50% of carrier mothers in Asia are highly infectious (HBeAg seropositive), compared with only 10% in Africa. The reasons for this difference are not known.

Childhood infection plays an important role in countries of both high and intermediate endemicity, whereas adult transmission is predominant in areas of low endemicity (Table 4). Perinatal transmission does occur in countries of low endemicity and is particularly important among migrants from highly endemic regions and their descendants. Adoption of carrier children from highly endemic countries can lead to intra-familial transmission (Christenson, 1986; Friede *et al.*, 1988).

Variation may be seen within countries, as in Nigeria, with high prevalences in the north of the country but intermediate levels in the south (Fakunle *et al.*, 1980; Nasidi *et al.*, 1986); in Italy, with a low prevalence of infection in the north but an intermediate prevalence in the south (D'Amelio *et al.*, 1992); and in China, with a markedly higher prevalence of persistent infection in adults in the southeast of the country than in the northern inland areas (Beasley *et al.*, 1982). Variation in infection is also seen at the village level in Africa (Whittle *et al.*, 1983, 1990) and the Middle East (Toukan *et al.*, 1990): adults in adjacent villages have significantly different prevalences of persistent infection which are associated with the age at infection of children. Urban–rural differences in infection vary, some countries having higher urban rates and some higher rural rates (Soběslavský, 1980). In some countries, minority groups have significantly different risks of infection from the general population. For example, Maoris in New Zealand have higher rates than Caucasians (Milne *et al.*, 1985), and Aborigines in Australia have intermediate to high rates of infection in comparison with the low rate in non-aboriginal Australians (Holman *et al.*, 1987).

1.4 Clinical diseases (other than cancer)

The natural history and clinical manifestations of HBV infection are highly variable. In industrialized societies, about 45% of all HBV infections result in acute disease, and 1% have a fatal outcome. Chronic infections develop in 5% of infected people, and the remaining 50% of cases follow an asymptomatic course. There are multiple subtypes of the virus, but there is no known difference between the subtypes with respect to pathogenesis. In contrast, recently described HBV mutants may play a role in the clinical manifestations and natural history of HBV infection.

Whereas HBV replication and gene expression in infected individuals do not appear to be directly cytopathic, hepatic injury appears to be immune-mediated. Cytotoxic T cells are directed against HBcAg (Mondelli *et al.*, 1982; Ferrari *et al.*, 1987; Milich *et al.*, 1989) and

Table 3. Hepatitis B seroprevalence in children and adults in selected countries

Country	Children[a] HBsAg-positive %	No. tested	Any HBV marker-positive %	No. tested	Adults HBsAg-positive %	No. tested	Any HBV marker-positive %	No. tested	Reference
Senegal	9.0	2212	52.6	2212	13.3	765	89.3	683	Barin et al. (1981)
Zambia	7.6	264	36.0	264	5.1	356	68.8	356	Tabor et al. (1985)
Argentina	0	104	–		0.7	922	–		Soběslavský 1980
Brazil (Amazon)	6.7	210	51.0	210	7.1	238	68.5	238	Bensabath et al. (1987)
Canada[b]	0.6	322	0.4	452	0.7	1788	4.6	1855	Soběslavský (1980)
USA	0	150	–		0.2	570	–		Soběslavský (1980)
USA	–		0.8	3304	–		6.6	10 971	McQuillan et al. (1989)
India	4.9	144	12.9	179	6.5	556	32.2	661	Soběslavský (1980)
Japan	2.2	552	5.3	552	2.2	1357	21.0	1357	Soběslavský (1980)
Former Czechoslovakia	0.3	324	6.2	324	2.1	668	14.4	667	Soběslavský (1980)
Germany (eastern)	0.7	294	12.7	157	1.6	626	17.3	458	Soběslavský (1980)
Greece	7.2	470	10.2	609	9.9	2150	41.3	2672	Soběslavský (1980)
Romania	13.3	218	18.0	206	9.7	484	53.6	491	Soběslavský (1980)
United Kingdom	–		–		0.1	871	9.7	871	Soběslavský (1980)
Former USSR	3.8	131	40.5	131	3.7	347	46.4	347	Soběslavský (1980)
Jordan	9.5	505	[18.0]	505	10.2	610	51	610	Toukan et al. (1990)

[a]Under 15 years of age
[b]Urban population only

Table 4. Endemicity of chronic infection with HBV by area of the world and predominant mode of transmission

Endemicity	Geographical area	Predominant time of infection
High, ≥ 8%	China, Southeast Asia, Pacific Basin, sub-Saharan Africa, Amazon Basin	Perinatal, childhood
Intermediate, 2–7%	East, central and southern Europe, Middle East, South Asia, Japan	Perinatal, childhood, adulthood
Low, < 2%	North America, western Europe, Australia, southern Latin America	Adulthood

HBeAg (Ferrari *et al.*, 1992; Tsai *et al.*, 1992) but not against HBsAg (Mondelli *et al.*, 1982), and the exact nature of the target antigens for cytotoxic immune reactions is unknown (Ferrari *et al.*, 1987; Vento & Eddleston, 1987; Ferrari *et al.*, 1992). Conversely, immune suppression by co-infection with human immune deficiency virus or by treatment for organ transplantation reduces inflammatory reactions in the liver and frequently results in normalization of biochemical parameters, with no resolution of liver disease (Davis, 1989; Todo *et al.*, 1991; Martin *et al.*, 1992; McNair *et al.*, 1992).

1.4.1 *Acute infection*

The lag between exposure to HBV and onset of hepatitis B is 2–26 weeks, and the clinical expression of this infection is heterogeneous. Subclinical episodes of acute hepatitis are common, as indicated by the large number of chronically infected patients with no history of acute hepatitis B (Redeker, 1975). The usual clinical attack of hepatitis caused by HBV in adults is more severe than that in either children or patients with hepatitis caused by hepatitis A or C virus. The self-limited bout of icteric hepatitis usually lasts less than three months and only occasionally has a prolonged or cholestatic course. A minority of patients become jaundiced and have symptoms and signs of hepatitis, such as fever, fatigue, hepatosplenomegaly and dark urine. Fulminant hepatic failure is an occasional result of acute hepatitis (Junge & Deinhardt, 1985; Krogsgaard *et al.*, 1985).

In uncomplicated hepatitis, HBV DNA is the first serum marker to appear, during the first four weeks of exposure, followed by HBsAg (Fig. 4a) (Krogsgaard *et al.*, 1985). In acute self-limited hepatitis, HBsAg persists for several weeks. After a variable time (window period), anti-HBs appears. Detection of IgM antibodies to anti-HBc, another early marker of HBV infection, is useful in differentiating acute hepatitis B from other forms of acute liver damage which could also be present in healthy carriers of HBsAg (Chau *et al.*, 1983; Perrillo *et al.*, 1983). HBeAg appears concurrently with HBsAg as a fourth marker in the serum (Krugman *et al.*, 1979). Recovery from acute hepatitis is heralded by clearance of serum HBV DNA, HBsAg and HBeAg and sequential appearance of anti-HBe and anti-HBs (Fig. 4).

1.4.2 *Chronic infection*

Chronic HBV infection may follow acute symptomatic or asymptomatic infection but is more frequent after asymptomatic infection. It occurs more frequently in men than in

Fig. 4. Serological patterns of acute infection (a) and chronic infection (b) with HBV

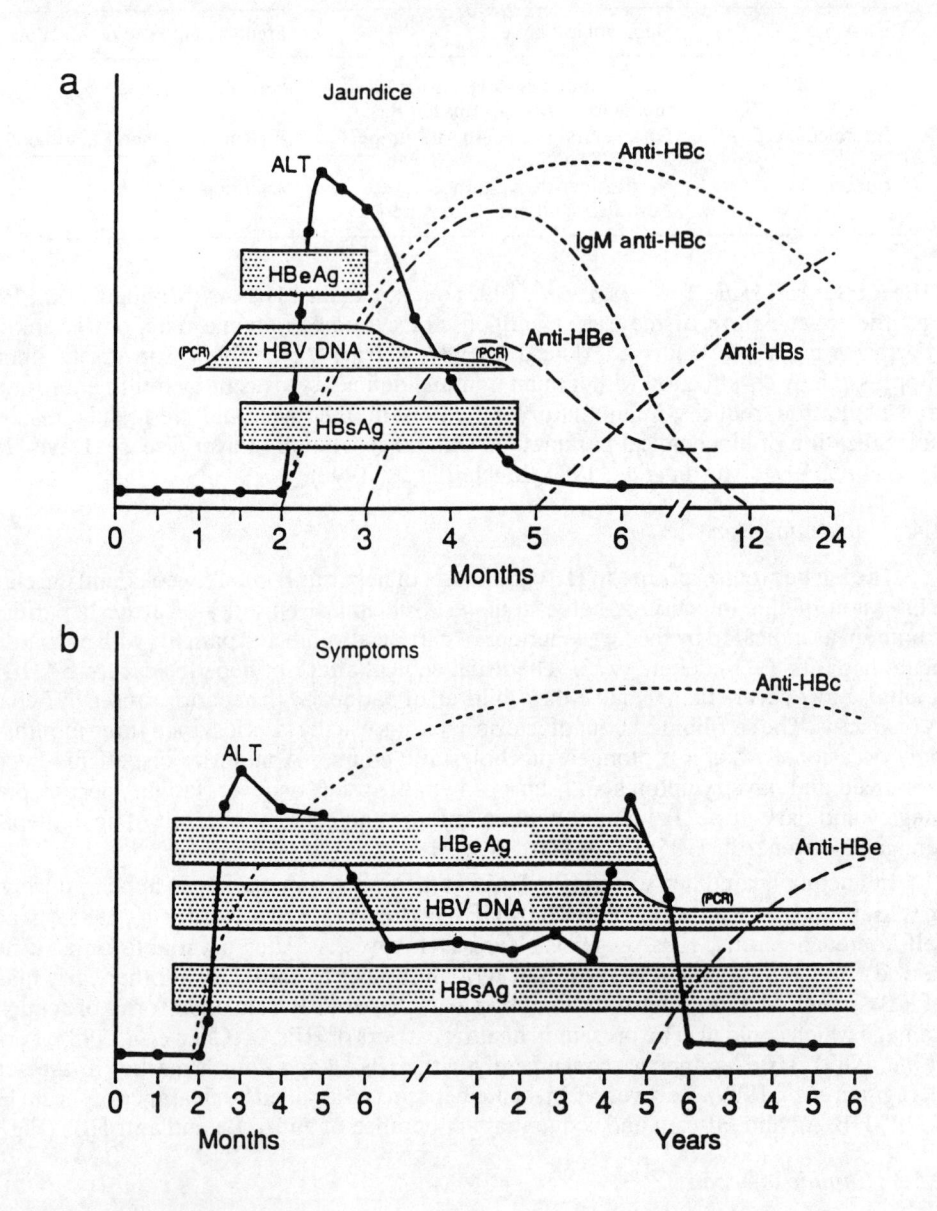

Modified from Dusheiko *et al.* (1992)
(PCR), period in which HBV DNA can be detected by the polymerase chain reaction; ALT, alanine aminotransferase

women, in children than in adults and in immunocompromised patients than in immunocompetent patients (Taylor et al., 1988) (see section 1.3.2). The risk of chronicity declines from 80–90% following perinatal infection to 0–10% in older children and immunocompetent adults (McMahon et al., 1985; Edmunds et al., 1993).

Persistence of HBV infection is associated with variable degrees of hepatic inflammation; seroconversion to anti-HBe is paralleled by exacerbation of hepatitis caused by immune-mediated liver-cell necrosis and progressive clearance of infected hepatocytes and serum HBV DNA (Fig. 4). After seroconversion to anti-HBe, many patients show long-term, non-replicating, latent HBV infection. An important molecular process in HBsAg carriers is integration of HBV DNA into the liver-cell genome, and the majority of such carriers show no evidence of replication (De Franchis et al., 1993). Patients with replicating HBV display various degrees of liver damage—from no histological change to benign forms of chronic lobular hepatitis to more severe forms of active hepatitis and cirrhosis. Chronic active hepatitis is the result of host immune attacks on infected liver cells.

The annual rate of HBeAg/anti-HBe seroconversion and disease remission was 10–15% in adult Italian patients (Fattovich et al., 1986), but the rate varies by geographical location and age at infection. Children do not show reactivation of replication of HBV after anti-HBe seroconversion (Bortolotti et al., 1990). Although HBeAg to anti-HBe seroconversion in adults was accompanied by clinical, biochemical and histological remission of disease, in a study of 88 patients followed-up for a mean of five years, 10 (22%) had transient spontaneous reactivation of HBV infection and exacerbation of disease (Fattovich et al., 1990). Thus, seroconversion from HBeAg to anti-HBe during adulthood is not always stable, in contrast to infantile HBV infections (Lok et al., 1987). HBV reactivation may lead to deterioration of the underlying liver disease, from quiescent chronic hepatitis to active cirrhosis (Fattovich et al., 1990). Reactivation of a latent HBV infection occurs more frequently in immunocompromised patients infected with human immunodeficiency virus (Vento et al., 1989) and in patients receiving cytotoxic therapy (Lok et al., 1991).

HBV replication is instrumental in progression of the disease to cirrhosis. In 105 Italian patients with chronic hepatitis B (Fattovich et al., 1991) who were followed prospectively for a mean of 5.5 years, cirrhosis was documented in 34% of patients with persistent serum HBV DNA but in only 15% of those without serum HBV DNA. In these patients, bridging hepatic necrosis was another important predictor of cirrhosis. In 43 Dutch patients with compensated cirrhosis, five-year survival was 72%, but the risk of death was decreased by a factor of 2.2 when HBeAg seroconversion occurred during follow-up (De Jongh et al., 1992).

1.4.3 *Extrahepatic manifestations*

Extrahepatic clinical disease is infrequent during hepatitis B and has often been associated with circulating immune complexes containing viral antigens. Some patients in the prodromal phase of acute hepatitis have symptoms indicating immune complex disease, such as serum sickness-like syndrome, fever, urticarial skin lesions and symmetrical arthropathy. Systemic necrotizing vasculitis (polyarteritis) affecting the gastrointestinal tract (Shusterman & London, 1984), peripheral or central nervous system has been reported (Tabor, 1987). The presence of circulating complexes correlated well with disease activity. Membranous or membrano-proliferative glomerulonephritis due to HBeAg immunocomplexes has been found either alone or as part of a generalized vasculitis (Shusterman & London, 1984). The Guillain–Barré syndrome was reported, with HBsAg-containing immunocomplexes in serum and cerebrospinal fluid (Penner *et al.*, 1982). Aplastic anaemia complicating hepatitis B is extremely uncommon and shows typical features of refractory marrow failure or hepatitis-dependent pancytopenia (McSweeney *et al.*, 1988).

1.5 Therapy and immunoprophylaxis

1.5.1 *Therapy*

(a) *Acute or fulminant HBV infection*

Most cases of acute HBV infection are asymptomatic and do not require medical attention. In case of malaise and fatigue, bed rest is advised. In symptomatic acute or fulminant HBV infection, therapy is given to relieve the signs and symptoms associated with the acute phase of the disease. Therapy includes parenteral nutrition in cases of dehydration and inanition due to nausea and vomiting, replacement of coagulation factors in cases of bleeding due to impaired synthetic liver function and liver transplantation in cases of advanced liver failure and hepatic coma (Maddrey & Van Thiel, 1988). Except for anecdotal reports (Halevy *et al.*, 1990), no trial of antiviral agents in acute HBV infection has been published.

(b) *Chronic HBV infection*

Because of the severe natural course of HBV infection, several therapeutic strategies have been explored in patients: plant extracts (Thyagarajan *et al.*, 1988; Blumberg *et al.*, 1990), the immunomodulator AM3 (Villarrubia *et al.*, 1992), steroids (Tygstrup *et al.*, 1986), thymosin (Mutchnick *et al.*, 1991), adenine arabinoside monophosphate (Garcia *et al.*, 1987), dideoxyinosine (Catterall *et al.*, 1992; Fried *et al.*, 1992) and interferon-α, interferon-β and interferon-γ. Interferon-α or prednisone followed by interferon-α and interferon-β are the only regimens of some value for treating chronic active hepatitis B (Alexander *et al.*, 1987; Hoofnagle *et al.*, 1988; Perrillo *et al.*, 1990; Janssen *et al.*, 1992; Lok *et al.*, 1992). Response is usually defined as seroconversion from HBeAg to anti-HBe, decrease or loss of HBV DNA and normalization of serum transaminase. Long-term follow-up of HBV carriers who responded to interferon therapy indicated that the improvement is sustained over a long time (Carreño *et al.*, 1992).

The parameters that predict a response to interferon-α therapy in HBsAg- and HBeAg-seropositive patients are: high levels of transaminases, low level of HBV DNA, short duration of disease, female sex and seronegativity for human immunodeficiency virus (Brook *et al.*, 1989). The ethnic origin of patients may have some influence on the efficacy of interferon-α therapy, in that Chinese patients appear to respond less well than patients of Caucasian extraction (Lok *et al.*, 1986). Any differences may be attributable in part to the age at infection. Like people infected with human immunodeficiency viruses, patients under immunosuppression after organ transplantation respond poorly to interferon-α therapy (Davis, 1989; Degos & Degott, 1989; Wright *et al.*, 1992).

Interferon treatment seemed to favour the emergence of pre-C stop codon mutants in some studies (Takeda *et al.*, 1990; Santantonio *et al.*, 1991b; Günther *et al.*, 1992) but not in others (Xu et al., 1992); this phenomenon does not seem to affect virus elimination and thereby the efficacy of interferon. The persistence of HBV in peripheral blood mononuclear cells of patients with chronic hepatitis B after HBsAg clearance may, however, pose a real clinical problem and set the stage for reinfection of the liver (Mason et al., 1992).

Therapeutic trials in HBeAg-seronegative, anti-HBe-seropositive and HBV DNA-seropositive patients have yielded conflicting results (Fattovich et al., 1992; Pastore et al., 1992). Further, combined therapy of chronic active hepatitis B with interferon-β and interferon-γ seems to hold some promise (Caselmann et al., 1989); the usefulness of this regimen has not been confirmed, however. In contrast, interferon-γ therapy alone is clearly ineffective (Ruiz-Moreno et al., 1992). The only effective therapy for chronic active hepatitis B is thus administration of interferon-α, which gives a long-term response rate of 30–50% in selected individuals.

Interferon therapy has, however, several limitations. It must be given by injection over long periods, has very significant side-effects in many patients and is expensive, reducing its availability to patients in developing countries.

1.5.2 *Immunoprophylaxis*

Krugman et al. (1970) first demonstrated that serum containing HBsAg could be inactivated by heat but retain its immunogenic properties. This finding led to the development of hepatitis B vaccines by purification and inactivation of HBsAg from the plasma of HBV carriers (Hilleman et al., 1975; Maupas et al., 1981). These vaccines are administered intramuscularly, but gluteal injection is less effective than into other muscles (McLean et al., 1985). Although reduced doses can be given intradermally (Whittle et al., 1987), the results are variable. Three doses are generally required: during the first month of age, then at two, four and nine months of age; however, these intervals are not crucial (Inskip et al., 1991). The vaccine is immunogenic in newborns, and the immunogenicity is not affected by maternally derived passive antibody. Immunogenic HBsAg can also be produced by yeast and mammalian cells using recombinant technology. Both plasma-derived and recombinant vaccines are now widely available and licensed.

Local reactions at the injection site occur in about 10% of vaccinees; long-term sequelae are very rare (Whittle et al., 1991). In addition to active vaccination, a passive immunoprophylaxis is available which can be used in children born to infectious mothers and after accidental occupational exposures. As immunoglobulin does not affect the response to vaccine, a combination of the two will protect in both the short and long term (Mitsui et al., 1989). Many studies (for example, Beasley et al., 1983; Wong et al., 1984) have demonstrated the protective effect of a combination of vaccine and immunoglobulin or vaccine alone in preventing perinatal transmission of hepatitis B in the short term.

Nine trials of immunoprophylaxis involved sufficient follow-up to assess protection against acute hepatitis and persistent infection. Three of these (one in China, two in the USA) were designed to prevent perinatal infection, three (one in Senegal, two in the Gambia) to prevent horizontal childhood infection, one to prevent childhood and adult infection (in Inuits) and two to prevent adult, primarily sexual, transmission (in the USA).

Beasley et al. (1983) assessed the efficacy of hepatitis B immunoglobulin in neonates of HBeAg-seropositive carrier mothers in Taiwan, China. When immunoprophylaxis was given at birth and after three and six months, it had a protective efficacy of 71%. The protection persisted until 24 months of age, with no further follow-up available. Because children become susceptible to HBV infection after passive immunoprophylaxis wanes, however, hepatitis B immunoglobulin is no longer used alone.

Children recruited into two studies of perinatal vaccination were followed up for four to nine years to assess long-term protection. In the first study (Stevens *et al.*, 1985), 113 children of HBeAg-seropositive carrier Asian–American women were treated with 0.5 ml hepatitis B immunoglobulin and three intramuscular doses of 20 µg plasma-derived vaccine according to various schedules. In the second study (Stevens *et al.*, 1987), 122 infants of HBeAg-seropositive carrier Asian–American mothers were given plasma- or yeast-derived vaccine according to various schedules after a dose of 0.5 ml hepatitis B immunoglobulin at birth. Only 8.2% of children in these two studies became persistently infected; as the rate expected on the basis of historical controls was 70%, the protective efficacy was approximately 88%. Of 104 children who were seronegative for HBV markers at 9–18 months of age (Stevens *et al.*, 1992), none developed hepatitis, although 6.7% were seropositive for anti-HBc and anti-Hbs, indicating past infection with the virus. Very few lost vaccine-induced antibody.

Three of four studies of vaccination in populations with high rates of 'horizontal' transmission were carried out in West Africa and the fourth among Alaskan Inuits. In Senegal, Coursaget *et al.* (1986) followed up 135 infants who had received four doses of plasma-derived vaccine in the first year of life and 143 who had received no vaccine by the age of seven years, which represented a small fraction of the original children in the vaccination programme. Four children in the vaccine group and 20 in the control group developed HBsAg. As samples were taken at only one point in time, at seven years of age, it is not possible to determine if these children were persistently infected. The protective efficacy against HBsAg-positive events was 85%.

Two studies were conducted in the Gambia: the first was limited to two villages in which hepatitis B was well documented in 1980 and 1984 (Whittle *et al.*, 1983, 1990) and in which trials of intramuscular and intradermal (Whittle *et al.*, 1987) vaccination with plasma-derived vaccine were carried out in 1984. All children under five subsequently born in the villages received intramuscular plasma-derived vaccine in the first year of life, and a complete cross-sectional survey of people under 20 years of age was made in 1989, five years after the initial vaccine trials. Vaccination was 97% effective in preventing chronic infection in comparison with the rate in historical controls, although 5.3% of 264 vaccinees in one village and 19.1% of 94 in the other had evidence of past infection with the virus. The dose, route and schedule of vaccination did not influence protective efficacy in this study. None of the children with 'breakthrough' infection (seroconversion to anti-HBc) had evidence of acute hepatitis (Whittle *et al.*, 1991). The second study was initiated in 1986 to evaluate the protective efficacy of vaccination against chronic liver disease in a 'stepped-wedge' design (The Gambia Hepatitis Study Group, 1987). A cohort of 1041 vaccinees was followed up to four years of age by examining serum samples taken annually. At four years, a cross-section of 816 unvaccinated children was studied as a control group. The efficacy of the vaccine against infection was 84% (95% confidence interval [CI], 78–89%), and that against persistent infection (defined as HBsAg seropositivity on two occasions one year apart) was 94% (95% CI, 84–98%) (Fortuin *et al.*, 1993). In the vaccinated cohort, four children were found to be chronic carriers; two of three who had had HBsAg-seropositive mothers were also HBeAg seropositive, and both became infected during the first year of life.

The fourth study in populations in which horizontal childhood transmission is common was carried out in Alaska (McMahon et al., 1987; Wainwright et al., 1989). All 1693 susceptible people in a population of 3988 Inuits in 17 villages were vaccinated in 1981–82 with three doses of plasma-derived vaccine. No persistent infection had occurred after five years of follow-up, giving a vaccine efficacy of 100%. Four subjects developed anti-HBc, indicating natural infection, but did not develop acute hepatitis (Wainwright et al., 1989). The annual incidence of acute clinical HBV infection in the entire population declined from 215/100 000 per year before the study to 14/100 000 per year after vaccination (McMahon et al., 1987).

Two large-scale, randomized trials involving adult US homosexual men reported long-term follow-up of vaccinees. In the first (Szmuness et al., 1980), 1083 homosexual men known to be at high risk of HBV infection were recruited and randomized to placebo or plasma-derived vaccine. The protective efficacy against infection at 18 months was 92%. Subgroups of the vaccinees in this trial were followed up for longer periods. Among 138 followed for up to eight years (Taylor & Stevens, 1988), three cases of HBV infection occurred between five and eight years, to give a life-time attack rate of 2.6%.

In a multicentre trial of hepatitis B vaccination among homosexual US men conducted by the Centers for Disease Control, those in the placebo group who remained susceptible at the time of the first analysis were vaccinated (Francis et al., 1982; Hadler et al., 1986). Some of these and the vaccinated group are still being followed up. A total of 733 men were followed for five years after completion of vaccination; 15% of 635 participants with detectable antibody lost it within this time. The duration of antibody persistence was related to the peak antibody response. HBV infection occurred in 55 men; in eight, infection was associated with raised liver enzyme levels and HBsAg seropositivity. The risk for infection was highest in men with the lowest antibody responses. The only two individuals who became persistently infected with HBV did not respond to the vaccine (Hadler et al., 1986). More information is expected from further follow-up of these cohorts. Early indications of the effect of vaccination on chronic liver disease are also expected from studies under way in China (Sun et al., 1986, 1991) and from the mass programme of immunization in Taiwan, China (Chen et al., 1987).

Immunogenicity is reduced in immunosuppressed individuals infected with human immunodeficiency virus (Laukamm-Josten et al., 1987; Collier et al., 1988; Bruguera et al., 1992), in dialysis patients (Jilg et al., 1986) and in individuals immunosuppressed after organ transplantation (Sokal et al., 1992). HBsAg-seropositive individuals (Dienstag et al., 1982) and some patients with anti-HBc as the only marker of HBV infection (McMahon, B.J. et al., 1992) do not respond to vaccination. In such cases, vaccination is not harmful, however. The small proportion of people who do not respond to HBV vaccination, with anti-HBs levels of < 8 radioimmunoassay units, may be determined partly genetically (Craven et al., 1986; Kruskall et al., 1992).

2. Studies of Cancer in Humans

Reports of epidemiological studies of liver cancer relevant to these monographs have employed a variety of terms to describe this disease, for example, liver cancer, primary liver cancer, primary hepatocellular carcinoma and hepatocellular carcinoma. We chose to use only the term hepatocellular carcinoma (HCC) in describing these studies. This choice was made because most of the studies have specified primary cancer of the liver or HCC, and the vast majority of primary liver cancers in most areas of the world are HCC (Colombo, 1992). A large number of case–control studies and fewer cohort studies have been conducted on the association between HBV and HCC. The many case reports, case series and descriptive studies are therefore not described in detail.

HBsAg is the marker of infection with HBV most often measured in epidemiological studies of HBV infection and HCC. While it is not often measured twice, six months apart (as required by the strict definition of carrier status), its presence in adults without acute hepatitis has generally been taken to indicate chronic infection with the virus.

The presence of other markers of HBV infection has also been documented in many studies, but most studies in which these markers were measured were not analysed with the intention of estimating their relationship with HCC. In addition, in some countries, the large majority of the population may have been exposed to HBV, and most have some marker of infection. Thus, an appropriate—uninfected—reference population of sufficient size may not be available for comparison with individuals with anti-HBc or anti-HBs alone or in combination. Lastly, in populations in which a suitable reference group may exist, it has usually not been reported separately.

2.1 Case series and case reports

2.1.1 *Hepatocellular carcinoma*

Payet *et al.* (1956) appear to have been the first to have suggested that HCC is a consequence of chronic viral hepatitis. Within five years of the identification of HBsAg (then called Australia antigen) by Blumberg *et al.* (1965), its significance as a marker of chronic viral hepatitis had been appreciated, and case reports and case series had given rise to the suspicion that it was linked to liver cancer. Okochi and Murakami (1968) appear to have been the first to have found HBsAg in a case of liver cancer (one of 19), but they made no specific comment as to its relevance. Wright *et al.* (1969) found no HBsAg-seropositive patients among 11 with liver neoplasms in the United Kingdom. In reporting the presence of HBsAg in sera from 2 of 42 cases of HCC in Hong Kong but not in 11 East African or 12 US cases, Smith and Blumberg (1969) stated the hypothesis that the antigen and its underlying viral infection were linked to HCC. Sherlock *et al.* (1970) reported HBsAg seropositivity in five male patients with HCC, three from Greece, one from the United Kingdom and one from Sierra Leone; Hadziyannis *et al.* (1970) found HBsAg in sera from 4 of 13 Greek patients with HCC superimposed on active cirrhosis and in six other cases of HCC.

With the development and application of more sensitive tests for HBsAg, case series of HCC have consistently shown apparently high proportions seropositive for the antigen

(Blumberg & London, 1982, 1985). The earlier reports were comprehensively reviewed by Szmuness (1978). Reports of HBsAg seropositivity in the rare cases of HCC in children also appeared (Shimoda *et al.*, 1980), often linking the infection in the child to chronic infection in the mother (Ohaki *et al.*, 1983). Instances of multiple HCC have been reported in families, often with an apparently high prevalence of HBsAg in the serum in both the cases and unaffected members of the family (Tong *et al.*, 1979; Tong & Govindarajan, 1988; Alberts *et al.*, 1991).

HbsAg, and sometimes HBV DNA, have also been reported in liver tissue from patients with HCC (see, for example Tanaka & Mori, 1985; Tanaka *et al.*, 1986), usually in non-neoplastic hepatocytes and rarely in the cancer cells (Tanaka & Mori, 1985).

2.1.2 *Other cancers*

In several case series of patients with cholangiocarcinoma, the prevalence of HBsAg (Okuda *et al.*, 1980) or of markers of HBV in liver tissue (Bunyaratvej *et al.*, 1979; Suwangool, 1979) appeared to be lower than that among cases of HCC and similar to that reported in subjects without HCC.

In two early studies of the presence of HBsAg in sera from patients with a range of cancers (e.g. leukaemias, Hodgkin's disease, breast cancer, lymphoma, multiple myeloma), prevalences of 1.1–2.8% were observed (Viola *et al.*, 1972; Al-Sarraf *et al.*, 1973). In a study of pancreatic tissue from patients who had undergone surgery, immunoperoxidase staining revealed HBsAg in five (7%) patients with pancreatic cancer (Hohenberger, 1985). Planes *et al.* (1976) noted that the prevalence of HBsAg in the sera of patients with malignant lymphoma was related to treatment and that infection with HBV may have occurred as a result of chemotherapeutic immunodepression, parenteral injection, transfusion or a prolonged stay in a hospital environment. In several reports of high prevalences of HBV markers in children with cancer, mainly lymphatic and haematopoietic cancers (Mikhailov *et al.*, 1986; Pontisso *et al.*, 1987; Jackowska *et al.*, 1990), it was considered possible that infection had occurred after the cancer developed.

2.2 Descriptive studies

A strong geographical correlation has been found between the incidence of HCC and the prevalence of HBsAg seropositivity (see, for instance, Szmuness, 1978; Maupas & Melnick, 1981; Lin *et al.*, 1986; Hsing *et al.*, 1991). A number of studies have also shown a high prevalence of HBsAg seropositivity in migrants from countries where the risk for HCC is high (see, for example, Szmuness *et al.*, 1978b).

2.3 Cohort studies

Cohort studies of HBV and HCC can be divided into three broad groups: studies of general population groups, studies of blood donors and studies of populations with pre-existing disease.

2.3.1 *Prospective studies of general population groups* (Table 5, p. 73)

Beasley and colleagues recruited 22 707 male Government employees in Taiwan, China, to evaluate their risk for HCC (Beasley & Lin, 1978; Beasley *et al.*, 1981; Beasley & Hwang,

1991). Subjects were recruited at the time of routine physical examinations offered by the Government between March 1976 and June 1978. Study subjects were Chinese men aged from their twenties to over 70; 82% were 40–59 years of age. Follow-up for cancer incidence and mortality from all causes was conducted through medical and life insurance records and also by annual physical examinations of both HBV carriers and a subset of non-carriers. At the time of enrolment into the study, 3454 of the 22 707 men were HBsAg seropositive, 15 570 were anti-HBs seropositive and anti-HBc seropositive, 2411 were only anti-HBc positive and 1272 had no HBV marker. As at 30 June 1989, none of the HBsAg-seronegative men who were re-tested had become HBsAg seropositive. All HBsAg-seropositive men were re-tested annually; about 1% per year became HBsAg seronegative. At 30 June 1989, 194 cases of HCC had occurred, 184 (95%) in the HBsAg seropositive men, conferring a relative risk (RR) of 103 (95% CI, 57–205) as compared with HBsAg-seronegative subjects. The remaining 10 cases of HCC all occurred among the 17 981 anti-HBc-seropositive men. Among HBsAg-seronegative men, the difference in risk between those who were anti-HBc seropositive and those with no marker of HBV infection was not significant. The occurrence of HCC in the entire population was related to age, evidence of cirrhosis, HBeAg seropositivity and IgM anti-HBe seropositivity. The only causes of marked excess mortality found in relation to HBV markers were HCC and cirrhosis.

Tu et al. (1985) studied all men over the age of 40 from four communes on Chongming Island, China, for development of HCC; 98% (12 222 men) of those eligible participated and were followed for three years. Of the 12 222 men, 1971 (16.1%) were classified as HBV carriers (defined as being either HBsAg seropositive or anti-HBs seronegative and anti-HBc seropositive at the time of the survey). Thirty-seven of the 70 deaths from HCC occurred among the HBV carriers and 33 occurred among the non-carriers, giving an RR of 6.7 [95% CI, 4.2–10.7]. The authors also studied the effects of water source, cigarette smoking, maize consumption (as a measure of exposure to aflatoxin B_1) and alcohol consumption on the risk for HCC. A significantly higher rate of HCC was seen among carriers who smoked 20 cigarettes or more per day. None of the other factors had a significant effect.

Yeh et al. (1989) conducted a prospective study of the effects of HBV and aflatoxins on risk for HCC in the southern Guangxi Autonomous Region, China. The entire cohort consisted of 7917 men who were between the ages of 25 and 64 at enrolment, lived in one of five communities and did not have HCC at the initiation of the study. The cohort was assembled between July 1982 and June 1983, at which time demographic information was collected and a blood sample was drawn; the sera were banked. In 1987, the sera of 2072 men were tested for HBsAg. The 2072 men included 149 men who had died as of 31 July 1986, of whom 76 had died of HCC, and a 25% random sample of the men (1923) still alive. Four live controls were matched to each death from HCC. Of the 76 cases, 69 had occurred in HBsAg-seropositive men (90.7%), whereas 68 of the 304 matched controls were HBsAg seropositive (22.4%) (RR, 39; 95% CI, 16–117). In a geographical analysis of these data, mortality from HCC was not correlated with the mean prevalence of HBsAg seropositivity by commune, but the range of HBsAg seropositivity was narrow (19.5–24.8%). A positive correlation was found between the estimated mean level of aflatoxin B_1 consumed in food and the rate of HCC by commune, and the range of aflatoxin B_1 levels was broad (0.3–51.8 mg/person per year).

Ding et al. (1988) carried out a prospective investigation of residents of the Guangxi Autonomous Region, China. A total of 22 830 people [sex distribution unspecified] over the age of 20 years were stratified on the basis of HBsAg status, hepatic enlargement, alanine aminotransferase levels and residence in an area with a high or low rate of HCC. The average period of follow-up was 6.8 years. The highest RR for HCC occurred in HBsAg-seropositive people with evidence of both liver enlargement and abnormal liver function, regardless of place of residence. In the group from the high-rate area, 30.6% who were HBsAg seropositive and 2.7% who were HBsAg seronegative developed HCC. In the group from the low-rate area, 10% of the HBsAg-seropositive and 2.4% of the HBsAg-seronegative people developed HCC. In the total population, the RR for HCC, adjusted for age, was 8.2 [95% CI, 4.5–15] in HBsAg-seropositive as compared with HBsAg-seronegative subjects.

In a study in Shanghai, China, an association between HBsAg seropositivity and HCC was reported among men participating in a prospective study of diet and cancer (Ross et al., 1992). Between January 1986 and September 1989, 18 244 male subjects aged 45–64 were enrolled in the cohort; 22 cases of HCC had occurred by 1 March 1990. A nested case–control study was conducted with 140 controls matched by age (within one year), sample date (within one month) and residence, who had no history of liver cancer when the case was diagnosed. Five cases have been confirmed by biopsy. Conditional logistic regression, controlling for education, urinary aflatoxins, smoking and alcohol use, yielded an RR of 8.5 (95% CI, 2.8–26) for HBsAg seropositivity as compared with HBsAg seronegativity. The RR associated with detectable urinary aflatoxins was 3.8 (1.2–12), adjusted for educational level, HBsAg seropositivity, smoking and alcohol use; the RR associated with both HBsAg seropositivity and detectable urinary aflatoxins was 60 (95% CI, 6.4–562).

In the Japan–Hawaii Cancer Study of 7498 men of Japanese ancestry born between 1900 and 1919 and living in Hawaii, sera were collected in 1967–70 and stored. From 1967 through 1980, 18 histologically confirmed incident cases of HCC were identified; serum was available for 16. In a case–control analysis (Nomura et al., 1982), each of the 16 cases was matched to three controls from the study cohort by age and serum collection date. Ten of the cases were seropositive for HBsAg as compared with none of the controls ($p < 0.0001$). Another indicator of persistent infection, anti-HBc without anti-HBs, was detected in 7 of the 16 patients and in two of the 48 controls.

Iijima et al. (1984) and Sakuma et al. (1988) studied prospectively two overlapping cohorts of male Japanese employees of Japan National Railways. The first cohort was identified in 1973 and 1978. A total of 6918 men, 126 of whom were found to be HBsAg seropositive at the time of the study (1.8%) were followed to March 1985. Average follow-up was 8.5 years (range, 6.5–11.5 years) and was conducted using annual health examinations, self-reported disease (mandatory for any illness lasting more than six days), follow-up of all men who failed to report for an annual examination, and death certificates. Four HCCs developed in the HBsAg-seropositive group and six in the HBsAg-seronegative group, giving an RR of 30 [95% CI, 8.1–77]. The second cohort consisted of 25 547 men who were identified in 1977–79; the purpose of this study was to determine whether HBeAg status among HBsAg-seropositive men ($n = 513$) was associated with the risk for developing HCC. Average follow-up to 1985 was 7.3 years. RRs were calculated in relation to the risks for HBsAg-seronegative men. HCC was observed in 21 HBsAg-seronegative and 9 HBsAg-seropositive individuals. The RR was 50 [95% CI, 0.66–280] for the 30 HBsAg-seropositive, HBeAg-seropositive men (one HCC), 9.5 [1.1–34] for the 238 HBsAg-seropositive, anti-HBe-seropositive carriers (two HCCs) and 29 [11–63] for the 245 HBsAg-seropositive, HBeAg- and anti-HBe-seronegative carriers (six HCCs).

A population-based study of risk for HCC was conducted among Alaskan natives (Alward et al., 1985; Heyward et al., 1985; McMahon et al., 1990a,b). About two-thirds of the Alaskan native population was classified according to HBV infection status in a statewide screening programme begun in 1983 with the establishment of a HBV carrier registry. The authors identified 1400 HBV carriers (824 men, 576 women) and followed them up until 1 July 1987 (when 1292 were left) for a total of 7815 person-years. The study cohort comprised people of all three Alaskan native groups (85% Inuit, 7.5% Indian, 7.5% Aleut). Review of HBV sequelae from January 1975 to July 1987 showed that 20 cases of HCC had occurred, 19 of which were histologically confirmed. The annual incidence among men was 387/100 000, and that among women was 63/100 000. The incidence of HCC in HBsAg-seronegative people was estimated from the prevalence of HBsAg seronegativity in the Alaskan native population (97%) and the seven HCCs diagnosed in HBsAg-seronegative Alaskan natives between 1975 and 1987, to give an RR of 148 [95% CI, 59–305] for carriers *versus* non-carriers (McMahon et al., 1990a).

2.3.2 *Prospective studies of blood donors* (Table 5)

Oshima et al. (1984) followed a cohort of 8646 HBsAg-seropositive male Japanese blood donors in the Osaka Red Cross Blood Center, who were found to be HBsAg seropositive in 1972–75. Follow-up was conducted by examining data in the Osaka Cancer Registry and the death certificate files of Osaka Prefecture through the end of 1980. The mean length of follow-up was 6.2 years (range, 5–8.5 years). The expected number of cases was based on the age-specific incidence rates among the general population of Osaka. The study cohort developed 20 HCCs during the follow-up period, with 3.0 expected, giving a significant RR of 6.6 [95% CI, 4.0–10]. In a nested case–control analysis, alcohol drinking was significantly related to the risk of developing HCC, with RRs of 5.5 (95% CI, 1.2–26) for moderate drinkers and 8.0 (95% CI, 1.3–50) for heavy drinkers in comparison with non-drinkers.

Fukao (1985) identified 1000 HBsAg-seropositive and 10 000 HBsAg-seronegative blood donors from blood donation records in Miyagi Prefecture, Japan. All cohort members were men over the age of 30 years who had donated blood between 1971 and 1977. The HBsAg-seronegative group was matched 10:1 to the HBsAg-seropositive group by age, district of residence and month of blood donation. Cancer incidence was determined from the records of the Migayi Prefectural Cancer Registry for the years 1971–80. Three HCCs were detected in the HBsAg-seropositive group and one in the HBsAg-seronegative group, giving an RR of 30 [95% CI, 6.0–88] in carriers as compared with non-carriers.

Tokudome et al. (1987, 1988) estimated the risk for HCC among HBV carriers in Japan. A cohort of 3769 HBsAg-seropositive women was identified from among blood donors at the Fukuoka Red Cross Blood Center by examining Red Cross records of donations between the years 1977 and 1982. Mortality follow-up was completed until 1985; vital status was determined by checking against each donor's home residence card. Death certificates were obtained for each donor known to be dead. The 220 women (5.8%) who were lost to follow-up were assumed in the analysis to be alive at the end of the study. The average period of follow-up was five years. Seventeen deaths occurred during the study period, four of which were due to HCC. In comparison with the age-adjusted mortality rates among all women in Fukuoka Prefecture in 1980, the RR for HCC was 5.6 [95% CI, 1.5–14] (Tokudome *et al.*, 1987). In a cohort of 2595 HBsAg-seropositive male blood donors identified during 1977–79 and followed up to 1983 (9.2% lost to follow-up; average length of follow-up, six years), 15 HCCs developed as compared with 2.1 expected on the basis of age-specific mortality rates for Fukuoka Prefecture in 1980. The RR in HBsAg-seropositive men in relation to the general male population was 7.3 [95% CI, 4.1–12] (Tokudome *et al.*, 1988).

Prince and Alcabes (1982) identified a cohort of HBsAg-seropositive men from four sources in the USA: the health departments of New Jersey, New York State and New York City and blood donors in the Greater New York Blood Program. The three health departments maintain lists of HBsAg-seropositive people, most of whom are blood donors who were found to be HBsAg seropositive during routine testing. Men identified as being HBsAg seropositive between 1971 and 1979 and who were residents of either New York City ($n = 5353$) or New York State ($n = 1497$) were included. Causes of death were determined by record matching with the New York State and New York City health departments. Four deaths from HCC occurred (three in New York City), as compared with 0.40 expected on the basis of mortality rates for the general populations of New York City and New York State [RR, 10; 95% CI, 2.7–25].

Dodd and Nath (1987) conducted a mortality study of people who had given blood during 1971–80 in the national Red Cross Donor Deferral Registry and identified 15 166 HBsAg-seropositive and 18 144 HBsAg-seronegative people. Vital status was determined by matching records with those of the Social Security Administration, and cause of death was determined from death certificates. The mean length of follow-up for the HBsAg-seropositive group was 3.7 years and that for the HBsAg-seronegative group, 3.3 years. Men comprised 70% of the HBsAg-seropositive group and 63% of the HBsAg-seronegative group. Six HCCs occurred in the HBsAg-seropositive group and none in the HBsAg-seronegative group. The authors give a standardized mortality ratio (SMR) for HCC of 27 [95% CI, 10–39] on the basis of mortality rates in the general population.

A prospective mortality study of HBsAg-seropositive people who donated blood in England and Wales between 1971 and 1981 (Hall *et al.*, 1985) comprised 2880 men and 1054 women, of whom more than 92% could be followed for death to the end of 1983. Seventy-seven cohort members died during the period. Five deaths from HCC were reported among men in contrast to the 0.1 expected, giving a RR of 42 (95% CI, 13–98). No death from HCC occurred among the female cohort members (0.02 expected).

2.3.3 *Prospective studies of populations with pre-existing disease*

The incidence of HCC in HBsAg-seropositive and HBsAg-seronegative subjects has been studied among patients with pre-existing liver disease, as indicated variously by abnormal liver function, 'chronic hepatitis' and cirrhosis. The RRs for HCC associated with HBsAg seropositivity in these studies were generally small, e.g. [RR, 2.1 (95% CI, 0.3–17)] (Liaw *et al.*, 1986). Their interpretation is complicated by the fact that causes of liver disease other than HBV may also be associated with an increased risk for HCC (Liaw et al., 1986; Dodd & Nath, 1987; Colombo et al., 1991; Johnson, 1991; Kato et al., 1992).

2.4 Case-control studies

2.4.1 Hepatocellular carcinoma

Many case-control studies have been published on the relationship between HCC and HBV infection. The prevalences of seropositivity are summarized in Table 6 (p. 90). In all studies, tests for HBV markers were performed on one occasion only, and 'carriers' were taken to be subjects in whom HBsAg was detected at that time. Unless otherwise noted in the Table, testing for HBV markers was done by radioimmunoassay. RRs, as measured by the odds ratio (OR) and 95% Cornfield confidence intervals (CIs), were calculated by the Working Group wherever the data reported in the original papers allowed it. In general, only ORs and p values are reported in the text, while ORs and CIs are reported in Table 6. Studies of clinical series (typically, patients with liver disease) in which cases of HCC were a subgroup but in which there was no specifically defined control group were not included.

(a) Africa

Prince et al. (1970) reported a comparison of patients with HCC and other chronic liver diseases with various control groups in relation to the prevalence of HBsAg seropositivity. They tested sera from subjects from Senegal, Uganda and the USA using two serological assays—agar-gel diffusion and high-voltage immunoelectroosmophoresis; the latter was 10 times more sensitive than the former. The prevalences of HBsAg seropositivity among the subjects examined were: in Senegal, 42% of 210 HCC patients, 9% of 201 adult males and 12.7% of 959 army personnel; in Uganda, 12% of 34 HCC patients, 23% of 26 with cirrhosis and 2% of 311 healthy subjects [OR for HCC, 6.8; 1.8-25]; in the USA, 4% of 55 HCC patients, 29% of 42 with chronic active hepatitis, 8% of 124 with cirrhosis and 0.1% of 55 956 blood donors. The authors remarked that, although the controls were not matched to the cases by age, sex or place of residence, hepatitis virus appeared to play an important role in at least a proportion of the cases of chronic liver disease.

Vogel et al. (1972) reported the results of a study conducted among in-patients at Mulago Hospital, Kampala, Uganda, or the Solid Tumour Centre in Uganda between October 1969 and May 1970 (Vogel et al., 1970) and January 1970 to May 1971. The 90 HCC cases (in 73 men and 17 women) had a significantly higher frequency of HBsAg in their sera (40%) than the 224 (149 non-neoplastic and 75 neoplastic) controls combined (151 men, 73 women) (3%; $p < 0.001$). Control patients with cirrhosis or hepatitis were excluded; histological confirmation was available for 71 of the HCC cases. There was no difference between cases and controls with respect to anti-HBs seropositivity (28-37%). A nonsignificant association was noted between HBsAg seropositivity in HCC patients and the presence of cirrhosis (44% in comparison with 27% without cirrhosis). Serum was tested by complement fixation, counter immunoelectrophoresis and passive haemagglutination.

Kew et al. (1974) investigated 75 male Bantu miners in South Africa with HCC confirmed at necropsy. The control group of 18 377 healthy miners was comparable with respect to age and tribal distribution. Testing of sera for HBsAg by complement fixation and

Table 5. Prospective studies of HBV surface antigen (HBsAg)-seropositive people for the development of hepatocellular carcinoma (HCC)

Region, reference, location	Subjects (age)	HBsAg seroprevalence	Mean duration of follow-up (years)	No. of cases of HCC	Annual incidence (cases/100 000)	RR (95% CI)
America						
Nomura et al. (1982) Hawaii, USA	Men of Japanese ancestry (born 1900–19) Controls	7498 HBsAg+ 16 HCCs (10 HBsAg+) 48 (0 HBsAg+)	11.8	16	[18]	[∞], $p < 0.0001$ Nested case-control analysis
Prince & Alcabes (1982) New York, USA	Blood donors; men (20–>50 years)	6850 HBsAg+	4.4	4	[13, crude]	[10; 2.7–26] SMR using HCC mortality in New York
Dodd & Nath (1987) USA	Red Cross blood donors (age at death from HCC, 30–64 years)	15 166 HBsAg+ 18 144 HBsAg–	3.68 3.26	6 0	11 0	27 [10–39] SMR using HCC mortality in US population in 1975
McMahon et al. (1990a) Alaska, USA	Alaskan native population; men, women; average age, ~22 years	1400 HBsAg+; 59% male	5.58	20	Men, 387 Women, 63	148 [59–305] Compared with estimated incidence in general population
Asia						
Oshima et al. (1984) Osaka, Japan	Blood donors; men (more than half < 30 years)	8646 HBsAg+	6.2	20	[37]	6.6 (4–10) Compared with incidence in Osaka general population
Fukao (1985) Miyagi, Japan	Blood donors; men (> 30 years)	1000 HBsAg+ 10 000 HBsAg– Matched by age, residence, month of donation	NR	3 1	45	30 [6.0–88]

Table 5 (contd)

Region, reference location	Subjects (age)	HBsAg seroprevalence	Mean duration of follow-up (years)	No. of cases of HCC	Annual incidence (cases/100 000)	RR (95% CI)
Asia (contd)						
Tu et al. (1985) Chongming Island, China	Men (> 40 years) from 4 communes	1971 HBsAg+ or anti-HBc+ and anti-HBs− 10 251 HBsAg−	3	37 33	651 (carriers) 98.6 (non-carriers)	6.7 [4.2–11]
Tokudome et al. (1987) Fukuoka, Japan	Blood donors; women (age, NR)	3769 HBsAg+	5.05	4	[21]	5.6 [1.5–14] Ccompared with adjusted mortality in Fukuoka population
Tokudome et al. (1988) Fukuoka, Japan	Blood donors; men (age, NR)	2595 HBsAg+	5.86	15	[98.6]	7.3 [4.1–12] Compared with adjusted mortality in Fukuoka population
Ding et al. (1988) Guangxi, China	Men and women (> 20 years)	1839 HBsAg+ 9233 HBsAg−	6.8	[41] [39]	NR	[5.3; 3.8–7.2]
Sakuma et al. (1988) Japan	Railway workers; 6918 men	126 HBsAg+ 6792 HBsAg−	8.5 8.5	4 6	[374] [10]	30 [1–77]
Sakuma et al. (1988) Japan	Railway workers; men (40.55 years)	513 HBsAg+ 25 034 HBsAg−	7.3 7.3	9 21	[240] [12]	[21; 9.6–40]
Yeh et al. (1989) Guangxi, China	Men (25–64 years) from 5 communes	2072 tested for HBsAg 76 HCC (69 HBsAg+) 304 controls (68 HBsAg+)	3.8	69 HBsAg+ 7 HBsAg−	NR	39 (16–117) Nested case-control analysis
Beasley & Hwang (1991) Taiwan, China	Government employees; men (82% 40–59 years)	3454 HBsAg+ 19 253 HBsAg−	[11.25] [10.28]	184 10	474 [52]	103 (57–205)

Table 5 (contd)

Region, reference, location	Subjects (age)	HBsAg seroprevalence	Mean duration of follow-up (years)	No. of cases of HCC	Annual incidence (cases/100 000)	RR (95% CI)
Asia (contd)						
Ross et al. (1992) Shanghai, China	Men (45–64 years)	18 224 men 22 HCCs (12 HBsAg+) 140 controls (15 HBsAg+)	1.9 years	12 HBsAg+ 10 HBsAg−	NR	8.5 (2.8–26) Nested case-control analysis
Europe						
Hall et al. (1985) United Kingdom	Blood donors (age, NR)	2880 HBsAg+ men 1054 HBsAg+ women	NR	5 0	NR	42 (13–98)

NR, not reported

counter immunoelectrophoresis revealed a difference in the prevalence of persistent HBV infection: 40% versus 7% [$p < 0.05$]. No significant relationship was noted between HBsAg seropositivity and the presence of cirrhosis (46% in comparison with 31% without cirrhosis) among cases. [No information was provided as to how and when cases and controls were identified.]

A study conducted at Le Dantec Hospital, Dakar, Senegal, between October 1972 and July 1974 involved 165 cases of HCC (in 127 men and 38 women), 154 controls with other cancers (102 men, 52 women) and 328 non-cancer controls (226 men, 102 women) (Michon et al., 1975; Prince et al., 1975). A diagnosis of HCC was histologically confirmed for 80 cases. Controls were matched to cases on sex, age (within 10 years) and admission date (within 30 days) and were of similar ethnicity and religion; non-cancer controls were free of liver disease. A higher frequency of HBsAg seropositivity was reported among the cases than in each control group: 61.2% versus 11.8 and 11.3% in the two control groups, respectively [$p < 0.05$]. The prevalence of anti-HBs seropositivity (tested by passive haemagglutination) alone was lower among cases (18.2%) than controls (45.4 and 42.1%, respectively) (Michon et al., 1975). In 94 documented cases of HCC, the presence of cirrhosis was not related to HBsAg seropositivity but was related to anti-HBs seropositivity (6% versus 20%; $p < 0.05$) (Prince et al., 1975).

Larouzé et al. (1976) matched 28 cases of HCC (in 22 men and 6 women) from Le Dantec Hospital, Dakar, Senegal, to healthy individuals from the same urban neighbourhood or rural village, of the same sex, age and ethnic group. Blood was also collected from parents and siblings. Histological confirmation was obtained in 24 cases. Although no significant association was observed between the presence of HBsAg (by radioimmunoassay) and HCC (79% in cases, 57% in controls; $p = 0.15$ [OR, 2.8]), the prevalence of HBsAg among the controls was very high. Cases were markedly less likely to be seropositive for anti-HBs (by passive haemagglutination) (25% versus 64%; $p = 0.006$) and more likely to be seropositive for anti-HBc (by counter immunoelectrophoresis and immunodiffusion) (89% versus 64%; $p = 0.05$). [Neither the time frame nor the case selection method was described.]

In a study in Addis Ababa, Ethiopia, HBsAg seroprevalence was compared in 46 HCC cases (in 31 men and 15 women) and 90 healthy hospital employees without a history of liver disease, blood transfusion, leprosy, leukaemia or Down's syndrome (Tsega et al., 1976; Tsega, 1977). The cases from whom serum was collected were a subset of 100 consecutive HCC patients admitted to St Paul's or Haile Selassie I hospitals between June 1972 and November 1974. The diagnosis of HCC was confirmed by biopsy in 25 cases. HBsAg seropositivity was significantly associated with the occurrence of HCC: 50% among cases, 7% among controls [OR, 14, $p < 0.001$].

Tabor et al. (1977) analysed serum samples from 47 cases of HCC confirmed by biopsy in Uganda (previously studied by Vogel et al., 1972), 19 in Zambia and 27 in the USA; the controls were 50 in-patients with melanoma or Kaposi's sarcoma in Uganda, 40 healthy Zambian villagers (from the same geographic region as the cases) and three US blood donor groups (6726 total), respectively. Evidence of active HBV infection (HBsAg seropositivity with or without anti-HBs seropositivity or anti-HBc seropositivity with anti-HBs seronegativity) was significantly associated with HCC in each comparison: 72% of cases in Uganda, 68% in Zambia and 41% in the USA. Anti-HBs was tested by radioimmunoassay and passive haemagglutination and anti-HBc by complement fixation and counter immunoelectrophoresis.

In a study involving blood donor controls, 32 histologically confirmed cases of HCC in 19 men and 13 women in Mozambique were studied (Reys et al., 1977). Their 60% HBsAg seropositivity was significantly higher than the 3-15% [9% overall] observed in 231 male African blood donors from the Hôpital Central de Maputo by subgroup ($p < 0.01$). Anti-HBs was measured by radioimmunoprecipitation (12% compared with 33-49% had anti-HBs). [Neither the methods of subject selection nor the time period were further specified in either study.]

Van Den Heever et al. (1978) conducted a study at H.F. Verwoerd Hospital in Pretoria, South Africa, during 1973-76 of 92 histologically confirmed cases of HCC from the Pretoria area (in 75 men and 17 women) matched to 92 orthopaedic out-patients from the same area, of the same age and sex with no history of liver disease; all subjects were black. The association between seropositivity for HBsAg and HCC status was significant (34% of cases, 9% of controls; $p < 0.01$) [RR, 5.3].

In another case-control study in South Africa (Kew et al., 1979), a 62% seroprevalence of HBsAg was found among 289 blacks (280 men, nine women) with histologically confirmed HCC over a four-year period; the prevalence in the 213 healthy controls (gold miners matched by age, sex and ethnic group) was significantly lower, 11% ($p < 0.001$). The cases had been referred consecutively to the South African Primary Liver Cancer Unit from mine hospitals or admitted to two teaching hospitals; most were miners, and the majority were not from South Africa. A significant inverse association was observed for anti-HBs reactivity and HCC (17% in cases, 42% in controls; $p < 0.001$) [OR, 0.28]. In a subset of 74 cases and 104 controls tested for anti-HBc, a significant difference was found (89% versus 38%; $p < 0.001$). A detailed serological analysis of 131 HBsAg-seropositive (98 cases, 33 controls) and 222 HBsAg-seronegative (50 cases, 172 controls) male miners was performed (Kew et al., 1981), using the more sensitive radioimmunoassay to detect HBeAg, anti-HBe and anti-HBc. Significant positive correlations with HCC were observed for anti-HBc ($p < 0.01$) and anti-HBe ($p < 0.05$) among the HBsAg-seronegative subjects, and significant inverse relationships for anti-HBe ($p < 0.02$) among HBsAg-seropositive individuals and for anti-HBs ($p < 0.05$) among HBsAg-seronegative subjects. No relationship was observed between HBsAg seropositivity and the presence of cirrhosis among HCC cases (Kew et al., 1979). [The case identification period was not further specified. The later study (Kew et al., 1981) may have included additional subjects not in the earlier one.]

Seventy-six cases of HCC (in 60 men and 16 women) and 33 controls matched for age, sex and tribe were studied by Bowry and Shah (1980) in Nairobi, Kenya. The cases attended Kenyatta National Hospital between January 1976 and April 1979; histological or cytological confirmation was obtained for 56. Of the controls, 28 were relatives of hospital patients and five were hospital patients. HBsAg was detected (by passive haemagglutination) in 51% of cases and 6% of controls [$p < 0.05$]. A report published a year later by the same group (Bowry et al., 1981) probably involved a subset of 60 of these HCC cases [subject selection was not described]. Seropositivity only for anti-HBc was found in eight [13%] of the 60 HCC cases, 15% of 20 matched hospital controls and 4% of 104 volunteer blood donors;

the prevalence was higher among the 13 HCC patients with known cirrhosis (31%). [The blood donors were younger than the cases.]

Coursaget et al. (1981) conducted a study in Senegal of 134 cases of HCC (in 114 men and 20 women) diagnosed at Le Dantec Hospital and 100 blood donor controls from the National Blood Center of Dakar, in which anti-HBc was measured by counter immuno-electrophoresis. A significant association was found between HCC and active HBV infection [OR, 14] (67% versus 13%; $p < 10^{-6}$). A significantly lower frequency of past infection (HBsAg seronegativity and anti-HBs seropositivity or anti-HBc seropositivity by radio-immunoassay) was noted for cases (33%) in comparison with controls (74%; $p < 10^{-6}$). HBsAg was detected in 63% of the HCC patients and in 12% of the 100 blood donors [OR, 12], 14% of 833 rural country dwellers (72 men, 761 women) [OR, 11] and 25% of 560 leprosy patients from the Pavillon de Malte (410 men, 150 women) [OR, 50]. Two earlier reports of this study (Maupas et al., 1977; Coursaget et al., 1980) showed consistent findings. [Little detail could be found as to subject selection.]

Gombe (1984) found a significantly higher prevalence of HBsAg seropositivity among 65 cases of HCC (in 47 men and 18 women) (74%) than among 120 blood donors (115 men, five women) (9% [$p < 0.05$]) or 71 other cancer controls (13 men, 58 women) (3%; $p < 0.05$) in the Congo. The blood donors were tested in two centres by radioimmunoassay and passive haemagglutination, and the HCC cases and cancer controls from the Brazzaville General Hospital by passive haemagglutination. [The process for selecting subjects was not clear.]

Sebti (1984) in Rabat, Morocco, reported a significant but weaker association between HCC and HBsAg seropositivity (17% in 46 cases and 5% in 379 controls) [OR, 4.2]. The HCC patients were a subset of 63 cases hospitalized at Avicenne Hospital between 1976 and 1983; the controls were healthy subjects and people with non-hepatic disease. [The process for selecting subjects was not clear.]

Another study by Kew et al. (1986a) focused on southern African blacks living in an urban environment. Markers of HBV infection were assayed in 62 urban-born patients with histologically confirmed HCC (41 men, 21 women) and in pair-matched urban-born hospital controls, matched according to race, sex, age, tribe (when possible), hospital and ward. Subjects were identified from two large general hospitals, Baragwanath in Soweto and Hillbrow in Johannesburg. HBsAg was detected significantly more frequently among the cases (40%) than the controls (3%) ($p < 0.001$). No difference was observed with regard to past infection (HBsAg seronegativity and anti-HBs or anti-HBc seropositivity). [Information about the period of subject selection was not provided.]

Otu (1987) studied 200 consecutive, histologically confirmed cases of HCC (in 180 men and 20 women) at the University of Calabar Teaching Hospital, Nigeria, between January 1978 and December 1982. Two symptomless controls matched for sex and age (within five years) were selected per case from the general out-patient department. HBsAg was detected in 49% of the cases and 8% of the controls ($p < 0.01$). [Little detail was provided about selection of controls.]

Gashau and Mohammed (1991) compared the prevalence of HBV markers in 65 HCC patients (57 men, eight women) and 69 sex- and age-matched healthy controls in Nigeria. The cases of HCC were examined consecutively at the University of Maiduguri Teaching Hospital between 1986 and 1987; needle biopsy was used for diagnosis in 21. The controls were examined at the hospital during the same period; most were blood donors. The cases had a significantly higher rate of HBsAg seropositivity (65%), measured by ELISA and reverse passive haemagglutination, than the controls (35%) [OR, 3.2]. Seropositivity for anti-HBc, measured by ELISA, was about the same in those tested in the two groups; HBeAg seropositivity was higher and that of anti-HBe lower in the cases. [Few details were provided about the controls.]

Mohamed et al. (1992) examined the prevalence of current (HBsAg seropositivity) and past (seronegative for HBsAg and seropositive for anti-HBs or anti-HBc) infection among 101 black South Africans with HCC, matched for ethnic origin, sex, age (within two years) with patients from the wards of Baragwanath Hospital, Johannesburg (77 men, 24 women). Controls were excluded if they had a disease caused by alcohol abuse or were unable to answer questions. Histological confirmation was obtained for 85 cases of HCC. Among men, 35% of cases and 5% of controls were currently HBsAg seropositive; the OR, adjusted for alcohol and smoking, was 7.5 (95% CI, 2.2–25). Among women, HBsAg seropositivity was 25% for cases and 4% for controls, with an adjusted OR of 12 (95% CI, 1.0–154). [The time frame for subject selection was not given.]

At the Parirenyatwa Teaching Hospital in Zimbabwe, Tswana and Moyo (1992) studied 182 HCC cases (in 128 men and 54 women) and 100 non-liver disease patient controls (50 men, 50 women). Pregnant women, cigarette smokers and alcohol consumers were excluded from the study. The diagnosis of HCC was made clinically and confirmed by α-fetoprotein level. Controls were selected randomly and were comparable to the cases with respect to age and sex; subjects were 20–65 years old. A significant correlation ($p < 0.0001$) was reported between HBsAg seroprevalence and HCC [OR, 10] (56% in cases versus 11% in controls); anti-HBc was detected in 54% of cases and 4% of controls [OR, 29; $p < 0.05$]. Among HBsAg-seropositive subjects, the seroprevalence of HBeAg was 20% among cases and 9% among controls. HBV markers were determined by ELISA. [The time frame for the study was not given.]

Ryder et al. (1992) studied HCC and HBV infection in the Gambia between 1 December 1981 and 30 November 1982. In a community-based surveillance system, they identified 70 cases (in 61 men and nine women); 44 were confirmed histologically. Patients were interviewed within one month of diagnosis in their village, at which time the person living closest to the case, of the same sex and age (within five years) was identified as a control. All potential subjects agreed to participate, and the two groups were not significantly different with respect to length of residence, alcohol consumption, smoking habits or family size. After adjustment for age, the following associations were reported: HBsAg (64 cases and 67 controls tested), OR, 6.9 ($p < 0.01$); anti-HBs (63 cases and 68 controls tested), OR, 0.31 (not significant); HBeAg (63 cases and 68 controls tested), OR, undefined ($p < 0.001$); and anti-HBe (62 cases and 66 controls tested), OR, 2.3 (not significant). The prevalence of HBsAg seropositivity was 63% among cases and 21% among controls; that of HBeAg was 17% among cases and 0 among controls. In all instances, the relationships were strongest among people under 50 years of age.

Serological HBV markers were investigated by the immunoperoxidase procedure in 40 cases of HCC selected in 1985 among 223 cases collected at the Department of Pathology of the University Hospital and Medical School of Kinshasa, Zaire, and in 68 age- and sex-matched controls selected from among blood donors (Kashala et al., 1992). The proportion of seropositive individuals among cases of HCC was significantly higher for HBsAg (57.6% vs 7.35%) and for anti-HBeAg (27.5% vs 16.2%) but was significantly lower for anti-HBs (25% vs 63%), and no significant difference was observed for anti-HBc, HBe or HBV DNA.

(b) *Americas*

Yarrish et al. (1980) analysed sera collected from patients attending hospitals in Philadelphia, USA, between 1968 and 1977. The sera from 34 HCC cases (in 28 men and six women) were then matched to those of 38 patients (30 men, eight women) with colon cancer, 45 (36 men, nine women) with lung cancer and 56 blood donors (48 men, eight women) matched for age (within five years) and sex. All but one HCC case was histologically confirmed. Blood donor samples were collected prior to routine screening for HBsAg and were stored on average 39 months longer than the sera from HCC cases; the sera of the colon cancer controls were stored for four months less and those of the lung cancer controls for 17 months less than those of the HCC cases. Five HCC cases (15%) were seropositive for HBsAg (assayed by radioimmunoassay), which was significantly higher than in any control group ($p < 0.05$). Seropositivity for anti-HBs, as assayed by passive haemagglutination, was not significantly different between cases and controls. [The details of subject selection were not provided.]

In the Japan–Hawaii Cancer Study, described in detail on p. 69, Nomura et al. (1982) found a significant excess of HBsAg in HCC patients in Hawaii (63%, with none in controls).

Austin et al. (1986) performed a multicentre study of 67 HCC patients (45 men, 22 women), aged 18–84, from 12 US hospitals, for whom HBsAg status was known (49 assayed by radioimmunoassay, 18 from medical records). The 18% (all in men) HBsAg prevalence among these cases was significantly higher ($p = 0.0002$) than the 0 prevalence for the 63 controls, who had no liver disease or a condition related to tobacco use and were matched by sex, year of birth (within five years), race and current residence (59 assayed by radioimmunoassay, four from records). Of the people seronegative for HBsAg who were tested, 7/40 (18%) of cases and 5/58 (9%) of controls were seropositive for anti-HBs [not significant]. [Details were not given about the time and method of case selection.]

Yu et al. (1990) described a study of black and white residents of Los Angeles County, USA, 18–74 years of age. Histologically confirmed incident cases of HCC were identified between January 1984 and August 1989; 392 cases were eligible, but only 51 (12 blacks, 39 white; 35 men, 16 women) were analysed, either because of death (290), refusal (29), inability to locate (9), incorrect diagnosis (7) or serum sample depletion (6). Controls were selected from among 404 community control subjects used in a case–control study of lymphoma from 1978 to 1982; 128 of 404 controls were randomly selected to be frequency matched by sex and age (10-year intervals) to the cases (1 black, 127 white; 81 men, 47 women). All interviews were performed in the subjects' homes. The age- and sex-adjusted ORs for the various HBV markers, tested by radioimmunoassay with no markers as the reference level, were: HBsAg, infinity ($p = 0.002$); anti-HBc, 7.3 ($p < 0.0005$); anti-HBs, 5.2 ($p < 0.0005$). Neither adjustment for level of education nor a separate analysis of US-born or white subjects affected the results.

In a study conducted in Baltimore, USA, 99 consecutive histologically confirmed HCC patients at the Johns Hopkins Oncology Center were compared between January 1987 and May 1988 with 98 consecutive patients with other malignancies seen at the same centre between November 1987 and January 1988 (Di Bisceglie *et al.*, 1991). The cases were from the eastern half of the USA and were referred for inclusion in therapeutic radiation trials. No significant difference was reported between the two groups with regard to age, sex or race. HBsAg and IgM anti-HBc were detected only in the cases (7% and 8%, respectively), at significantly higher prevalences than in the controls ($p = 0.009$ and 0.004). Cases and controls were similar with regard to the presence of the other HBV markers measured. Anti-HBc was determined by enzyme immunoassay. [The fact that the patients had advanced disease might have affected HBsAg levels.]

(c) Asia

In Taiwan, China, Tong *et al.* (1971) examined the prevalence of detectable antigen in 55 cases of HCC (in 52 men and three women) and 943 male personnel at the Tsoying Naval Base. The cases were from the Chinese Veterans' Hospital, and 25 diagnoses were confirmed by needle biopsy or autopsy. No subject had Down's syndrome, leprosy, leukaemia or a recent transfusion (within 12 months); the controls had no past or present liver disease. A significant difference in HBsAg seropositivity was found by a modified immunodiffusion technique: 80% among cases and 15% among controls ($p < 0.001$) [OR, 23]. The cases were older than the controls (mean, 48 *versus* 30 years). [No details were provided concerning the timing or selection of subjects.]

Simons *et al.* (1972) studied HBsAg seroprevalence among 156 Chinese HCC patients in Singapore; 114 (87 men, 27 women) had been reported previously (Simons *et al.*, 1971). The control groups consisted of 1516 male blood donors, 260 women attending antenatal clinics and 207 patients investigated for suspected nasopharyngeal carcinoma at one of the hospitals; all controls were Chinese. HBsAg seropositivity was markedly higher among the HCC cases (35%) than in any of the control groups (8%, 2% and 6%, respectively). [The associations calculated by the Working Group were all statistically significant; the blood donors and women attending antenatal clinics are combined in Table 6 as 'normal controls'. No details were found concerning selection of controls.]

Lee (1975) compared the prevalence of HBsAg seropositivity in 100 cases of HCC (in 85 men and 15 women) and 120 patient controls (98 men, 22 women) in Hong Kong with no history of liver disease or blood transfusion; the diagnosis of HCC was confirmed by biopsy in 81 cases. Testing by immunoelectroosmophoresis and complement fixation showed a significant difference (49% *versus* 9%; $p < 0.001$). [No data were provided on the timing or process of subject selection or on the gender distribution of the cases.]

Chainuvati *et al.* (1975) reported a higher frequency of HBsAg seroprevalence, measured by crossover immunoelectrophoresis, among 49 HCC patients with cirrhosis (16%) than among 87 hospitalized controls (74 men, 13 women) without liver disease (2%) in Thailand ($p < 0.005$). No HBsAg was found in eight HCC patients without cirrhosis. The cases in this study had been identified between August 1972 and April 1973 and were histologically confirmed.

Kubo *et al.* (1977) studied 124 cases of HCC (in 107 men and 17 women) seen at Kurume University and Chiba University Schools of Medicine, Japan; the diagnosis was histologically confirmed in 108 cases. Healthy employees of the Japan National Railways (290 men, nine women) seen at regular physical check-up were used as controls. The difference in seroprevalence of HBsAg between cases and controls was significant (46% *versus* 4%; $p < 0.01$) [OR, 20], as were smaller differences in anti-HBc seropositivity (73% *versus* 30%; $p < 0.01$) [OR, 6.2] and the presence of any marker (81% *versus* 34%; $p < 0.01$) [OR, 8.1]. No difference between cases and controls was observed for anti-HBs, as tested by passive haemagglutination. Immune adherence haemagglutination was used to detect anti-HBc. [No details were given as to when subjects were diagnosed.]

In Taiwan, China, 127 HCC cases admitted to the National Taiwan University Hospital between May 1974 and December 1976 were compared with 729 healthy controls (Chen & Sung, 1978). The controls comprised 241 40–67-year-old adults from a cancer education programme and 488 18–22-year-old university students receiving a regular check-up in 1975. HCC was histologically confirmed in 63 cases. HBsAg (assayed by reverse passive haemagglutination) was found in 83% of cases and 15% of controls [OR, 28; $p < 0.05$], and anti-HBs (detected by passive haemagglutination) in 14% and 45%, respectively [OR, 0.21; $p < 0.05$]. An analysis of 68 HCC cases with and without cirrhosis revealed no association with HBsAg seropositivity (81% in each group). [The gender breakdown for the subjects was not given.]

Chien *et al.* (1981) conducted a study among Chinese HCC patients seen at the Taiwan Veterans General Hospital (Tong *et al.*, 1971). The 102 cases (in 97 men and five women) were matched by age and sex to 100 healthy controls from the out-patient clinic; histological confirmation was obtained for 36 cases. A larger proportion of cases than of controls were seropositive for HBsAg (71% *versus* 12%) [OR, 18] or anti-HBc (98% *versus* 84%) [OR, 4.7], and a lower proportion for anti-HBs (27% *versus* 54%). HBsAg-seropositive patients had higher levels of HBeAg and lower levels of anti-HBe than controls. All differences except those for HBeAg and anti-HBe were significant [$p < 0.05$].

Lam *et al.* (1982) performed a study in Hong Kong which included 107 Chinese cases (in 95 men and 12 women) of HCC at the Queen Mary Hospital, who were matched by sex and age (within five years) to 107 control (94 men, 13 women) trauma patients in the orthopaedic ward of the same hospital; 106 cases were histologically confirmed. Between March 1977 and September 1980, 149 Chinese HCC patients were admitted to the hospital, 72% of whom were interviewed; controls were interviewed within one month of the index case. After adjustment for age and sex, the OR for HCC associated with the presence of HBsAg was 21 (95% CI, 10–46).

In the Republic of Korea, Sjøgren *et al.* (1984) reported an HBsAg seroprevalence of 82% among 110 histologically confirmed HCC cases (in 90 men and 20 women) and 14% among 63 controls with other cancers matched for sex and age ($p < 0.001$). Subjects were identified between 1973 and 1981 at St Mary's Hospital in Seoul; the control patients had no evidence of liver disease, although five had metastatic liver cancer (Chung *et al.*, 1983). IgM anti-HBc was present in 74 cases (67%) and one control (2%) ($p < 0.001$) [OR, 127]; the association between HCC and presence of IgM anti-HBc was also seen among the HBsAg-seropositive subjects (81% versus 11%; $p < 0.005$). [No details of subject selection methods were given.]

A report from Yamanashi Prefecture, Japan (Inaba et al., 1984), described a matched analysis of 62 cases (in 49 men and 13 women) of HCC from seven hospitals between April 1977 and August 1979. Patient controls with no hepatic disease were selected by sex, age (within five years) and hospital. Confirmation of the diagnosis in liver biopsies was obtained for 36 of the HCC cases. There was a significant, 10-fold increase in risk for liver cancer associated with HBsAg seropositivity, assayed by reverse passive haemagglutination (36% in cases versus 3% in controls) ($p < 0.01$), and a weaker association with anti-HBs (27% versus 18%) ($p < 0.05$) [crude OR, 1.7].

A matched analysis of cases of HCC in Guangxi Autonomous Region, China, revealed a high OR (17; 95% CI, 4.3–99) for the relationship between HBsAg seropositivity and HCC (Yeh et al., 1985a,b), based on 50 cases (in 47 men and three women) and 49 controls without liver disease matched by sex, age (within five years) and ward/clinic; 86% of the cases were seropositive for HBsAg versus 22.45% of the controls. Case identification began on 1 July 1982 and continued until 50 cases were obtained at the College Hospital; only four diagnoses were based on histological examination. In the HBsAg-seropositive subjects assayed, HBeAg reactivity was not significantly greater in HCC patients (31%) than in controls (18%); the seroprevalence of anti-HBe was lower among cases than controls (50% versus 64%) (Luo et al., 1988).

In Riyadh, Saudi Arabia, a significant difference ($p < 0.001$) was found between cases of HCC and local population controls for HBsAg seropositivity [60% versus 12%] (Arya et al., 1988). The 30 histologically confirmed cases (in 25 men and five women) were a subset of cases in 75 local HCC patients hospitalized at King Fahad Central Hospital from September 1984 to October 1985, from whom serum was available. The control group comprised 326 patients aged 20–> 40 treated for minor ailments in the area. Among the HBsAg-seropositive subjects, a significant inverse association was reported between HCC and anti-HBe seroprevalence [OR, 0.15] (24% in cases versus 67% of controls; $p < 0.01$), but no significant association was seen for HBeAg [OR, 2.7]. ELISA was used to assay all HBV markers. [Little detail was available about control selection.]

A matched analysis by Lu, C.Q. et al. (1988) of 30 HCC patients and 60 matched controls with other tumours or anorectal diseases in the same hospital in Tianjin, China, showed significant associations with reactivity to HBsAg ($p < 0.001$) (OR, 5) and anti-HBc ($p < 0.05$) (OR, 39). The prevalences among the cases were 57% and 83%, respectively, and those among controls were [17%] and [20%]. HBV markers were assayed by passive haemagglutination and ELISA.

Lingao (1989) conducted a study in the Philippines of 340 HCC cases (in 288 men and 52 women) individually matched by age and sex to asymptomatic population-based controls from five rural areas. About 90% of the diagnoses of HCC were confirmed histologically. The presence of HBsAg was evaluated by reverse passive haemagglutinin, radioimmunoassay and ELISA only in patients with HBV infection and was significantly higher for HCC patients than for the controls [75% versus 14%; $p < 0.0001$; OR, 19 (12–29)]. Among the HBsAg-reactive subjects, a significant association was found between HCC and anti-HBe seropositivity (73% versus 52%; $p < 0.01$) [RR, 2.6] but not with HBeAg; these markers were determined by gel diffusion followed by radioimmunoassay and ELISA. Among 99 cirrhosis patients studied, the HBsAg seroprevalence was 58%. In a preliminary study of 104 histopathologically confirmed HCC cases (in 88 men and 16 women), which probably represented a subset of the larger case group (Lingao et al., 1981), the control group consisted of 84 asymptomatic controls (42 men, 42 women). [No details of subject selection were provided.]

In the study of Yeh et al. (1990) in southern Guangxi Autonomous Region, China (see p. 68), 91% of 76 HCC cases were HBsAg seropositive compared with 22% of 304 controls (OR, 39; 95% CI, 16–117).

In a study by Tsukuma et al. (1990) in Japan, of 229 (192 men, 37 women) newly diagnosed HCC patients admitted to the Center for Adult Diseases in Osaka between November 1983 and June 1987, 221 (96.5%) were interviewed; 87 cases were histologically confirmed. One control per male case and two per female case (266 in all) were selected from among patients admitted for gastroenterology, people admitted for health check-ups and those admitted for gastroenterological endoscopy. People with liver disease, malignancy, smoking- and alcohol-related disease, and lack of HBsAg testing were excluded. All subjects were interviewed at admission or at the time of endoscopic examination. In the analysis, confounding by sex, age, history of blood transfusion, heavy drinking, cigarette index and family history of liver cancer was controlled by unconditional logistic regression; the OR for HBsAg seropositivity was 14 (95% CI, 5.7–36; $p < 0.0001$). HBsAg was determined by reverse passive haemagglutination; the results were abstracted from medical records.

Lin et al. (1991) studied cases of HCC and hospital controls at the Chang-Gung Memorial and Kaohsiung Medical College Hospitals in Taiwan, China, and interviewed them between 20 February 1985 and 20 December 1986. Preliminary results were reported previously (Lu, S.N. et al., 1988). The subjects were 243 hospitalized or out-patient cases of HCC (in 218 men and 25 women) and 302 orthopaedic and ophthalmic in-patient controls (260 men, 42 women). Two controls were matched to each case by age (within three years) and sex, but some subsequently refused to have blood drawn; the authors stated that no significant difference was found between cases and controls with regard to age or sex. Adjustment for age, sex and hepatitis markers yielded significantly increased risks in association with seropositivity for HBsAg (OR, 10; 77% in cases versus 19% in controls) and HBeAg (OR, 3.2; 18% versus 2%) and significantly decreased risks in association with seropositivity for anti-HBs (OR, 0.1; 28% versus 78%) and anti-HBc (OR, 0.1; 97% versus 100%). [No information was given about how many subjects refused to have blood drawn or how many cases were histologically confirmed.]

Chen et al. (1991) examined 200 male HCC patients from the same two hospitals in Taiwan who were recruited consecutively between September 1985 and July 1987. Healthy community controls were matched individually to cases by age (within three years), ethnic group and residence, using a roster from household registration offices. Seventeen female pairs had also been identified but were excluded owing to their small number. Only two cases and three controls were seronegative for markers of HBV infection; thus, the authors focused on detection of HBsAg and HBeAg. In comparison with those seronegative for both antigens, those only seropositive for HBsAg had a 17-fold higher risk for HCC (95% CI, 7.4–38) and those seropositive for both had an OR of 58 (95% CI, 27–124). [Refusal rates were not provided. The cases of HCC overlapped with those analysed by Lin et al. (1991); the number of histologically confirmed diagnoses was not stated.]

Srivatanakul et al. (1991) studied subjects from three hospitals in several areas of northeast Thailand as part of a larger study of liver cancer (Parkin et al., 1991). Sixty-five cases (in 47 men and 18 women) were compared with 65 controls matched by sex, age (within five years), residence and hospital. Controls were either in-patients or clinic patients with nonmalignant, nonhepatic diseases and diseases unrelated to tobacco or alcohol. All subjects were under 75 years, were recruited during 1987–88 and were interviewed in hospital; histological confirmation was obtained for 20 HCC cases. Conditional multivariate analysis, controlling for consumption of alcohol, shrimp paste, powdered peanuts and fresh vegetables and for betel-nut chewing gave a significant OR of 15 (95% CI, 2.3–103) for the relationship between HCC and seropositivity for HBsAg ($p < 0.001$); 42% of the cases were HBV carriers versus 8% of the controls. HBV markers were determined by ELISA.

A study in Japan involved 204 patients with HCC (31 were not studied 'for logistic reasons') admitted to Kyushu University Hospital between December 1985 and June 1989 (Tanaka, K. et al., 1988, 1992). The cases were diagnosed within one year of identification, were aged 40–69 and were residents of Fukuoka or Saga Prefecture (168 men, 36 women). The diagnosis of HCC was confirmed by histology in 82 cases. The 410 controls selected were residents of Fukuoka City, had undergone a health examination between January 1986 and July 1989 at a nearby public health centre, did not have chronic liver disease and had had a blood specimen taken; they were frequency-matched by sex and age to the cases (291 men, 119 women). Cases and controls were similar with respect to education and occupation and were interviewed in the hospital wards or at the health centre. The OR for HBsAg seropositivity as a risk factor for HCC was 14 (95% CI, 5.9–33) after adjustment for sex, age, history of blood transfusion, family history of liver disease, alcohol consumption and smoking (19% prevalence in cases versus 2% in controls). Case sera were tested by radio-immunoassay or reverse passive haemagglutination and control sera by the latter method.

In Kaohsiung Medical College Hospital, Taiwan, China, Chuang et al. (1992) studied 128 histologically or cytologically confirmed cases of HCC (in 112 men and 16 women) and 384 community controls (336 men, 48 women) matched for age (within five years) and sex; no significant difference was found in age and sex distributions. HBsAg was detected in 77% of the cases, which was significantly higher than in controls (28%) ($p < 0.001$). Using these data, Leandro and Duca (1993) calculated an OR of 14 for HBsAg seropositivity (95% CI, 7.8–25).

A case–control study of HCC was carried out in Hanoi, Viet Nam, between 1989 and 1992 (Cordier et al., 1993). A total of 152 male cases were recruited from two hospitals and frequency-matched on sex, age, hospital and residence to 241 controls admitted to the abdominal surgical departments of the same hospitals. HBsAg status was investigated using a second-generation ELISA test. One hundred and thirty-eight (93%) cases and 44 (18%) controls were seropositive for HBsAg (OR, 62; 95% CI, 30–128). The effect of alcohol consumption was significant only among HBsAg-seronegative individuals.

(d) Europe

Trichopoulos et al. (1978) reported the findings of a study of 80 HCC patients (69 men, 11 women; 47 histologically confirmed cases) admitted to one of eight large hospitals in

Athens, Greece, between April 1976 and June 1977. Two control patients were matched by sex and age (within five years) to each case, who had diagnoses exclusive of neoplasm and liver disease. After Mantel–Haenszel adjustment for age and sex, the OR for an association between HCC and active HBV infection (HBsAg seropositivity or anti-HBc seropositivity and anti-HBs seronegativity) was 10 ($p < 0.001$) by comparison with people with no evidence of active infection. No relationship with any antigen was observed in 40 metastatic liver cancer patients (OR, 1.2). In addition, the presence only of anti-HBs did not confer a greater risk for HCC than the absence of HBV markers (OR, 0.8; 95% CI, 0.3–2.1). Among the HCC cases, the prevalence of active HBV infection was significantly higher in the 45 with cirrhosis (67%) than in the 35 without cirrhosis (26%) ($p < 0.001$).

The prevalence of active HBV infection (HBsAg seropositivity or anti-HBc seropositivity and anti-HBs seronegativity) was determined in 34 cases of HCC (22 with cirrhosis) and 100 healthy general population controls of similar age and sex in Barcelona, Spain (Pedreira et al., 1980). Eighteen cases were verified by biopsy. A strong association was observed, with 52% of cases and 5% of controls having this HBV status [OR, 21; $p < 0.05$]. The prevalence was somewhat higher for HCC cases without cirrhotic liver (58%) than for those with (50%); 38% of 139 cirrhotic patients (47 alcoholics, 92 not) had active HBV infection. HBsAg was determined by reverse passive haemagglutination. [No details of subject selection methods were given.]

Goudeau et al. (1981) reported the prevalence of HBV markers in 46 histologically confirmed cases of HCC (in 39 men and seven women) and in 10 000 blood donors in Tours, France. All subjects were Caucasian. Significant differences were found for HBsAg seroprevalence (4% versus 0.5%; $p < 0.01$) and the seroprevalence of anti-HBc alone (15% versus 2%; $p < 10^{-6}$). [No information was given on the timing and method of subject selection.]

De Franchis et al. (1982) studied 42 subjects with HCC (33 men, nine women) and two groups of controls matched for age (within five years) and sex, comprising 42 patients with chronic liver disease and 84 patients with diagnoses other than neoplasm or liver disease. Subjects were identified from 1974 at the University Hospital in Milan, Italy, and histological examination was used to diagnose HCC. The cases were significantly different from the other hospital controls with respect to all HBV markers analysed, the greatest differences ($p < 0.0005$) being for the presence of HBsAg (36% versus 2%) [OR, 23], of anti-HBc (95% versus 51%) [OR, 19], of HBeAg (19% versus 0%) and of active infection (seropositivity for HBsAg or a high titre of anti-HBc alone; 44% versus 2%) [OR, 32]. The only significant associations ($p < 0.05$) for HCC cases in the comparison with chronic liver disease controls were for HBsAg seropositivity (12% of controls) [OR, 4.1], anti-HBs seropositivity (43%) [OR, 0.14] and active infection (17%) [OR, 3.9]. The direction of the associations between HCC and markers of HBV infection was the same in comparison with both control groups. [No information was given about the timing of subject selection.]

In a multicentre case–control study in Italy (Pagliaro et al., 1982), a significant OR of 14 (1.4–∞) was reported for HBsAg seropositivity in relation to HCC (80% confirmed histologically) in a matched analysis of 50 case–control pairs (37 men, 13 women). Consecutive prevalent cases were collected from 23 hospitals and university medical departments from December 1974 through December 1976; controls were diagnosed with non-surgical diseases other than liver disease. Matching was by sex, age (within five years), hospital and admission date (within six months). HBsAg seropositivity was assayed by the same method for each case–control pair, by radioimmunoassay, counter electroimmunophoresis or reverse passive haemagglutination.

A study from 17 centres in Italy of patients newly diagnosed with HCC during 1979–80 (Pagliaro et al., 1983) comprised 286 HCC cases with cirrhosis (in 250 men and 36 women), who were compared with 3629 patients with cirrhosis (2340 men, 1289 women), and 64 HCC cases without cirrhosis (in 52 men and 12 women), who were compared with 1545 patients with chronic, non-hepatic disease (1038 men, 507 women). The latter control group represented a random sample of non-surgical disease. Among the cirrhotic subjects, cases were significantly different from controls for seropositivity for all HBV markers except HBeAg and anti-HBe: HBsAg, 30% versus 17% ($p < 0.0005$); anti-HBs, 26% versus 37% ($p < 0.005$); anti-HBc alone, 26% versus 16% ($p < 0.005$). Among those without liver cirrhosis, a significant difference was reported for seropositivity for HBsAg (33% versus 2%; $p < 0.0005$). HBsAg was detected by radioimmunoassay or ELISA; anti-HBs and anti-HBc were assayed by radioimmunoassay in a subset of the sample that was similar to the whole group with respect to sex, age and HBsAg reactivity. [The data were incompletely reported.]

In London, United Kingdom, 27 consecutive HCC patients (20 men, seven women) who had undergone liver biopsy between 1979 and 1981 were compared with 112 hospital in-patient and staff controls (60 men, 52 women) (Bassendine et al., 1983); the subjects were Caucasian. The cases had significantly higher frequencies than the controls of HBsAg (15%; controls, 0.9%; $p < 0.005$), anti-HBc (48%; controls, 11%; $p < 0.005$) and anti-HBe (26%; controls, 7%; $p < 0.001$). [Details about the control selection process were not available.]

An association with HBsAg seropositivity was reported by Pirovino et al. (1983) in Switzerland: 31% in 65 HCC cases and 17% in 115 liver cirrhosis controls ($p < 0.05$) [RR, 2.3]. The cases were a subset of 75 histologically confirmed HCC cases diagnosed between 1975 and 1982 at the City Hospital Waid in Zurich on whom HBV testing was done. [Although all of the controls had cirrhosis, it is not known what proportion of cases did.]

Filippazzo et al. (1985), in Palermo, Italy, enrolled 120 consecutive in-patients with HCC (99 men, 21 women) between December 1980 and December 1983 and three controls from the same hospital matched for sex and age (within five years), who had either cirrhosis, solid tumour or chronic non-neoplastic disease. Biopsy or laparoscopy was used to verify the diagnosis in 62 cases of HCC. The difference in HBsAg prevalence between cases (17%) and controls was greater for the two non-cirrhotic control groups (2–3%) than for the cirrhotic controls (15%). [The prevalences reported in the paper did not correspond exactly to those calculable from the data given. No information was provided on how HBsAg status was determined.]

Colloredo Mels et al. (1986) conducted a study in Bergamo, Italy, which included 72 histologically confirmed HCC cases (in 60 men and 12 women), 57 of whom also had cirrhosis. Cases were identified between January 1980 and December 1984, as were two control groups from the same hospital: 199 without liver disease (159 men, 40 women) and 156 with liver cirrhosis (114 men, 42 women). The OR for the relationship between seropositivity for HBsAg and HCC was 11.5 among the non-cirrhotic patients ($p < 0.001$) and 1.0 among the cirrhotic patients: 47% of the HCC cases without cirrhosis, 7% of their controls and 28% of those with cirrhosis and 26% of their controls were seropositive for HBsAg. The authors calculated an overall OR of 4.6 on the basis of an HBsAg seroprevalence of 9.1% in the general population. Among the subset of HBsAg-seronegative subjects assayed, no significant difference was found for the prevalence of past HBV infection in either comparison. [The sample sizes were small, and the means of subject selection could not be determined.]

A case–control study in Greece (Trichopoulos et al., 1987) involved 194 cases of HCC (in 81 cirrhotic subjects out of 173 men and 21 women) and 456 in-patient controls (400 men, 56 women). Cases admitted to eight hospitals in Athens between April 1976 and October 1984 were interviewed in hospital; 113 were confirmed by histology. Controls with diagnoses other than neoplasm or liver disease were selected from the same hospitals (as well as the hospital for accidents and orthopaedic disorders) and were also interviewed in hospital. All subjects were Caucasians of Greek nationality and were comparable with respect to education and birthplace. Data on about one-third of these subjects were analysed previously (see above: Trichopoulos et al., 1978; 1980a), but all assays were repeated for this study. Multiple logistic regression was used to control for age, sex and anti-HCV status (Kaklamani et al., 1991). A significant, 11-fold association was observed between HBsAg seropositivity (46% in cases; 7% in controls) and HCC on the basis of 185 cases (in 166 men and 19 women; 108 confirmed by histology) and 432 controls (381 men, 51 women). This estimate was slightly lower than the earlier one, in which HCV infection was not controlled for (OR, 14; 95% CI, 8.0–24); the association with HBsAg seropositivity was stronger in comparison with subjects with no HBV marker (OR, 19; 95% CI, 10–38) (Trichopoulos et al., 1987). An additional analysis of these cases according to the presence of cirrhosis (Tzonou et al., 1991) revealed a stronger association with HBsAg seropositivity among 78 cases with cirrhosis (65% positive; OR, 33) than those 107 without (32% positive; OR, 6.7), after control for age, sex, anti-HCV seropositivity and smoking.

Vall Mayans et al. (1990) investigated 96 cases of HCC (in 67 men and 29 women; 83 cases with cirrhosis) admitted to the University Hospital in Barcelona, Spain, between October 1986 and March 1988; 74 cases were confirmed histologically or cytologically. Two controls were chosen for each case from the same hospital and matched for sex and age (within five years), within one month after identification of the case; controls with diagnoses related to the risk factors of interest (HBV infection, alcohol consumption, smoking and oral contraceptive use) were not eligible, leaving 199 controls for analysis. Cases and controls were Caucasian and had comparable histories of occupation and blood transfusion. All interviewing took place in hospital. A significant, nearly five-fold association was observed for HBsAg seropositivity after adjustment for age and sex (OR, 4.9, exact 95% CI, 1.3–22); the seroprevalence of HBsAg was low (9% in cases, 2% in controls). The OR for anti-HBc seropositivity (2.3; 95% CI, 1.3–3.9) was also significant, 50% of cases and 31% of controls being seropositive. The authors reported that adjustment for alcohol drinking did not change the association with HBV infection.

Leandro et al. (1990) studied 457 patients with liver cirrhosis in Italy: 140 (117 men, 23 women) had confirmed cases of HCC, and 317 without HCC (209 men, 108 women) were used as controls. HCC patients were diagnosed in 1980–88 at a hospital in either Bari or Bergamo; the controls were admitted to the same centres between 1 January 1984 and

3 December 1985. After control for age and sex by logistic regression, the association with HBsAg seropositivity was significant ($p < 0.05$), with an OR of 2.3 [similar to the crude estimated OR of 1.8 (95% CI, 1.1–3.1)]. [The ORs are related to the probability of developing HCC given the presence of pre-existing cirrhosis.]

A study was carried out in four cities in Italy (Stroffolini et al., 1992) to investigate HBsAg seropositivity in 65 incident cases of HCC with underlying cirrhosis (in 47 men and 18 women) admitted to four teaching hospitals during 1990. Patients with chronic nonhepatic disease, matched for age (within five years) and sex and admitted consecutively to the same hospitals in the same year were selected as controls (75 men, 23 women). Multiple logistic regression methods were used to control for age, sex, anti-HCV status and HBV markers. A significant OR of 12 (95% CI, 3.1–41) was found for the association between HBsAg reactivity and HCC; 25% of cases and 6% of controls were seropositive for the antigen. HBV markers were determined by ELISA. [Not all cases were confirmed histologically.]

(e) International collaborative studies

Not included in Table 6 are the results of two large collaborative studies. In one, patients with liver disease (including HCC) were compared with healthy subjects in Burma, China, Hong Kong, India, Indonesia, Japan, Kenya, Papua New Guinea, the Philippines and Thailand (Nishioka et al., 1975). HBsAg was determined by immune adherence haemagglutination and anti-HBs by passive haemagglutination. The seroprevalence of HBsAg ranged from 33 to 80% among HCC patients and from 3 to 18% among healthy controls; that for anti-HBs was 0–26% among HCC patients and 12–43% among controls. In each country, HBsAg seropositivity was always higher and anti-HBs lower among HCC cases than among controls.

In the other collaborative study, data on blacks in Senegal, Burundi and Mali were combined (Coursaget et al., 1984, 1985) to give a total of 453 HCC patients, 221 cirrhotic patients and 7051 adult controls. HBsAg seropositivity was 58–65% among HCC cases, 4–17% among controls and 63% among cirrhotic patients. HBeAg was detected in 25% of cases and 13–19% of controls, and anti-HBe was detected in 60% of cases and 75% of controls. An analysis of HBsAg-seropositive Senegalese subjects (Coursaget et al., 1986a) revealed an OR of 6.2 (95% CI, 4.1–9.6) for HCC; HBsAg/IgM complexes were detected in 14% of controls, 40% of cirrhotics and 50% of HCC cases. [No details were provided about subject selection.]

Some studies have addressed immunohistochemical identification of HBV antigens in liver tissues and detection of HBV DNA in serum or liver tissue. Their results are important in elucidating pathogenetic mechanisms but cannot provide directly interpretable estimates of effect parameters like the OR, since it is inherently difficult to assess the suitability of the comparison groups. These studies provide strong support for the hypothesis that HBV is an important factor in the etiology of HCC (Nayak et al., 1977; Tan et al., 1977; Turbitt et al., 1977; Omata et al., 1979; Bréchot et al., 1981a, 1985; Röckelein & Hecken-Emmel, 1988; Sjøgren et al., 1988; Guan et al., 1989).

Table 6. Summary of results of case–control studies of hepatocellular carcinoma and presence versus absence of hepatitis B surface antigen (HBsAg)

Reference and location	Subjects	Seroprevalence of HBsAg				OR	95% CI	Comments[a]
		Cases		Controls				
		No.	%	No.	%			
Africa								
Prince et al. (1970); Uganda	Sex unspecified	4	12	6	2	[6.8]	[1.8–25]	Blood donor controls
Vogel et al. (1972); Uganda	Women and men	90	40	224	3	[19]	[7.6–45]	Adjusted for age and sex; testing by CF, CEP and PHA
Kew et al. (1974); South Africa	Men	75	40	18 377	7	[8.7]	[5.3–14]	Mineworkers; testing by CEP and CF
Michon et al. (1975); Prince et al. (1975); Senegal	Women and men Controls with other cancer	165	61	154	12	[11]	[5.8–19]	Adjusted for age
	Controls without cancer	165	61	328	11	[14]	[8.7–24]	
Larouzé et al. (1976); Senegal	Women and men	28	79	28	57	[2.8]	[0.74–10]	
Tsega et al. (1976); Tsega (1977); Ethiopia	Women and men	46	50	90	7	[14]	[4.6–44]	
Tabor et al. (1977)	Women and men							
Uganda		47	47	50	6	[14]	[3.8–51]	
Zambia		19	63	40	8	[21]	[4.7–96]	
USA		27	30	6726	0.02	[134]	[53–337]	
Reys et al. (1977); Mozambique	Women and men	32	60	231	9	[15]	[5.9–37]	Male controls; solid-phase RIA + CEP
Van Den Heever et al. (1978); South Africa	Women and men	92	34	92	9	[5.3]	[2.2–14]	Blacks
Kew et al. (1979); South Africa	Women and men	289	62	213	11	[13]	[7.6–21]	Blacks; solid-phase RIA
Bowry and Shah (1980); Kenya	Women and men	76	51	33	6	[16]	[3.4–106]	Testing by PHA

Table 6 (contd)

Reference and location	Subjects	Seroprevalence of HBsAg					OR	95% CI	Comments[a]
		Cases		Controls				
		No.	%	No.	%			

Africa (contd)

Reference and location	Subjects	No.	%	No.	%	OR	95% CI	Comments[a]
Coursaget et al. (1981); Senegal	Women and men Blood donor controls	134	63	100	12	[12]	[5.9-26]	
	Rural controls	134	63	833	14	[11]	[6.9-16]	
	Leprosy patient controls	134	63	560	25	[5.0]	[3.3-7.5]	
Gombe (1984); Congo	Women and men Blood donor controls	65	74	120	9	[32]	[11-87]	Adjusted for sex; testing by RIA or PHA
	Other cancer controls	65	74	71	3	[55]	[12-256]	Adjusted for sex
Sebti (1984); Morocco		46	17	379	5	[4.2]	[1.6-11]	
Kew et al. (1986a); South Africa	Women and men	62	40	62	3	[20]	[4.3-132]	Blacks
Otu (1987); Nigeria	Women and men	200	49	400	7.5	[12]	[7.3-19]	
Gashau & Mohammed (1991); Nigeria	Women and men	65	65	69	36	[3.2]	[1.5-7.0]	Testing by ELISA and reverse PHA
Mohamed et al. (1992); South Africa	Men	77	35	77	5	7.5	2.2-25	Adjusted for alcohol intake and smoking; blacks
	Women	24	25	24	4	12	1.0-154	
Tswana & Moyo (1992); Zimbabwe	Women and men	182	56	100	11	[10]	[5.0-22]	Testing by ELISA
Ryder et al. (1992); Gambia	Women and men	70	63	70	21	6.9		Adjusted for age; $p < 0.01$; 64 cases, 67 controls tested
Kashala et al. (1992); Zaire	Women and men	40	57.6	68	7.4	[17]	[5.7-51]	Testing by immunoperoxidase

Table 6 (contd)

Reference and location	Subjects	Seroprevalence of HBsAg Cases No. / %	Seroprevalence of HBsAg Controls No. / %	OR	95% CI	Comments[a]
Americas						
Yarrish et al. (1980); USA	Women and men Controls with colon cancer	34 / 15	38 / 0			$p < 0.05$; control sera stored 4 months less than case sera
	Controls with lung cancer	34 / 15	45 / 0			$p < 0.05$; control sera stored 17 months less than case sera
	Blood donor controls	34 / 15	56 / 0			$p < 0.02$; control sera stored 39 months longer than case sera
Nomura et al. (1982); Hawaii, USA	Men	16 / 63	48 / 0			$p < 0.0001$; subjects of Japanese ancestry
Austin et al. (1986); USA	Women and men	67 / 18	63 / 0	—	3.8–∞	$p = 0.0002$
Yu et al. (1990); USA	Women and men	51 / 10	128 / 0	—	3.8–∞	Adjusted for age and sex
Di Bisceglie et al. (1991); USA	Women and men	99 / 7	98 / 0			$p = 0.009$
Asia						
Tong et al. (1971); China	Women and men	55 / 80	943 / 15	[23]	[11–49]	Male controls; testing by modified ID
Simons et al. (1972); Singapore	Women and men Normal controls	156 / 35	1776 / 7	[7.6]	[5.1–11]	Controls were male blood donors and female antenatal clinic attendees; testing by immune adherence HA
	Suspected cancer controls	156 / 35	207 / 6	[8.9]	[4.4–18]	
Lee (1975); Hong Kong	Women and men	100 / 49	120 / 9	[9.5]	[4.4–21]	Testing by immunoelectroosmophoresis and CF
Chainuvati et al. (1975); Thailand	Women and men Cases with cirrhosis	49 / 16	87 / 2	[8.3]	[1.5–59]	Testing by cross-over immunoelectrophoresis
	Cases without cirrhosis	8 / 0	87 / 2	Not significant		

Table 6 (contd)

Reference and location	Subjects	Seroprevalence of HBsAg Cases No. / %	Controls No. / %	OR	95% CI	Comments[a]
Asia (contd)						
Kubo et al. (1977); Japan	Women and men	124 / 46	299 / 4	[20]	[9.9–43]	RIA + reverse PHA + CEP
Chen & Sung (1978); China	Women and men	127 / 83	729 / 15	[28]	[17–46]	Testing by reverse PHA [$p < 0.05$]
Chien et al. (1981); China	Women and men	102 / 71	100 / 12	[18]	[8.0–40]	
Lam et al. (1982); Hong Kong	Women and men	107 / 82	107 / 18	21	10–46	Adjusted for age and sex
Chung et al. (1983); Sjögren et al. (1984); Republic of Korea	Women and men	110 / 82	63 / 14	[27]	[11–70]	Solid-phase RIA
Inaba et al. (1984); Japan	Women and men	62 / 36	62 / 3	10		Matched-pairs analysis; $p < 0.01$; 59 controls tested; testing by reverse PHA
Yeh et al. (1985a,b); Luo et al. (1988); China	Women and men	50 / 86	49 / 22	17	4.3–99	Matched analysis
Arya et al. (1988); Saudi Arabia	Women and men	30 / 60	326 / 12	[11]	[4.6–27]	ELISA
Lu, C.Q. et al. (1988); China	NR	30 / 57	60 / 17	5		Matched analysis; $p < 0.001$
Lingao (1989); Philippines	Women and men HBV-infected subjects	329 / 75	238 / 14	[19]	[12–29]	Adjusted for sex
Yeh et al. (1989); China	Men	76 / 91	304 / 22	39	16–117	Matched analysis

Table 6 (contd)

Asia (contd)

Reference and location	Subjects	Seroprevalence of HBsAg Cases No.	Cases %	Controls No.	Controls %	OR	95% CI	Comments[a]
Tsukuma et al. (1990); Japan	Women and men	229	19	266	2	14	5.7–36	Adjusted for sex, age, history of blood transfusion, heavy drinking, cigarette index and family history of liver cancer; testing by reverse PHA
Lin et al. (1991); China	Women and men	243	77	302	19	10		Adjusted for age, sex and other hepatitis markers; $p < 0.05$
Chen et al. (1991); China	Men	200	20	200	2	58	27–124	Matched-pair analysis; HBsAg(+) and HBeAg(+)
		200	64	200	19	17	7.4–38	Matched-pair analysis; HBsAg(+) and HBeAg(−)
Srivatanakul et al. (1991); Thailand	Women and men	65	42	65	8	15	2.3–103	Adjusted for alcohol, shrimp paste, powdered peanut and fresh vegetable consumption, betel-nut chewing, by conditional multivariate regression; ELISA
Tanaka et al. (1992); Japan	Women and men	204	19	410	2	14	5.9–33	Adjusted for sex, age, history of blood transfusion, family history of liver disease, alcohol consumption and smoking amount; testing by RIA or reverse PHA
Chuang et al. (1992); China	Women and men	128	77	384	28	[9.9]	[5.9–17]	Adjusted for anti-HCV status
Cordier et al. (1993); Viet Nam	Men	152	93	241	18	62	30–128	Testing by second-generation ELISA

Table 6 (contd)

Reference and location	Subjects	Seroprevalence of HBsAg Cases No.	%	Controls No.	%	OR	95% CI	Comments[a]
Europe								
Trichopoulos et al. (1978); Greece	Women and men	80	49	160	8	10	5.2–21	Adjusted for age and sex; $p < 0.001$; HBsAg seropositivity or anti-HBc seropositivity and anti-HBs seronegativity
Pedreira et al. (1980); Spain	Women and men	34	52	100	5	[21]	[7–66]	Testing by reverse PHA; $p < 0.005$; HBsAg seropositivity or anti-HBc seropositivity and anti-HBs seronegativity
Goudeau et al. (1981); France	Women and men	46	4	10 000	0.5	[10]		$p < 0.01$
De Franchis et al. (1982); Italy	Women and men Controls with chronic liver disease Other hospital controls	42	36	42 84	12 2	[4.1] [23]	[1.2–15] [4.5–155]	
Pagliaro et al. (1982); Italy	Women and men	50	NR	50	NR	14	1.4–∞	Matched analysis; testing by RIA, CEP or reverse PHA
Pagliaro et al. (1983); Italy	Women and men Subjects with cirrhosis Subjects without cirrhosis	286 64	30 33	3629 1545	17 2	[2.1] [24]		$p < 0.0005$; testing by RIA or ELISA $p < 0.0005$
Bassendine et al. (1983); UK	Women and men	27	15	112	0.9	[19]	[1.9–476]	
Pirovino et al. (1983); Switzerland	Women and men	65	31	115	17	[2.3]	[1.0–4.9]	
Filipazzo et al. (1985); Italy	Women and men Controls with cirrhosis Controls with solid tumour Controls with chronic disease	120 120 120 120	18 18 18 18	120 120 120 120	14 3 4	[1.4] [6.8] [5.3]	[0.68–2.9] [2.2–20] [1.9–15]	Adjusted for age Adjusted for age Adjusted for age

Table 6 (contd)

Reference and location	Subjects	Seroprevalence of HBsAg Cases No. / %	Controls No. / %	OR	95% CI	Comments[a]
Europe (contd)						
Colloredo Mels et al. (1986); Italy	Women and men Subjects without cirrhosis Subjects with cirrhosis	15 / 47 57 / 28	199 / 7 156 / 26	12 1		$p < 0.001$ NS
Kaklamani et al. (1991); Greece	Women and men	185 / 46	432 / 7	11	6.7–19	Adjusted for age, gender and anti-HCV status
Trichopoulos et al. (1987); Tzonou et al. (1991); Greece	Cases with cirrhosis	78 / 65 of 81	432 / 7	33	15–70	Adjusted for age, gender, anti-HCV status and smoking (percentages calculated from the data of Trichopoulos et al.; no. with cirrhosis from Tzonou et al.)
	Cases without cirrhosis	107 / 32 of 113	432 / 7	6.7	3.6–12	Adjusted for age, gender, anti-HCV status and smoking
Vall Mayans et al. (1990); Spain	Women and men	96 / 9	190 / 2	4.9	1.3–22	Adjusted for age and sex
Leandro et al. (1990); Italy	Women and men	140 / 23	317 / 14	2.3		Adjusted for age and sex; $p < 0.05$
Stroffolini et al. (1992); Italy	Women and men	65 / 25	98 / 6	11	3.1–41	Adjusted for age, gender, anti-HCV and HBV markers; testing by ELISA

OR, odds ratio; CI, confidence interval; NR, not reported. The estimates in square brackets were calculated by the Working Group and are unadjusted unless otherwise indicated in the comments.

[a] Serological testing for HBV markers was by radioimmunoassay (RIA), unless otherwise specified. ID, immunodiffusion; HA, haemagglutination; CF, complement fixation; CEP, counter immunoelectrophoresis; PHA, passive HA, ELISA, enzyme-linked immunosorbent assay; NS, not significant; HCV, hepatitis C virus; HBeAg, hepatitis B envelope antigen

(f) Factors that modify the risk for HCC associated with HBV

Male HBsAg carriers are more likely to develop HCC than female carriers (Anthony, 1984; Coursaget *et al.*, 1987), and there is some evidence that establishment of the carrier state prenatally or early in life is associated with a higher OR for HCC than establishment of a similar state in adulthood (Larouzé *et al.*, 1976; London, 1981; Hsieh *et al.*, 1992).

Several factors other than HBV have been evaluated as causally associated with HCC. In particular, aflatoxins, drinking of alcoholic beverages and oral contraceptives have been determined to be human carcinogens (IARC, 1987, 1988, 1993). Whether these factors modify the effect of HBV in the causation of HCC is inconclusive. The modifying effect of concurrent infection with HCV on the action of HBV is discussed in the monograph on HCV (p. 165).

2.4.2 *Cholangiocarcinoma*

Two case–control studies found no association between HBsAg seropositivity and the occurrence of cholangiocarcinoma. Parkin *et al.* (1991) conducted a case–control study in north-east Thailand involving 103 cases and 103 hospital controls matched for sex, age and hospital; patients with tobacco- and alcohol-related disease and other liver disease were excluded. No association was found with HBsAg seropositivity (OR, 1.0; 95% CI, 0.4–2.7). In Taiwan, China, Chen and Sung (1978) reported that of seven cases one (14%) was HBsAg seropositive, giving a similar rate to that seen among 729 controls (15%).

2.4.3 *Other cancers*

The relationship between HBsAg seroprevalence (as measured by reverse passive haemagglutination) and the occurrence of oral and uterine cervical cancer was examined in one study (Vijayakumar *et al.*, 1984). The subjects analysed were 350 oral cancer patients (232 men, 118 women), 150 cervical carcinoma patients and 100 healthy controls (50 men, 50 women); all were 40–60 years old and had no history of jaundice. Significant differences ($p < 0.001$) were found for all sex-specific comparisons between cases and controls: the seroprevalence of HBsAg was 11% in male and 12% in female oral cancer cases, 13% in cervical cancer cases and 4% in both male and female controls. [No data were provided on social class, nor was it clear whether the carrier state preceded treatment of the disease.]

3. Studies of Cancer in Experimental Animals

3.1 Primates

3.1.1 *Infection with HBV*

(a) Chimpanzee

Chimpanzees (*Pan troglodytes*) have been used for many years to test for the presence of pathogens in biological products derived from human serum. Chimpanzees inoculated with HBV (Barker *et al.*, 1975) or cloned HBV DNA (Sureau *et al.*, 1988) express HBV antigens in liver and blood and can develop a carrier state. Chimpanzees chronically infected with HBV can develop a mild chronic hepatitis resembling chronic persistent hepatitis in human patients infected with HBV. The extent of inflammation in chronically infected chimpanzees appears to be milder than that seen in human patients, and chronic active hepatitis (Shouval *et al.*, 1980) and cirrhosis have apparently not been reported in HBV-infected chimpanzees. HCC has not been seen in chimpanzees infected with HBV, except in one brief report of the occurrence of a liver tumour in a 15-year-old male (Muchmore *et al.*, 1990). This animal had been under surveillance since 1978 after developing seropositivity for anti-HBs and anti-HBc (HBsAg seronegativity) two years after inoculation of human serum thought to be infectious for non-A, non-B hepatitis. The chimpanzee's serum did not transmit non-A, non-B hepatitis to another susceptible animal [details not presented]. HCC was found 10 years later during investigation of liver disease associated with elevated serum alanine aminotransferase and gamma glutamyl transpeptidase. The HCC was composed of neoplastic hepatocytes arranged in trabeculae and plates, and the surrounding non-neoplastic liver was infiltrated by amyloid. The authors reported that hybridization showed free HBV genomes in the liver but no HBV sequences in tumour cells [data not presented]. [Limited details were reported, and there was limited evidence that HBV was causally involved.]

[No other report of HCC developing in chimpanzees with HBV in serum was available to the Working Group. The Group noted the limited reporting of studies on chimpanzees observed for many years after infection with HBV. Little published evidence is available to suggest that HBV-infected chimpanzees develop progressive liver disease.]

(b) Monkey

Five monkeys (three male and one female rhesus and one female cynomolgus), ranging in age from less than one month to 19 months, were inoculated intravenously with a single dose of 2 ml of a pool of five human sera each containing HBsAg titres ranging from 1:640 to 1:2560. Between 22 and 26 months later, three monkeys (two male and one female rhesus) were given a second inoculation of a single human serum with a complement fixing titre of 1:1280, containing 'abundant HBV particles'; all animals were killed three years after the first inoculation. Another group of 12 monkeys (six rhesus and six cynomolgus) [sex and age unspecified] served as uninoculated controls. All monkeys were HBV seronegative before initiation of the study, and all survived up to three years. None of the monkeys was seropositive for HBsAg three to four weeks after inoculation, but HBV core particles were occasionally observed in hepatocytes by electron microscopy. Gross and histological examination of the animals at the end of the study showed no tumour in the livers of those inoculated with HBV, but there was mild persistent hepatitis in the livers of three monkeys. No liver tumour was observed in uninoculated controls (Gyorkey *et al.*, 1977). [There was no evidence that the monkeys were infected with HBV, and the observation period after the second inoculation was brief.]

Seven of 10 monkeys (*Macaca assamensis*; nine males and one female, 6–12 months of age) were inoculated with serum from patients seropositive for HBsAg, anti-HBs, anti-HBc, anti-HBe, HBV DNA or Dane particles [viral titres not stated], and three served as controls. Liver biopsy samples were taken to establish histopathological evidence of hepatitis and hepatic neoplasia and were analysed for the presence of HBsAg, HBcAg, HBeAg, anti-HBs, anti-HBc, anti-HBe and HBV DNA and also for alanine aminotransferase four to six times over a period of 2.5 years. Alanine aminotransferase levels were elevated after inoculation and were still persistently high in five of seven animals 137 weeks after inoculation. Two animals died of other causes during the course of the study. HBsAg, anti-HBs, anti-HBc and HBV DNA were found in sera of all seven treated monkeys. Histopathological changes consistent with hepatitis, including hepatocellular degeneration, necrosis, inflammatory cell infiltration, bile-duct proliferation and fibroplasia, were seen. Liver lesions in some animals progressed to cirrhosis, and one of them developed a mucin-producing, well-differentiated tumour described as an HCC (Ge *et al.*, 1991). [The reporting was limited, and the statement that the HCC secreted mucin and arose from bile ducts was noted.]

3.1.2 *Infection with HBV with concomitant administration of chemical carcinogens*

Monkey

In a study described in section 3.1.1 (Gyorkey *et al.*, 1977), three groups of animals were used. Nine monkeys in group 1 (four male and two female rhesus, one male and two female cynomolgus), ranging in age from less than one to 20 months, were given intraperitoneal injections of 20 mg/kg bw *N*-nitrosodiethylamine (NDEA) [vehicle unspecified] twice a week for two years. Six of the monkeys (two male and one female rhesus, one male and two female cynomolgus) were given a single intravenous injection of 2 ml of serum containing HBV (see section 3.1.1) 25–33 months after the NDEA injections were started, and three were killed three to six months after inoculation and the remaining three 11 months after inoculation. The three animals that were not inoculated were killed three years after the start of the experiment. A second group of 11 monkeys ranging in age from one to 20 months (four male and five female rhesus, one male and one female cynomolgus) were given a single intravenous injection of 2 ml of the pooled HBV serum (see section 3.1.1), followed one month later by the same NDEA treatment as animals in group 1. Five of the 11 monkeys in group 2 (three male and two female rhesus) received a second inoculation of the individual HBV serum (see section 3.1.1) approximately two years after the initial inoculation and were killed one year later. Animals in group 3 (seven monkeys aged 1–21 months: one male and three female rhesus, two male and one female cynomolgus) were given intraperitoneal injections of 20 mg/kg bw NDEA twice a week for two weeks. One month after the first injection of NDEA, each monkey received a single intravenous injection of 2 ml of the pooled HBV serum, followed two weeks later by re-institution of the twice-weekly NDEA treatment, which was continued for two years. Three of the seven animals received a further inoculation with the individual HBV serum about 21 months after the first HBV inoculation. All surviving animals were killed three years after the start of the experiment. The livers of all animals in group 1 had large invasive HCCs with central haemorrhagic necrosis; some animals also had cirrhosis. Six had metastases to the lung. The incidence and time of onset of liver tumours in monkeys given injections of NDEA in combination with HBV were not different from those in animals that received NDEA alone. All monkeys in group 2 that survived to the end of the experiment developed cirrhosis and invasive multifocal HCC; six developed metastases to the lung. Reinoculation with HBV of monkeys in group 3 failed to affect tumour outcome. [No evidence of viral infection was observed, and the study was inadequately designed to allow demonstration of an enhancing effect of HBV on hepatocarcinogenicity.]

3.2 Transgenic mice

3.2.1 *With no concomitant administration of chemical carcinogens*

The expression of various HBV gene sequences in livers of transgenic mice has been examined in several studies (for reviews, see Chisari, 1991; Slagle *et al.*, 1992). Only those transgenic models in which hepatic neoplasia was the end-point are included in this section (for a discussion of gene expression and mechanisms of tumour induction, see also section 4.3.2).

Male mice of three transgenic lineages producing the HBV large surface antigen were back-crossed with normal C57Bl/6J females (see Table 7). Mice from the first generation (36 animals from lineage 50-4, 12 from lineage 45-2, eight from lineage 45-3 and four non-transgenic controls) were observed for two years for the development of liver injury (as indicated by increased levels of serum glutamic and pyruvic transaminases) and neoplasms (determined by abdominal palpation and serum levels of α-fetoprotein). Variable expression of large surface antigen (as measured by western blot of total liver protein) was correlated with lineage, being highest in lineage 50-4, medium in lineage 45-2 and lowest in lineage 45-3. Lineages that expressed the highest levels of large surface antigen and filamentous protein in hepatocytes had the highest level of liver injury, and liver tumours developed in animals that had hepatocellular injury. Tumours were first detectable in lineages 50-4 and 45-2 at 9-12 months after the onset of injury, and virtually all mice of the 50-4 lineage with pre-existing chronic liver-cell injury developed HCC by 18-21 months of age. One or two large tumours (1.0-2.0 cm) usually predominated, and numerous smaller tumours were scattered throughout the livers. Thirty-eight animals (25 males and 13 females) [lineage unspecified] with palpable abdominal masses were examined histologically at necropsy. Males developed more palpable liver tumours and displayed more HCCs (18/25) than did females (4/13). Adenomas predominated (5/7) in younger males (10-15 months) and carcinomas (13/18) in older males (16-21 months). All tumours occurred concurrently with hepatocellular injury, characterized by ground-glass hepatocytes, necrosis and inflammation. Neither metastases nor fibrosis or cirrhosis were observed (Chisari *et al.*, 1989). [The Working Group noted that the terms 'hepatoma' and 'hepatocellular carcinoma' appear to have been used interchangeably.]

A group of 59 male and female transgenic mice (lineage 50-4; see Table 7) were examined for abdominal masses every four months for 24 months. Selected animals were killed at monthly intervals from 1 to 23 months, and nine control nontransgenic animals were killed at 3, 11, 18 and 24 months [exact number of animals killed at each time point not specified]. Liver sections were examined histologically for the presence of hepatocellular adenomas and carcinomas. Livers of nontransgenic mice were normal histologically at all time points. Starting at two months, mice progressively developed liver injury and inflammation, including hepatocellular necrosis, Kupffer-cell hyperplasia and mononuclear-cell infiltration, with concurrent preneoplastic lesions which appeared by seven months of age. Preneoplastic lesions consisted of hepatocellular dysplasia and foci of altered hepatocytes, which progressively developed into larger compressive nodular masses. Seventy-five adenomas, characterized by masses of neoplastic hepatocytes which compressed adjacent parenchyma, occurred in 18 mice from eight months and peaked in incidence around the 17th month of the study. HCC (29 in all) had occurred in all surviving transgenic mice by 20 months of age (Dunsford et al., 1990).

Table 7. Transgenic mice that express hepatitis B surface antigen as the major product

Founder strain	Crossing strain	Lineage	Promoter	HBV sequence Pre-S S X C P	Reference
C57Bl/6J × SJL/J	C57Bl/6J	50-4[a]	Albumin	+ + +	Dunsford et al. (1990); Chisari et al. (1989)
C57Bl/6J × SJL/J	C57Bl/6J	45-2[b]	Albumin		Chisari et al. (1989)
C57Bl/6J × SJL/J	C57Bl/6J	45-3[c]	Albumin		Chisari et al. (1989)
C57Bl/6 × SJL/J	C3H/He	E36	HBV	+ + + +	Babinet et al. (1985); Dragani et al. (1990)
CD1	CD1	C11 H9 E1	X	+	Kim et al. (1991)

[a]Current designation: Tg (Alb-1 HBV)Bri 44
[b]Current designation: Tg (Alb-1 HBV)Bri 43
[c]Current designation: Tg (Alb-1 HBV)Bri 141

Transgenic mice containing the entire coding region of the HBx gene, including the X promoter, the principal RNA start sites, transcriptional enhancer and polyadenylation site, were created by microinjecting embryos from outbred CD_1 mice (see Table 7). Six transgenic mice, each with at least one intact, stably expressed copy of the X gene, were identified by Southern blot analysis, and three animals with a high level of expression were bred into permanent lines (lineages C11, H9 and E1) [strain and sex of crosses and total numbers of transgenic and nontransgenic offspring from all three lineages unspecified]. Livers were examined histologically at various times. At four months, preneoplastic lesions consisting of multifocal areas of altered hepatocytes were observed in progeny from all three lines of transgenic mice but not in nontransgenic littermates. Neoplastic nodules [sizes unspecified], which occurred by 8–10 months of age, compressed surrounding hepatocytes and accumulated high levels of HBx protein. The authors reported that fewer than 10% of control male CD_1 mice develop hepatic neoplasms during an average lifespan of 24 months [no data shown]. HCCs were observed in 19/21 males and 12/20 females of line C11, in 8/10 males and 4/6 females of line H9 and in the E_1 line [details not given]. Most males of the C11 line died with HCC between 11 and 15 months of age, and most females between 17 and 21 months of age. There was no difference in the incidence of liver tumours in male and female mice. Liver damage, determined by concentration of serum alanine aminotransferase, was not observed, and the levels were consistently within normal range (Kim et al., 1991). [Detailed data on liver lesions in nontransgenic littermates were not provided.]

In another study of a transgenic lineage expressing the X gene driven by the α-1-antitrypsin promoter, mice did not exhibit liver disease or tumour development. This lineage exhibited an early but transient expression of the HBx protein (Lee et al., 1990).

3.2.2 *With concomitant administration of known chemical carcinogens*

The transgenic mouse strain E36 was derived from founder (C57Bl/6 × SJL/J)F$_1$ mice containing all of the HBV genome except for the core gene, allowing expression of HBsAg under control of the HBV promoter and enhancer sequences (see Table 7). Two hundred and four transgenic and nontransgenic mice (F$_1$ hybrids resulting from crosses of males of the transgenic strain E36 with C3H/He females) were allocated to three treatment groups. Animals of group 1 (23 HBV-seropositive males, 21 HBV-seropositive females, 19 HBV-seronegative males and 22 HBV-seronegative females still alive at 30 weeks) were treated at seven days of age by oral gavage with a single dose of 10 mg/kg bw NDEA in 0.9% saline solution. Animals of group 2 (12 HBV-seropositive and 22 HBV-seronegative males still alive at 30 weeks) were treated with a single dose of 150 mg/kg bw *para*-dimethylaminoazobenzene (DAB) in corn oil by gavage at seven days of age. Group 3 consisted of 52 untreated controls (15 HBV-seropositive males, 11 HBV-seropositive females, 14 HBV-seronegative males and 12 HBV-seronegative females still alive at 30 weeks). Survivors at 30 weeks were 92% of those treated with NDEA and 98% of those given DAB. Animals were killed at 30 weeks of age and examined both grossly and microscopically for the presence of liver tumours. No tumour was observed in the 52 control animals. Liver nodules > 220 μm in diameter were counted, and those 5 mm in diameter were classified as either adenomas or carcinomas by histological criteria. In NDEA-treated male groups, the total number of nodules per cubic centimetre of liver was about the same for HBV-seropositive and HBV-seronegative animals, but larger nodules (> 330 μm diameter) occurred at about twice the frequency in HBV-seropositive mice as compared with HBV-seronegative mice ($p < 0.05$, Wilcoxon test). The frequency of nodules in the DAB-treated group was much lower than that in NDEA-treated animals. The frequency of nodules per cubic centimetre of liver was 1.5–2 times higher in transgenic than in nontransgenic animals, but the increase was significant only for nodules ≤ 110 μm. The incidence of hepatocellular adenomas and carcinomas was higher in HBV-seropositive (18/56) than in HBV-seronegative (14/63) animals treated with either NDEA or DAB; this difference was not significant (Dragani et al., 1990).

Six groups of 10 female transgenic mice that produce the HBV large surface antigen (lineage 50-4; see Table 7) and of 10 nontransgenic littermates were treated as follows. Group 1 served as untreated controls; group 2 received five monthly intraperitoneal injections of 0.25 μg/g bw aflatoxin B$_1$ as a suspension in tricaprylin beginning at three or four months of age; group 3 received a single intraperitoneal injection of 0.25 μg/g bw aflatoxin B$_1$ suspended in tricaprylin at three or four months of age; group 4 received three weekly intraperitoneal injections of 2.0 μg/g bw aflatoxin B$_1$ suspended in tricaprylin at four months of age; group 5 received a single intraperitoneal injection of 50 μg/g bw NDEA dissolved in sterile saline at four or five months of age; and group 6 received 0.1% phenobarbital in powdered diet beginning at six months of age for one year. The study was terminated when the animals were 15 months of age. Survival rates were approximately 90%, except for group 6 in which survival was about 50%. Liver nodules and tumour masses were observed grossly *post mortem* and by histological examination. Nodules were classified by size into three categories: 0.1–1.9 mm, 2–4.9 mm and > 4.9 mm in diameter. Adenomas and HCCs were distinguished histologically. No gross or histological lesions were seen in the livers of nontransgenic control mice, whereas the livers of control transgenic mice contained multiple nodules of different sizes. Livers of transgenic mice treated with aflatoxin B_1 had 15–23 nodules (0.1–1.9 mm in diameter) per liver, as compared with 0.1–0.2 nodules of the same size per liver in nontransgenic aflatoxin B_1-treated mice and five nodules per liver in transgenic control mice not treated with aflatoxin B_1. Similar results were obtained for the incidence of larger nodules. Aflatoxin B_1-treated transgenic mice had 6.2–8.8 nodules (2.0–4.9 mm in diameter) per liver, whereas untreated transgenic mice had an average of 3.7 nodules per liver and aflatoxin B_1-treated nontransgenic mice had 0–0.1. Adenomas and HCCs were seen only in transgenic mice treated with aflatoxin B_1 or NDEA. In the three aflatoxin-treated groups (2, 3 and 4), a total of 20 adenomas and two HCCs were observed in 26 transgenic mice and none in 27 nontransgenic mice. In the NDEA-treated group (5), nine adenomas and two HCCs were seen in eight transgenic mice and none in nine nontransgenic mice examined. Livers of transgenic mice fed phenobarbital showed increased nodularity but no adenoma or HCC; however, survival was poor (Sell *et al.*, 1991).

3.3 Woodchucks (*Marmota monax*)

3.3.1 *Hepatocellular carcinoma in woodchucks naturally infected with woodchuck hepatitis virus*

The first non-human hepadnavirus was identified in woodchucks (*Marmota monax*) in a series of studies that began at the Philadelphia (USA) Zoo (for a review, see Paronetto & Tennant, 1990).

In the initial report, which appeared as an abstract (Snyder, 1968), a group of 50 woodchucks (42 males and eight females), trapped in the wild in the vicinity of Philadelphia when about five months of age, were held in captivity one or two per cage on tap-water and a standard feed. After about 72 months in captivity, 30 animals had died. HCC were observed in nine (six males and three females). In one of the nine animals, metastatic nodules were found in retroperitoneal fat. The author concluded that dietary carcinogens were probably not responsible, since other captive animals in the Philadephia Zoo fed on the same diet had not developed liver tumours; he proposed that a viral agent was involved in the etiology of liver cancer in woodchucks.

Ten years later, Summers *et al.* (1978) reported that post-mortem examination of 102 woodchucks that had been caught in the wild and kept at the Philadelphia Zoo for 18 years had revealed 23 HCCs (22.5%), which appeared at a mean age of 59 months. Three animals had acute hepatitis. About 15% of serum samples taken from captive woodchucks were found to contain DNA polymerase-containing particles in amounts comparable with those found in some human sera positive for HBsAg. Detailed investigations were carried out on three animals, two of which had died with HCC and one of which had died with a normal liver: Sera from the two animals with HCC, but not that from the control animal, had detectable levels of DNA polymerase-containing particles. When the particles were characterized and compared with particles from an HBV-infected human by caesium chloride equilibrium sedimentation, electron microscopy and electrophoresis, the particles from the woodchucks were found to be similar, but not identical. DNA of similar size and physical structure was found in sera and liver samples from the two animals with HCC. The authors concluded that the particles represented a distinct virus, which they called 'woodchuck hepatitis virus', which is phylogenetically related to HBV.

In a review, Summers (1981) reported that all 16 woodchucks in the colony at the Philadelphia Zoo that developed HCC also had chronic active hepatitis of varying severity and had been persistently infected with WHV from an early age, when they were obtained from the wild. No HCC had developed in groups of animals with anti-WHs and no marker of viral infection.

Seventy-three woodchucks from Pennsylvania and Delaware which had been trapped as yearlings or as adults and observed for at least one month in a colony established at the National Institute of Allergy and Infectious Diseases (NIAID) (Mitamura et al., 1982) were studied by Popper et al. (1981). Thirty-three selected animals, including all six animals that had developed HCC [criteria for selection of the remaining 27 animals not described], were studied in detail. The six animals with HCC were all seropositive for WHsAg, WHV DNA and WHV DNA polymerase. Of the remaining 27 animals, four were seropositive for all three markers and four for anti-WHs, three were seronegative for all markers and 16 were seropositive for one marker only or gave inconsistent or discrepant results. The authors pointed out that cirrhosis did not occur in animals with HCC. Furthermore, inflammation was generally characterized as mild, and chronic active hepatitis was seen in only two animals with HCC. The authors also noted the direct transition to HCC from neoplastic nodules in these woodchucks.

Mitamura et al. (1982) extended the observations on the NIAID colony of woodchucks and analysed markers of WHV infection among 62 animals that had died of various causes. Death from HCC occurred in 11 of 13 (85%) chronic carriers of WHV, in two of 33 (6%) animals with anti-WHs and no evidence of viral replication, and in none of 16 animals with no viral marker.

Of 113 woodchucks that had been trapped in different areas of Pennsylvania, Maryland and Delaware and kept in a colony at the New Bolton Center at the University of Pennsylvania, eight developed HCC between 44 and 88 weeks of captivity (Millman et al., 1984). Seven of the animals were seropositive for WHsAg at the time of capture; one animal that was seronegative at that time converted to WHsAg seropositivity after 33 weeks of captivity.

Nineteen WHsAg-seropositive woodchucks that had been trapped in Pennsylvania and Maryland were kept for up to two years at Cornell University, New York (Roth et al., 1985), and the livers of 16 animals were examined. HCC was found in 13, all of which had chronic active or persistent hepatitis. Metastases to the lung were observed in one animal. Among 149 WHsAg-seronegative woodchucks trapped in New York State and kept in captivity for four weeks or more, a single case of HCC was observed, although five had acute hepatitis.

3.3.2 *Hepatocellular carcinoma in woodchucks experimentally infected with woodchuck hepatitis virus*

(a) *Infection with woodchuck hepatitis virus*

A breeding colony of woodchucks consisting of the offspring of female woodchucks trapped in New York State and shown to be free of present or past WHV infection was established at Cornell University, New York (Popper *et al.*, 1987). Newborn animals were inoculated with $10^{5.5}$–$10^{6.5}$ 50% infectious doses of WHV one day after birth. Adult woodchucks with no evidence of active or past WHV infection, maintained in the NIAID woodchuck colony, were inoculated with $10^{5.8}$ 50% infectious doses. Animals were kept on tap-water and aflatoxin-free laboratory chow. A total of eight woodchucks, six infected at birth and two as adults, developed chronic infection, as indicated by the presence of WHsAg for one year or longer. All eight animals subsequently developed HCC 17–36 months after infection; no HCC was observed in 19 animals with virological markers of past infection or in 15 uninfected controls followed for 18–57 months. Mild hepatitis, characterized by lymphocytic infiltrates, was seen in the portal tracts of woodchucks infected as adults or newborns. In animals infected as adults, the portal inflammation regressed with time and the liver assumed the appearance of control livers. In woodchucks with HCC, the portal tract inflammation was more extensive, occasionally resembling that seen in human chronic active hepatitis. Furthermore, inflammation appeared to be most severe in the immediate vicinity of the HCC. Cirrhosis was not seen.

Two groups of 43 woodchucks were inoculated with infectious serum at birth or at eight weeks of age. Thirteen of those inoculated at birth (32%) became chronic carriers, 28 animals cleared the infection and two died within six months after birth. After three years, 11 of the chronic carriers and two of the animals with past infection had developed HCC. Of those inoculated at eight weeks of age, 23 developed acute WHV infection; three became chronic carriers (13%), while 20 animals recovered from the infection. Two of the three chronic carriers and eight of the 20 animals with past infection were followed for three years. Both chronic carriers but none of the eight woodchucks with past infection developed HCC. None of 46 uninfected, laboratory-born woodchucks followed for three years or more developed HCC (Tennant *et al.*, 1988).

Gerin *et al.* (1989) extended the analysis of HCC occurrence in experimentally infected woodchucks maintained at Cornell University: HCC developed in 61/63 chronic carriers (97%), 11/63 (17%) animals with past infection and in none of 108 concurrent, uninfected controls. Follow-up was for at least three years; the sex of the animal did not influence the occurrence of HCC. All three pair-wise comparisons between the three groups were significant at $p < 0.001$ by Fisher's exact test.

(b) *Infection with woodchuck hepatitis virus in combination with aflatoxin B_1*

In a study described in an extended abstract (Tennant *et al.*, 1990), 52 woodchucks [sex unspecified] were inoculated subcutaneously with WHV (5×10^6 50% infectious doses) at 1–3 days of age. A group of 27 of these animals received no further treatment; 25 inoculated and 29 uninoculated animals subsequently received aflatoxin B_1 in the diet (0.25–1.0 µg/kg) from three months of age for six months or comparable cumulative doses of aflatoxin B_1 in dimethyl sulfoxide solution by intraperitoneal injection (125 µg/kg bw, three times weekly) beginning at 1–4 months of age for 3–4 months. Twenty-three animals served as untreated controls. WHV-specific serological tests [unspecified] indicated that the rate of chronic infection (73%) at one year of age in the group given aflatoxin B_1 and WHV was similar to that of those infected with WHV alone (70%). Survival rates were 60% for woodchucks infected with WHV and given aflatoxin B_1 and 72% for those that received aflatoxin B_1 alone; no death occurred among animals infected with WHV alone. Histological analysis of livers from aflatoxin B_1-treated woodchucks revealed lesions consistent with hepatotoxicity due to that compound. Thirty-six months after initiation of the study, 6 of the 15 surviving animals (40%) given aflatoxin B_1 and WHV had HCC, in contrast to 21 of the 27 animals (78%) inoculated only with WHV. During the same period, 2 of 21 woodchucks that were treated with aflatoxin B_1 alone and survived more than one year developed HCC, while none of 22 untreated controls had hepatic tumours. [The high dose of aflatoxin B_1 compromised the interpretation of the results of this study by reducing the survival of the animals.]

3.3.3 *Hepatocellular carcinoma in woodchucks experimentally infected with ground squirrel hepatitis virus*

Seeger *et al.* (1991) reported experiments in which woodchucks were infected with Beechey ground squirrel (*Spermophilus beecheyi*) hepatitis virus (GSHV) or WHV. Three-day-old woodchucks from the breeding colony at Cornell University were inoculated subcutaneously with serum from infected woodchucks or from infected ground squirrels. Of 29 woodchucks infected with GSHV, 17 (59%) became chronic carriers; of 36 woodchucks inoculated with WHV, 27 (75%) became chronic carriers. Sixteen of these were selected for comparison with the 17 chronic carriers of GSHV. Two years after experimental infection, 7 of the 16 WHV-infected but none of the 17 GSHV-infected woodchucks had liver masses (detected by ultrasound imaging), all of which were verified histologically as HCC. Histological examination of all animals after 26 months revealed neoplastic lesions in two GSHV-infected woodchucks. At 51 months after infection, all 16 WHV carriers had developed one to five HCCs each (total, 41), and 6 of the 14 GSHV carriers that were tumour-free at 26 months and that survived laparotomy at that time developed one to four HCCs (total, 14). The median time to diagnosis of HCC in WHV-infected woodchucks was 32 months; the projected median time to diagnosis of HCC in GSHV-infected woodchucks was 55 months. The extent of non-neoplastic liver disease and chronic inflammation did not differ according to the virus inoculated.

3.4 Ground squirrels, ducks and other species

3.4.1 *Beechey ground squirrels*

GSHV infecting Beechey ground squirrels was discovered in 1979 in northern California, USA, as a result of a search for a virus similar to HBV in animals related to woodchucks (Marion *et al.*, 1980). The biology, genetic structure, gene products and viral replication of GSHV have been reviewed recently (Marion, 1991). The virus was originally detected in sera taken from apparently healthy animals. To date, the only known location of this virus is on the San Francisco Peninsula, although the virus that putatively infects

Richardson ground squirrels (*Spermophilus richardsonii*) (see section 3.4.2) (and viruses that possibly infect other ground squirrel species) may be a variant of the Beechey squirrel virus.

In an experiment described in a series of reports (Marion *et al.*, 1983, 1986, 1987), Beechey ground squirrels, estimated to be one to two years of age, were trapped live at various locations on the San Francisco Peninsula between 1980 and 1984. Animals were held individually in quarantine for one month, during which time their serum was tested for (i) surface antigen (GSHsAg), by a commercial solid-phase radioimmunoassay for cross-reacting HBsAg; (ii) anti-GSHs, by a virus-specific solid-phase radioimmunoassay; and (iii) virion-associated DNA polymerase activity, as a measure of virus load (Marion *et al.*, 1983). Animals with serum GSHsAg and DNA polymerase activity were housed in a room separate from GSHsAg-seronegative animals (Marion *et al.*, 1986). Marion *et al.* (1987) reported that 24/103 ground squirrels examined at necropsy had tumours at various sites; all tumour-bearing squirrels were 4.5–8 years of age and had been in captivity for a minimum of 2.4 years. Among animals under 4.5 years, no tumour of any kind was observed in 19 persistent carriers of GSHV, 22 seropositive for anti-GSHs or 19 with no serological marker of GSHV. Of the tumours observed in older squirrels, 11 were found in 17 GSHV carriers, eight in 11 squirrels seropositive for anti-GSHs and five in 15 GSHV marker-free squirrels. The predominant type of tumour observed in squirrels over 4.5 years of age was HCC, which was detected in 10/17 persistent GSHV carriers and in 3/11 squirrels seropositive for anti-GSHs, but in none of 15 GSHV marker-free squirrels in the same age range, resulting in a highly significant association between HCC and the GSHV carrier state ($p = 0.0005$, Fisher's exact test) and a weaker association with seropositivity for anti-GSHs. Development of HCC in carrier squirrels may be related either to age or to the length of the carrier state, as all animals appeared to have become carriers before 1.5 years of age. HCC was seen at necropsy in six of nine carrier squirrels (67%) over six years of age but in only three of nine carriers aged four to six years and none of 17 carrier squirrels less than four years of age. All HCCs except one were of the same histological type: a trabecular, highly differentiated liver carcinoma; the only non-trabecular HCC was seen in one of the three squirrels seropositive for anti-GSHs and was of the medullary type and less differentiated. The diameters of the major tumours were generally larger in squirrels that were older when the HCC was detected. Single nodules of HCC were commoner in the younger squirrels, while older squirrels usually had more than one nodule. Four of the five oldest squirrels with HCC also had metastases to or adhesions of the tumour in the spleen. While viral DNA was integrated into the host DNA of some of the HCCs examined, the majority of those from squirrels with GSHV markers did not have detectable integrated viral DNA. Chronic active hepatitis and cirrhosis were not seen (Marion *et al.*, 1986, 1987).

In a further assessment of the development of HCC in the squirrel colonies after nine years of observation (Marion & Cullen, 1992), 18 cases (45% of all neoplasms) were observed in the study population of 24 GSHV-infected, 20 anti-GSHs-seropositive and 26 GSHV marker-free ground squirrels over four years of age. Eleven of the liver tumours were seen in carrier animals, five in anti-GSHs-seropositive squirrels and two in GSHV marker-free animals. The association of HCC with the GSHV carrier state was significant ($p = 0.0016$). As in WHV-infected woodchucks, the incidence of HCC in animals that had recovered from infection was relatively high (20%). Anti-GSHs-seropositive squirrels that developed tumours experienced only a brief period of viraemia. No sex difference was noted. The average age of carrier squirrels at the time of detection of HCC was 6.5 years.

3.4.2 *Richardson ground squirrels*

HCC has been observed in Richardson ground squirrels from the southern half of the Canadian province of Alberta. The hepadnavirus thought to be associated with these tumours has not been characterized genetically or biologically, nor has it been transmitted experimentally to other animals. In a study by Minuk *et al.* (1986), animals were trapped and kept in captivity for less than one month. Two of 25 adult squirrels but none of 15 juveniles had HCC at necropsy (Table 8). Anti-GSHs was found in 7 of the 25 adult animals, and the serum of one animal reacted positively when tested with a commercial radioimmunoassay for HBsAg known to detect GSHsAg. Serum was not tested for the presence of virions. Anti-GSHs seropositivity was assayed with a commercial radioimmunoassay for anti-HBs. Of the animals in which HCC was found, one had GSHsAg reactivity in the serum, while the other was seropositive for anti-GSHs. No viral DNA was detectable in the HCC of the seropositive animal or in the DNA of adjacent liver tissue. [The assay to detect anti-GSHs was unspecific and insensitive.]

Table 8. Studies of hepatocellular carcinoma (HCC) in Richardson ground squirrels trapped or born in captivity in Alberta, Canada, according to age at necropsy

Age at necropsy	No. of animals	Location	GSHsAg-seropositive	Anti-GSHs-seropositive	Liver tumours	Reference
Adult	25	South of Calgary	1	7	2 HCC	Minuk *et al.* (1986)
Juvenile	15	South of Calgary	1	4	0	
1– ≥3 years	562	Picture Butte	ND	ND	0	Tennant *et al.* (1991)
3–4 months	56[a]	Picture Butte	ND	ND	0	
14–17 months	54[a]	Picture Butte	ND	ND	31 with nodules	
15 months	36	Cochrane	ND	ND	1 HCC, 4 with nodules	
≥3 years	5	Edmonton	0	} 10/12	2 HCC, 2 with nodules	
≥3 years	7[b]	Picture Butte	0		4 HCC	

GSHsAg, ground squirrel hepatitis surface antigen; ND, not determined
[a]Born in captivity
[b]Dams of 54 born in captivity

In a study by Tennant *et al.* (1991), several groups of Richardson ground squirrels were examined for the presence of masses in the liver at necropsy. The majority, collected at Picture Butte, Alberta, Canada, and not maintained in captivity, were not tested for hepadnavirus markers or examined histologically. None of 618 squirrels ranging in age from three to four months to three years or more had evidence of liver cancer (Table 8). Squirrels held in captivity for 14 months or longer for various experiments were also examined for HCC at necropsy; nodules or histological evidence of HCC were detected in some animals (Table 8).

HCCs were found in squirrels trapped at Picture Butte only after the animals had been maintained in captivity. Hepadnavirus markers were assayed in the sera of the five squirrels trapped near Edmonton and the seven from Picture Butte. None cross-reacted with HBsAg, but most had evidence of anti-GSHs. Viral DNA was detected in two of four HCCs; no anti-GSHc was detectable in any sample using an assay which readily detects this antibody. Non-neoplastic lesions in the livers of animals kept for three years in captivity included mild to moderate portal inflammation, with somewhat more severe inflammation adjacent to tumours. In the livers of six of seven animals with moderate portal inflammation, focal hepatocellular necrosis and inflammation were seen. [Limited data are available to support hepadnavirus infection *per se*.]

3.4.3 Ducks

Observations of liver tumours in domestic ducks (*Anas domesticus*) were first described in China by Wang *et al*. (1980), which led to the discovery of duck hepatitis B virus (DHBV) (Mason *et al*., 1980). The biology, genetic structure, gene products and viral replication of DHBV have been reviewed (Schödel *et al*., 1991).

Studies of the oncogenic potential of DHBV are of three types: (i) assessment of liver tumours and markers of DHBV in ducks collected on farms or free-ranging in communities; (ii) prospective studies of the development of HCC in ducks of known DHBV status and history; and (iii) experimental studies of the joint effects of DHBV infection and aflatoxin B_1 exposure in the development of HCC in ducks.

(a) Liver tumours and markers of duck hepatitis B virus in ducks collected on farms and in free-ranging flocks

After the initial discovery of DHBV in ducks with hepatitis and liver tumours in the Chinese Province of Qidong, several studies were carried out to determine whether the presence of HCC and hepatitis in domestic ducks was linked to current or past replication of DHBV in the same animals (see Table 9).

DHBV was found in 70/195 ducks from three of five locations in China but in none of 17 ducks from Chiba, Japan (Table 9); HCC was found only in four ducks from Qidong, and evidence of present or past DHBV infection was seen in three of them. Moderate to severe hepatitis was observed in both DHBV-seropositive and -seronegative ducks from Qidong, where there are known to be relatively high levels of aflatoxin B_1, a known cause of liver disease in ducks (IARC, 1993). Moderate hepatitis consisted of mild portal inflammation, with rare necrosis of hepatocytes. Severe hepatitis was associated with dense chronic inflammation of portal tracts, which extended into adjacent parenchyma and was accompanied by focal necrosis of hepatocytes. Severe hepatitis was sometimes accompanied by septal fibrosis, focal areas of parenchymal collapse and regenerative nodules; cirrhosis was seen in one duck with HCC (Marion *et al*., 1984). Three of the four HCCs were observed in Chinese ducks and none in white Pekin ducks. Overall, while there was concomitant presence of DHBV and HCC in some ducks from Qidong, the two have not been firmly linked, nor has the simultaneous presence of DHBV replication and liver inflammation been associated in these ducks.

Table 9. Presence of hepatocellular carcinoma (HCC) and duck hepatitis B virus (DHBV) infection in populations of ducks on farms and free-ranging

Age at necropsy (years)	Provenance	Breed	No. of ducks	No. with serum DHBV particles or serum or liver DHBV DNA	No. with HCC	Viral DNA in liver of ducks with carcinoma	Reference
1–2	Qidong, China	White Pekin	24	12	1[a]	ND	Omata et al. (1983)
1–2	Changchun, China	White Pekin	20	0	0		
1–2	Chiba, Japan	White Pekin	17	0	0		
3–5	Qidong, China	Chinese	14	7	2	1+, 1–	Marion et al. (1984)
1–3	Qidong, China	White Pekin	4	0	0		Yokosuka et al. (1985)
1–3	Qidong, China	Chinese	19	13	1	+	
1–3	Shanghai, China	White Pekin	17	1	0		Omata et al. (1987)
1–3	Shanghai, China	Chinese	10	7	0		
1–3	Xiamen, China	Chinese	28	14	0		
1–3	Qidong, China	White Pekin	4	1	0[b]		
1–3	Qidong, China	Chinese	19	15	0[b]		
1–3	Funan, China	White Pekin	36	0	0		

ND, not determined
[a]Cirrhosis was also seen.
[b]Seems to overlap with Yokosuka et al. (1985)

(b) *Prospective studies of hepatocellular carcinoma in ducks of known duck hepatitis B viral status*

Ducks infected either congenitally or by injection with DHBV as hatchlings were monitored for development of HCC in four studies (Table 10). HCC was seen in only 1/37 experimentally infected ducks aged 0.3–1.8 years and in none of eight congenitally infected and none of 26 uninfected ducks of similar ages. The single HCC observed was in a white Pekin duck similar to those used in all of the studies (Cullen et al., 1991).

Table 10. Presence of hepatocellular carcinoma (HCC) in ducks of known duck hepatitis B virus (DHBV) status

Age at necropsy (years)	Breed	Type of infection	No. of ducks	No. with DHBV markers in serum or liver	No. with HCC	Reference
0.6–1.0	Japanese	Experimental	20	17	0	Omata et al.
Not reported	Japanese		10	0	0	(1984)
0.8	Japanese	Experimental	2	2	0	Uchida et al. (1988)
0.3–1.8	White Pekin	Experimental	15	12	1	Cullen et al.
	White Pekin		16	0	0	(1989)
2.3	White Pekin	Congenital	8	8	0	Cullen et al.
2.3	White Pekin		16	0	0	(1989, 1990)

Inflammation of the liver was much less severe in two breeds of domestic ducks from California inoculated with known amounts of DHBV than in the free-range Chinese ducks (above). The majority of domestic birds (25/25 nonviraemic and 17/28 viraemic) showed only insignificant or mild inflammation; seven viraemic birds exhibited moderate inflammation (Marion et al., 1984).

[The relative absence of both inflammation and cancer in experimentally infected ducks is noteworthy. Further, the prospective experimental studies have been of limited duration relative to the lifespan of ducks.]

(c) *Synergy between infection with duck hepatitis B virus and treatment with aflatoxin B_1 in inducing hepatocellular carcinoma in ducks*

Ducks have been reported to be sensitive to the effects of aflatoxin B_1 and to the development of HCC as a consequence of treatment with this mycotoxin (IARC, 1993). Studies of the combined effect of DHBV infection and exposure to aflatoxin B_1 in the development of liver cancer all involved white Pekin ducks and a variety of dosing schedules (Table 11). Aflatoxin B_1 was highly toxic, increasing the mortality rate in treated over that in untreated ducks. The rate of appearance of HCC was not significantly different in DHBV-infected aflatoxin B_1-treated ducks from that in DHBV marker-free aflatoxin B_1-treated ducks, suggesting a lack of synergy between current viral infection and exposure to aflatoxin B_1. Integrated viral DNA was found in three of the eight DHBV-associated HCCs examined.

Table 11. Development of hepatocellular carcinoma (HCC) in ducks with and without duck hepatitis B virus (DHBV) infection treated with aflatoxin B_1 (AFB_1)

Treatment	Age at necropsy	No. of ducks	Effective number	No. with DHBV markers in serum	No. with HCC	Integrated viral DNA in carcinoma	Reference
Experimentally infected at hatch; AFB_1 soon after inoculation							Uchida et al. (1988)
0.1 mg/kg, 2 ×/week, oral, 54 weeks	54 weeks	22	22	22	0/8 surviving		
0.1 mg/kg, 2 ×/week, oral, 54 weeks	54 weeks	16	16	0	2/8 surviving		
0.1 mg/kg, 2 ×/week, oral, first 5 weeks only	54 weeks	5	5	4	1	−	
0.1 mg/kg, 2 ×/week, oral, first 5 weeks only	54 weeks	3	3	0	0		
0.1 mg/kg, 2 ×/week, oral, last 25 weeks only	41 weeks	5	5	5	0		
Solvent only	41 weeks	2	2	2	0		
Congenitally infected; AFB_1 started at three months of age							Cova et al. (1990)
0.08 mg/kg, 1 ×/week, i.p., 27 months	2.3 years	15	6	6	3	−	
0.08 mg/kg, 1 ×/week, i.p., 27 months	2.3 years	13	10	0	3	−	
0.02 mg/kg, 1 ×/week, i.p., 27 months	2.3 years	15	13	13	0		
0.02 mg/kg, 1 ×/week, i.p., 27 months	2.3 years	13	10	0	2	−	
None	2.3 years	16	15	15	0		
None	2.3 years	15	12	0	0		
Congenitally infected; AFB_1 started three days after hatch							Cullen et al. (1990)
0.2 mg/kg, 60 days, oral	28 months	12	8	8	4	3+	
0.2 mg/kg, 60 days, oral	28 months	10	4	0	3		
Solvent only	28 months	8	6	6	0		
Solvent only	28 months	9	6	0	0	NA	

[The existence of species-specific hepadnaviruses closely related to HBV, which produce HCC in two species (woodchuck and Beechey ground squirrels), strengthens the plausibility of the conclusion that HBV is carcinogenic.]

3.4.4 *Other species*

The DNA of a hepadnavirus that infects herons (HHBV) has been cloned and characterized genetically, but it has not been characterized biologically nor has infection with the virus been associated with the development of liver cancer (Sprengel *et al.*, 1988).

Evidence that a hepadnavirus infects tree squirrels (*Sciurus carolinensis pennsylvanicus*) was reported from studies of their livers, but viraemia has never been described in tree squirrels, and the virus remains uncharacterized both genetically and biologically (Feitelson *et al.*, 1986a,b). Liver cancer has not been observed in tree squirrels with evidence of hepadnaviral infection.

4. Other Relevant Data

4.1 Pathology

The pathology of infection by HBV involves an acute phase, which may be recognized clinically as acute viral hepatitis, and then a long chronic phase with development of chronic active hepatitis and often cirrhosis. HCC may evolve during some phase of chronic hepatitis, usually after cirrhosis has supervened but in some cases without cirrhosis. The majority of HCCs associated with HBV appear to arise in a clinically silent way, with few symptoms and no evidence of chronic hepatitis until the carcinoma is in a late stage.

4.1.1 *Acute hepatitis*

The histological features of acute viral hepatitis are highly variable, and hepatitis A, B, C, D and E viruses cannot be distinguished. They are also highly variable for the same agent in patients of different ages and immune status. In the neonate and other immuno-compromised individuals, the histological changes are usually very mild with no significant hepatocellular cytopathic change and no significant hepatocellular hydropic swelling, acidophilic necrosis or cholestasis. The typical histological changes in an adult with symptomatic, icteric acute viral hepatitis include: (i) portal expansion with lymphoid hyperplasia (as occurs in many systemic viral infections); (ii) lobular inflammatory reaction with proliferation of sinusoidal lining cells; and (iii) marked hepatocellular changes, including hydropic change (especially in the perivenular areas), acidophilic necrosis and hepatocellular dropout. In the most severe cases of acute viral hepatitis, extensive hepatocellular necrosis occurs (called submassive or massive acute hepatic necrosis), and this is usually fatal. Such severe viral reactions are rare in the very young. In young people with severe viral hepatitis and necrosis, regeneration of hepatocytes is rapid, and recovery occurs with no chronic sequelae (Peters, 1975). There are few histopathological data on the transition of acute viral to chronic hepatitis in large series of patients.

4.1.2 Chronic hepatitis

Chronic hepatitis B is defined as HBV infection for more than six months; the corresponding histological features are extremely variable. Many different terms are applied to the histological patterns, which range from nearly normal to mild inflammatory changes to progressive fibrosis to severe necrotizing reactions. The terminology has been based not on large series of patients with carefully documented courses, virological studies and multiple biopsies but often on small numbers of patients with a few years of observation.

Two commonly used categories of chronic hepatitis are chronic persistent hepatitis and chronic active hepatitis. Chronic persistent hepatitis is used for portal lymphoid hyperplasia and HBV infection without lobular degenerative and inflammatory features (which are required for application of the term chronic active hepatitis). A third term for chronic hepatitis, chronic lobular hepatitis, was redefined by Scheuer and Thaler (1977) as predominantly intralobular inflammation and necrosis with no significant portal lymphoid hyperplasia or piecemeal necrosis (which is periportal hepatocellular necrosis and lymphocytic infiltration).

The separation of chronic hepatitis B into chronic persistent hepatitis and chronic active hepatitis may be misleading and has been challenged (Scheuer, 1991). As a single patient may demonstrate both patterns at the same time or over time, neither pattern is prognostically valid. Since cirrhosis is a common outcome of chronic active hepatitis and because it is irreversible and is not associated with evolution from chronic progressive hepatitis alone, chronic active hepatitis is valuable as a category. In 1989, an international group indicated that many factors, such as age, immunocompetence, infection status, drug use and cirrhosis, can be used to predict the severity of chronic hepatitis (Sherlock, 1989). Scheuer (1991) called for a reassessment of the classification and indicated that the terms chronic persistent hepatitis and chronic active hepatitis were introduced in the absence of adequate knowledge about the natural history of HBV. Cirrhosis is the major form of irreversible severe chronic liver disease that is related to chronic infection with HBV. The number of patients with acute viral hepatitis that progress to cirrhosis is not clear, and the rate of progression is highly variable. Many patients acquire HBV in childhood, and the initial episode (acute viral hepatitis) is clinically silent (Bortolotti et al., 1990): of a series of 76 children with chronic hepatitis B, eight had a clinical event identified as acute viral hepatitis, but the rest were detected in screening programmes. Liver biopsy samples taken in this series showed a wide range of patterns, many having chronic persistent hepatitis and some having chronic active hepatitis. One of the patients had cirrhosis which subsequently became inactive (i.e. fewer inflammatory and hepatocellular degenerative changes). A few cases of cirrhosis resulting from HBV are detected in childhood, but the majority seem to be detected in late adult life. Clearly, many adults have chronic hepatitis B infection and do not progress to cirrhosis (Sugimura et al., 1991).

4.1.3 Cirrhosis

Cirrhosis is defined as irreversible hepatic fibrosis with regenerative nodule formation (Popper, 1977). The etiology of cirrhosis may be very difficult to discern by histological means. The pattern of inflammatory activity may be a clue to the underlying agent, but cirrhosis is often recognized at a late stage with little hepatocellular degeneration or inflammatory change. Hepatitis B viral cirrhosis is often identified on the basis of the presence of ground-glass cells, which are hepatocytes with a distinctive eosinophilic cytoplasmic change due to accumulated hepatitis B surface protein (Buendia, 1992), or by specific immunoperoxidase staining for HBV markers (Nayak & Sachdeva, 1975). The late stage of chronic hepatitis is associated with macronodular cirrhosis (formerly called postnecrotic cirrhosis). As cirrhosis progresses, the size of the nodules increases (Popper, 1977).

4.1.4 *Evolution of hepatocellular carcinoma from cirrhosis*

The strong correlation between HCC and cirrhosis is dependent on the etiology of the cirrhosis. Autopsy results suggest that HCC occurs with greatest frequency (38%) in association with cirrhosis due to chronic HBV infection, haemochromatosis and chronic HCV infection, with intermediate frequency (5–10%) in alcoholic cirrhosis and very low frequency in cirrhosis due to Wilson's disease, autoimmune chronic active hepatitis (< 5%) and primary biliary cirrhosis (Craig *et al.*, 1991).

The mechanism of progression of cirrhosis to HCC is much debated. Dysplastic hepatocellular changes have been described that may be associated with HCC in patients with HBV (Ho *et al.*, 1981). Liver-cell dysplasia is hepatocellular enlargement with nuclear pleomorphism and multinucleation; dysplastic cells occur in clumps or small nodules. Ho *et al.* (1981) reported that 60% of 558 cases of cirrhosis had liver-cell dysplasia and this change was strongly correlated with development of HCC; however, some nodules may be premalignant without liver-cell dysplasia. The transformation of regenerative nodules to atypical hyperplastic nodules and then to HCC is well described. The small regenerative nodule may have a 'nodule within the nodule' growth pattern, and some observers consider that such small nodules are precursors of carcinoma (Arakawa *et al.*, 1986).

Adenomatous hyperplasia (Takayama *et al.*, 1990), also called macroregenerative nodule, is a discrete nodule of hepatocytes that is apparent by gross examination because it is slightly larger and usually also has a different colour from the surrounding nodules of the cirrhotic liver. These nodules are usually 0.8–3.0 cm and not larger, as then the lesion is likely to be a small HCC. Light microscopy reveals that the nodule is composed of hepatocytes in regular trabeculae (not solid), lacks the overt features of carcinoma (such as acinar formation, mitosis and high nuclear:cytoplasmic ratios) and includes foci of small blood vessels and bile ducts. These 'trapped' bile ducts and vessels, usually at the periphery, distinguish adenomatous hyperplastic nodules from hepatocellular adenoma. Some enlarged nodules in cirrhotic livers are HCC, and other nodules demonstrate some features of both hepatocellular and adenomatous hyperplasia (and are thus called atypical adenomatous hyperplasia). These atypical nodules have small areas of acinar formation, an area of thicker cord development or focal hepatocytes with increased nuclear:cytoplasmic ratio. Additional levels of a tissue block and/or more sections of a single nodule reveal that some atypical nodules are small HCCs. The transition of benign hepatocytes to atypical hepatocytes to carcinoma has been observed in a few nodules of cirrhotic liver, whereas the usual histological examination of HCC reveals only masses of carcinoma with no transitional growth areas. In a series of 110 cirrhotic liver explants (of many etiologies, including HBV cirrhosis but excluding known HCC) examined carefully for distinctive (grossly apparent) nodules, 40 nodules were identified in 19 livers (Ferrell *et al.*, 1992). Microscopic examination allowed classification of 12 as small HCCs and 28 as adenomatous hyperplasia (some with atypia) and liver-cell dysplasia.

Several examples of atypical adenomatous hyperplasia have been shown to have the same clonal integration pattern as the HCC within the same liver. This clonal growth provides a link between atypical adenomatous hyperplasia and the evolution of HCC (Tsuda *et al.*, 1988). Furthermore, the same HBV DNA integration pattern detected in multiple nodules of HCC in the same liver with chronic hepatitis B has been interpreted as proof of clonal growth of HCC and consequent metastasis within the liver. The detection of an additional, new integration pattern in the tumour cells during its course suggests additional HBV-related mutagenesis (Hsu, H.-C. *et al.*, 1991). In experimental models of HCC, e.g. woodchuck with chronic WHV infection (Ogston *et al.*, 1982) and rats with various chemicals, oval cells are identified adjacent to the tumour which are considered to be possible stem cells for HCC. Similar oval cells were detected in human HCC associated with HBV in one laboratory (Hsia *et al.*, 1992).

4.1.5 *Hepatocellular carcinoma*

The morphological pattern of human HCC is usually a homogeneous tumour composed of cells resembling hepatocytes with a trabecular or solid growth pattern. Several other growth patterns are recognized, including spindle-cell, clear-cell and fibrolamellar carcinoma, which are not associated with HBV (Colombo, 1992). A few reports have been made, however, of coexistence of fibrolamellar carcinoma with HBV. Because this variant almost always arises in noncirrhotic, normal livers, the few HBV-infected patients are probably carriers of HBV. Cholangiocarcinoma, the other common primary hepatic carcinoma, does not have detectable HBV markers in the tumour or in the surrounding non-tumorous tissue (Peters *et al.*, 1977).

4.2 Molecular biology

The molecular biology of HBV in relation to HCC has been reviewed (Rogler, 1991; Buendia, 1992; Feitelson, 1992; Slagle *et al.*, 1992). The virus was first associated with HCC in epidemiological studies. During the last 10 years, the role of HBV in liver-cell transformation has been investigated by different approaches, either directly in human HCC or in experimental models, including human HCC cells in culture, transgenic mice carrying part or all of the viral genome (see section 3.2) and naturally occurring animal models of hepadnavirus infection (see sections 3.3 and 3.4). The studies have focused on three main subjects:

(i) integration of HBV: the integrated state of HBV DNA in human HCCs, integration of other hepadnaviruses, structure of viral inserts, cellular target sites for viral integration and insertional mutagenesis;

(ii) expression of HBV genes in human HCCs and their role in the tumorigenic process (mainly surface proteins and X transactivator); and

(iii) genetic alterations in human HCCs, activation of cellular oncogenes and inactivation of tumour suppressor genes.

4.2.1 Integration of HBV DNA

Viral integration has been detected only in hepatocytes, despite the presence of viral DNA in extrahepatic tissues (Bréchot, 1987).

(a) *Integrated state of HBV DNA in chronic hepatitis and hepatocellular carcinomas from hepatitis B surface antigen-seropositive patients*

Initial studies using Southern blot analysis showed the presence of integrated HBV sequences in cellular DNA of established HCC cell lines and in human HCCs from HBsAg-seropositive patients (Bréchot et al., 1980; Chakraborty et al., 1980; Edman et al., 1980).

It is at present uncertain whether or not integration occurs in the early stages of natural acute hepatitis. In contrast, multiple integrations have been observed in tissues from patients with chronic hepatitis (Bréchot et al., 1981b; Shafritz et al., 1981; Boender et al., 1985; Tanaka, Y. et al., 1988), indicating that viral integration takes place prior to tumour development. Analysis of 83 cirrhotic nodules from the livers of 11 HBV carriers with cirrhosis revealed discrete bands at a higher molecular weight region in 26 of 83 nodules (31.3%), indicating clonal outgrowth of altered hepatocytes with viral integration (Yasui et al., 1992). Single-site HBV insertions are common in childhood HCC but are less common later in life (Chang et al., 1991), suggesting that multiple-site integration occurring during the course of long-term HBV infections might accumulate within single cells, as indicated by sequence divergence among HBV inserts in the same tumour (Imai et al., 1987).

Integrated HBV DNA has been identified in HCC specimens from chronic HBV carriers in numerous other studies (Bréchot et al., 1981a; Shafritz et al., 1981; Hino et al., 1984, 1985; Horiike et al., 1989; Sakamoto et al., 1989), indicating that HBV DNA integration is present in more than 80% of HCCs developing in HBsAg-seropositive patients.

(b) *Presence of HBV DNA in hepatocellular carcinomas from hepatitis B surface antigen-seronegative patients*

The presence of serum anti-HBs and anti-HBc in HBsAg-seronegative HCC subjects has been reported (Kew et al., 1986b; Bréchot, 1987; Blum et al., 1990). In spite of the fact that these antibodies generally reflect past, resolved infection, HBV DNA sequences have nonetheless been detected in some tumours in this group (Bréchot et al., 1982, 1985; Hino et al., 1985; Bréchot, 1987; Tabor, 1989; Lai et al., 1990). Improvements in the sensitivity of assays for HBsAg and HBV DNA have made it possible to identify cases of chronic HBV infection with low viral replication (Bréchot et al., 1985; Liang et al., 1989; Bréchot et al., 1991; Kremsdorf et al., 1991; Liang et al., 1991b). The finding of HBV DNA in HCCs in HBsAg-seronegative patients (Pontisso et al., 1987; Paterlini et al., 1993) has been questioned because the estimated copy number of HBV DNA sequences per cell is only 0.001–0.1. The significance of these findings is unclear.

(c) *Integrated hepadnavirus DNA in animal models*

Integrated WHV sequences have been detected in chronically infected woodchuck liver and in a majority (> 90%) of woodchuck HCCs in chronic carriers (Ogston et al., 1982; Rogler & Summers, 1984; Hsu et al., 1990), although Korba et al. (1989) reported a lower frequency of integration. Viral integration appears to be less frequent in tumours associated with GSHV and even less in those associated with DHBV (Yokosuka et al., 1985; Marion et al., 1986; Imazeki et al., 1988; Transy et al., 1992).

(d) *Structure and expression of viral inserts*

Studies of the organization of cloned HBV inserts in liver tissues and HCCs show that HBV sequences are fragmented and rearranged and that integration and recombination sites are dispersed over the viral genome. These data indicate that HBV integration does not occur through a unique mechanism, as is the case for other retroelements and retroviruses. Virtually all HBV inserts consist either of linear subgenomic fragments or of rearranged fragments in different orientations, in the absence of a complete HBV genome, showing that these integrated sequences cannot serve as a template for viral replication. Integrated HBV sequences may be rearranged both during the integration process and after formation of viral inserts (Mizusawa et al., 1985; Nagaya et al., 1987; Tokino et al., 1987). Integrated forms, made up of a continuous genome or subgenomic fragment, which are frequent in tissues from children with HCC and chronic hepatitis (Yaginuma et al., 1987), are believed to represent primary products of integration.

Highly preferred integration sites have been mapped in the HBV genome within the 'cohesive end' region that lies between two 11-base pair direct repeats (DR1 and DR2) which are highly conserved in hepadnaviruses (Koshy et al., 1983; Dejean et al., 1984; Nagaya et al., 1987). A narrow region encompassing DR1 has been shown to be particularly prone to recombination (Yaginuma et al., 1987; Hino et al., 1989; Buendia, 1992; Quade et al., 1992). This region coincides with a short terminal redundancy of the minus-strand DNA, which confers a triple-stranded structure to the circular viral genome (Shih et al., 1987). Integration sites are tightly clustered at both the 5' and 3' ends of minus-strand DNA, suggesting that replication intermediates and specially relaxed circular DNA might be preferential preintegration substrates (Nagaya et al., 1987; Shih et al., 1987). Invasion of cellular DNA by single-stranded HBV DNA, using mainly free 3' ends, might take place through a mechanism of illegitimate recombination, also suggested by frequent patch homology between HBV and cellular sequences at the recombination breakpoints (Matsubara & Tokino, 1990). Different minor changes in flanking cellular DNA have been associated with viral integration, including microdeletions and short duplications (Yaginuma et al., 1985; Dejean et al., 1986; Berger & Shaul, 1987; Nakamura et al., 1988; Hino et al., 1989). The hypothesis that topoisomerase I might promote illegitimate recombination of hepadnavirus DNA *in vivo* has been proposed (Wang & Rogler, 1991). The mechanisms underlying HBV DNA integration have still not been fully identified. Analysis of a limited number of WHV and DHBV insertions suggests that a similar mechanism of integration occurs in these hepadnaviruses (Ogston et al., 1982; Rogler & Summers, 1984; Hsu et al., 1988; Imazeki et al., 1988; Fourel et al., 1990). No similar information is available for GSHV.

As a consequence of the viral integration process, sequences of the S and X genes and of the enhancer I element are present almost systematically in HBV inserts, whereas those of the C gene are less frequently represented (Buendia, 1992). It has been shown that the pre-S2/S promoter is transcriptionally active in its integrated form in human HCC (Freytag von Loringhoven et al., 1985; Caselmann et al., 1990) and that HBsAg might be produced from viral inserts (Zhou et al., 1987). Highly rearranged HBV inserts show virus–virus junctions scattered throughout the viral genome (Nagaya et al., 1987), and recombination breakpoints have been mapped in the S coding region of some of them (Buendia, 1992). Truncation of the S gene between residues 77 and 221 (Buendia, 1992) confers transcriptional activation activity on the mutated pre-S2/S products (Caselmann et al., 1990; Kekulé et al., 1990). Other studies have shown that a large percentage of virus–host junctions are located in the carboxy terminal of the viral X gene, predicting a fusion of the X open reading frame with flanking cellular sequences in a way that might preserve the functional capacity of the X transactivator. Transcripts have been demonstrated from integrated X sequences in tumours and chronically infected livers (Miyaki et al., 1986; Wollersheim et al., 1988; Takada & Koike, 1990; Hilger et al., 1991).

(e) *Cellular targets for viral integration in human hepatocellular carcinomas*

Studies of different viral insertions in many human HCCs have revealed that integration can take place at multiple sites on various chromosomes; insertion sites have been mapped on many different human chromosomes, with higher than average rates on chromosomes 11 and 17 (Tokino & Matsubara, 1991; Slagle et al., 1991; Quade et al., 1992). These studies did not demonstrate the presence of known dominant oncogenes or tumour suppressor genes in the immediate vicinity of any integration site. *Alu*-type repeats and minisatellite-like, satellite III and variable-number terminal repeat sequences have frequently been identified near HBV insertion sites (Shaul et al., 1986; Berger & Shaul, 1987; Nagaya et al., 1987; Buendia, 1992). A small cellular DNA compartment (H3), characterized by a base composition similar to that of HBV DNA and a high concentration of *Alu* repeats, has been designated as a major target for stable HBV integration (Zerial et al., 1986; Buendia, 1992).

In many tumours, large inverted duplications, deletions, amplifications and chromosomal translocations have been associated with HBV insertions, suggesting that HBV DNA integration may enhance chromosomal instability (Koch et al., 1984; Mizusawa et al., 1985; Rogler et al., 1985; Yaginuma et al., 1985; Hino et al., 1986; Tokino et al., 1987; Hatada et al., 1988). It has also been shown that HBV DNA promotes homologous recombination at a distance from the insertion site (Hino et al., 1991). Roles for most of these chromosomal abnormalities have not been assigned as yet, however, although amplification of *hst*-1 loci has been associated with HBV integration in the same chromosomal region (Hatada et al., 1988).

(f) *Insertional mutagenesis by HBV DNA*

Evidence for a direct *cis*-acting promoter insertion mechanism in HCC has been provided. In two cases, viral integration disrupted the structure of the gene (Dejean et al., 1986; de-Thé et al., 1987; Dejean & de-Thé, 1990; Wang et al., 1990) in early tumours that developed in non-cirrhotic livers from clonal proliferation of a cell containing a single, specific viral integration. In one case, the HBV insertion occurred in an exon of the retinoic acid receptor β gene (*RAR*β) and fused the amino terminal domain of the viral pre-S1 gene to the DNA and hormone binding domains of the gene (Dejean et al., 1986; de-Thé et al., 1987; Buendia, 1992). The predicted chimeric HBV/RARβ protein might have altered transcriptional capacity and thus participate in the tumorigenic process (Buendia, 1992). In the second case, HBV sequences were found to be integrated in an intron of the human cyclin A gene, resulting in production of spliced HBV/cyclin A fusion mRNAs initiated at the pre-S2/S promoter (Wang et al., 1990, 1992). In the deduced polypeptide, the amino terminal domain of cyclin A (a target for proteolytic degradation of cyclin A at the end of the M phase) was replaced by an amino acid sequence from the terminus of pre-S1. Cyclins are important in the control of cell division, and disruption of the cyclin A gene by viral insertion probably contributed to oncogenesis (Buendia, 1992).

In a third human HCC, integration of HBV DNA into a cellular gene related to the epidermal growth factor receptor (c-erbB) has been described (Zhang et al., 1992).

(g) *Insertional activation of* myc *family genes in woodchuck hepatocellular carcinoma*

The search for transcriptional activation of already known proto-oncogenes and for viral insertion sites in woodchuck HCCs has revealed that WHV acts as an insertional mutagen which activates myc family genes (c-myc and N-myc) in more than half of the tumours examined (Möröy et al., 1986; Hsu et al., 1988; Fourel et al., 1990). Analysis of the mutated c-myc alleles in two tumours showed integration of WHV sequences in the vicinity of the c-myc coding domain, either 5' of the first exon or in the 3' untranslated region (Hsu et al., 1988). Deregulated expression of the oncogene driven by its normal promoters resulted from deletion or displacement of c-myc regulatory regions known to exert a negative effect on c-myc expression and their replacement by viral sequences encompassing the enhancer I element (Buendia, 1992).

Insertional activation of N-myc genes was observed more frequently. In particular, the woodchuck N-myc2 gene (a functional processed pseudogene or 'retroposon') represents by far the most frequent target for WHV DNA integration. In about 40% of tumours, viral insertions were detected either upstream of the gene or in a short sequence of the 3' untranslated region (Fourel et al., 1990; Wei et al., 1992). The N-myc2 gene is also present in ground squirrels, although insertional mutagenesis has not been demonstrated in this animal model (Transy et al., 1992). Furthermore, woodchucks infected with GSHV do not show insertional mutagenesis (Hansen et al., 1993). Therefore, a direct role of WHV DNA integration in myc gene activation might account for the higher incidence and more rapid onset of HCC in the woodchuck model. Finally, there is no evidence that HBV integrates into myc family genes in human HCC (Buendia, 1992).

4.2.2 *Expression and potential oncogenic properties of HBV gene products*

The HBV genome encodes seven proteins from four open reading frames. Experimental evidence has been presented for an oncogenic role of two of the viral proteins, the large surface (HBs) protein and the transcriptional transactivator X.

(a) *Surface proteins*

In natural HBV infection, the production of infectious virions and HBsAg particles depends on tight regulation of the relative levels of the three envelope glycoproteins. Neither liver lesions nor HCCs have been observed in any of the published transgenic lineages that carry and replicate complete HBV genomes or produce the middle and major surface (HBs) proteins from HBV-derived regulatory sequences (Babinet et al., 1985; Chisari et al., 1985; Burk et al., 1988; Farza et al., 1988; Araki et al., 1989). The appearance and rate of development of preneoplasic nodules and liver tumours following administration of carcinogens are, however, slightly increased in HBsAg-seropositive transgenic mice over that in seronegative littermates, suggesting that HBsAg expression might enhance the effects of hepatocarcinogens (Dragani et al., 1990).

In contrast, when the endogenous pre-S1 promoter is replaced by an exogenous promoter (the metallothionein or albumin promoter), the production of roughly equimolar ratios of large HBs protein with respect to middle and major HBs proteins leads to intracellular accumulation of nonsecretable filamentous envelope particles within the endoplasmic reticulum of transgenic mouse hepatocytes (Chisari et al., 1986, 1987). This leads to histological and ultrastructural features similar to those of 'ground-glass' hepatocytes, which have been described in chronic hepatitis B in humans. Cell death follows, accompanied by mild persistent hepatitis, which is followed by the development of regenerative nodules and eventually HCC by 12 months of age (Chisari et al., 1989). The preneoplastic nodules and tumours display a marked reduction in transgene expression, suggesting that hepatocytes that express low levels of the large HBs polypeptide would have a selective survival advantage. Chemical carcinogens are not required for tumour induction in this model, but exposure of adult transgenic mice to hepatocarcinogens produced more rapid and extensive development of preneoplastic lesions and HCCs under conditions that do not alter the liver morphology of nontransgenic controls (Sell et al., 1991). These data show that inappropriate expression of the large HBs protein can be directly cytotoxic to hepatocytes and may initiate a cascade of events that ultimately progress to malignant transformation (Buendia, 1992).

Studies of integrated HBV sequences in human HCC suggest a possible role for abnormal expression of rearranged viral S genes in the development of HCC. Deletion of the carboxy terminal region of the S gene generates a novel transcriptional *trans*-activation activity (Caselmann et al., 1990; Kekulé et al., 1990; Lauer et al., 1992). Both integrated HBV sequences from a human tumour and from a hepatoma-derived cell line and different constructs bearing similarly truncated pre-S2/S sequences can stimulate the SV40 promoter in transient transfection assays; transactivation occurs at the transcriptional level and is dependent on the SV40 enhancer. The c-*myc* P2 promoter is also activated *in trans*. These findings support the hypothesis that accidental 3' truncation of integrated pre-S2/S genes could be a causative factor in HBV-associated oncogenesis (Buendia, 1992).

(b)   *HBx: a transcriptional transactivator*

Evidence for expression of the HBV *X* gene was obtained by Moriarty et al. (1985) and by Kay et al. (1985), who reported that the sera of HBV-related HCC patients recognize synthetic peptides made on X sequences. Expression of the *X* reading frame in prokaryotic and eukaryotic cells, using various vectors, allowed identification of a 17-kDa polypeptide that reacted with serum samples from a number of HBV-infected individuals (Elfassi et al., 1986; Meyers et al., 1986; Schek et al., 1991). Anti-HBx has been detected in a minor proportion of acutely infected patients about three to four weeks after the onset of clinical signs, and more frequently in chronic HBsAg carriers who have markers of active viral replication. Very few patients are seropositive for anti-HBx after seroconversion to anti-HBs or at the time an HCC is discovered (Levrero et al., 1991). Conflicting results have been obtained regarding the association between anti-HBx and other viral markers and with HCC. The problem may be related to the weak antigenicity of HBx protein or to its sequestration into cellular compartments that render it inaccessible to the host immune system. HBxAg has been detected in the livers of HBsAg carriers and has been correlated with current viral replication and chronic liver disease (Levrero et al., 1990; Haruna et al, 1991; Wang et al., 1991). The HBx protein is located mainly in the cytoplasm of cells infected in vivo, at or near the plasma membrane and at the nuclear periphery (Vitvitski et al., 1988; Levrero et al., 1990; Wang et al., 1991). The HBx protein has been detected in the nuclear compartment only in transfected cell lines (Höhne et al., 1990; Seifer et al., 1990).

The recent finding that the X gene product can *trans*-activate transcription from a number of HBV and heterologous promoters is of considerable importance in defining its role in the pathogenesis of HCC (for review, see Rossner, 1992). More clues to the possible role of HBx protein in HBV-associated pathogenesis were provided by three lines of evidence: in studies in vitro and in vivo and by direct analysis of biopsy samples of human liver and of HCC (Buendia, 1992).

High levels of expression of the X gene may induce malignant transformation of certain cultured cells, such as the mouse fibroblast NIH3T3 cell line (Shirakata et al., 1989) and immortalized hepatocytes that express the SV40 large tumour antigen (Höhne et al., 1990; Seifer et al., 1990). It has been shown that the c-*myc*, c-*jun* and c-*fos* proto-oncogene promoters can be *trans*-activated by the X gene product (Balsano et al., 1991; Seifer et al., 1991; Twu et al., 1993). Activation of protein kinase C (Kekulé et al., 1993) and formation of a p53-HBx protein complex have been reported (Feitelson et al., 1993).

Studies of transgenic mice carrying the X reading frame controlled by its natural HBV enhancer and promoter sequences or by heterologous liver-specific promoters have given rise to conflicting results. In three lines of mice (C11, H9 and E1) derived from the outbred CD1 strain (see Table 7) carrying a 1.15-kilobase HBV fragment (spanning the enhancer, the complete X coding region and the polyadenylation signal), preneoplastic lesions were observed in the liver, which were followed by carcinomas at 8–10 months of age (Kim et al, 1991). In contrast, a transgene in which the X coding domain was placed under the control of the α-1-antitrypsin regulatory region failed to induce tumours in ICR × B6C3F1 transgenic mice, although X mRNAs were detected in liver tissues (Lee et al., 1990).

Analysis of integrated viral sequences in tumour DNA has shed new light on one of the mechanisms leading to overexpression of the X gene in chronically infected livers and in HCCs. HBV sequences are frequently interrupted between or around the viral direct repeats DR1 and DR2 upon integration into host cell DNA (Buendia, 1992), and overproduction of hybrid viral and host transcripts may result from HBV DNA integration in a hepatoma cell line (Freytag von Loringhoven et al., 1985; Ou & Rutter, 1985). The presence of viral and host transcripts containing a 3′ truncated version of the HBx coding region fused with flanking cellular sequences and retaining *trans*-activating capacity was first described in a human HCC (Wollersheim et al., 1988). Moreover, enhanced *trans*-activating capacity of the integrated X gene product has been related to substitution of viral carboxy terminal residues by cellular amino acids (Koshy & Wells, 1991). *trans*-Activating ability of similarly truncated X gene products made from fusion of integrated HBV sequences with adjacent cell DNA has also been shown in many tissues from patients with chronic hepatitis (Takada & Koike, 1990).

This suggests that the integrated X gene might be essential for maintaining the tumour phenotype that develops at the early stages of carcinogenesis. Consistent with this model is the finding that viral and host junctions can be mapped in the carboxy terminal region of X in most human HCCs (Nagaya et al., 1987; Buendia, 1992).

4.2.3 Genetic alterations in hepatocellular carcinoma

Genetic alterations that cannot be associated clearly with a direct effect of viral infection have been observed in human HCCs. Such somatic changes include allele losses on several chromosomal regions, mutation and activation of cellular genes that show oncogenic potential and deletion or mutation of tumour suppressor genes.

(a) Chromosomal losses and tumour suppressor genes

Several groups have reported loss of heterozygosity in a large number of HCCs (for a review, see Buendia, 1992). Loss of heterozygosity on the distal 1p region and on chromosomes 4q, 11p, 13q and 16q has frequently been detected in human HCCs by restriction fragment length polymorphism (Pasquinelli et al., 1988; Wang & Rogler, 1988; Buetow et al., 1989; Tsuda et al., 1990; Simon et al., 1991). These studies showed no relation to tumour histology or grade, presence of HBV, cirrhosis or ethnic origin of the patient. Thus, it has been suggested that these parts of the human genome might contain genes, the functional loss of which might be involved in hepatocellular carcinogenesis. Allele loss of the short arm of chromosome 17p, which includes the *p53* gene, has also been observed frequently in human HCC (Fujimori et al., 1991; Slagle et al., 1991). Viral insertions at chromosome 17p in some HCCs are not physically linked to the *p53* gene (Hino et al., 1986; Tokino et al., 1987; Zhou et al., 1988). Accumulation of allelic loss on different chromosomes (e.g. 13q, 16q) has been associated with advanced stages of HCC (Nishida et al., 1992). Whether HBV DNA integration, which has been shown to promote genetic instabilily, contributes to these events has not been elucidated.

Tumour suppressor genes are identified on the basis of their loss or inactivation in tumour cells, as the product of such genes are negative regulators of cell growth (Marshall, 1991). Mutational inactivation of *p53* is the commonest known genetic alteration in human cancer (Hollstein et al., 1991). *p53* and retinoblastoma genes are the only genes known to be involved in HCC (Bressac et al., 1990, 1991; Hsu, I.C. et al., 1991; Murakami et al., 1991). The frequency of *p53* mutations in HCC was reported to be high ($\geq$ 45%) in Qidong, China (Hsu, I.C. et al., 1991; Scorsone et al., 1992; Li et al., 1993) and Mozambique (Bressac et al., 1991; Ozturk et al., 1991); intermediate (15–35%) in Japan (Murakami et al., 1991; Oda et al., 1992; Nishida et al., 1993) and in Shanghai (Buetow et al., 1992; Li et al., 1993), Xian (Buetow et al., 1992) and Taiwan, China (Hosono et al., 1991; Sheu et al., 1992); and low (0–15%) in Germany (Kress et al., 1992), the United Kingdom (Challen et al., 1992), Thailand (Hollstein et al., 1993) and Alaska, USA (Buetow et al., 1992). As shown in Table 12, the relationship between chronic infection with HBV (as determined by serum HBsAg) and the frequency of *p53* mutation in HCC was addressed directly in three studies, and *p53* mutations were shown to occur at similar frequencies in HbsAg-seropositive and HBsAg-seronegative patients.

Table 12. Frequency of *p53* mutations in patients seropositive and seronegative for hepatitis B surface antigen (HBsAg)

Location	All patients Total	With mutants No.	%	HBsAg seropositive Total	With mutants No.	%	HBsAg seronegative Total	With mutants No.	%	Reference
Japan[a]	140	46	33	30	10	33	98	32	33	Oda et al. (1992)
Taiwan, China	61	20	33	41	15	37	20	5	25	Sheu et al. (1992)
Thailand	15	2	13	7	2	29	6	0	0	Hollstein et al. (1993)
Total	216	68	31	78	27	35	124	37	30	

Numbers of seropositive and seronegative do not add up because the HBV status was not known for all patients.
[a]128 Japanese, six Korean, four Indonesian and two Taiwanese patients

A 'hot spot' mutation (Buendia, 1992) at the last guanine residue of codon 249 (AG*G* to AG*T*) was identified in more than 45% of HCCs from Mozambique and Qidong, China (Bressac *et al.*, 1991; Hsu, I.C. *et al.*, 1991). The codon 249 mutation (AGG→AGT) of *p53* is not a mutational hot spot in non-HCC tumours (Hollstein *et al.*, 1991). The presence of codon 249 mutations in HCC was reported in both HBsAg-seropositive and HBsAg-seronegative patients (Ozturk *et al.*, 1991; Buetow *et al.*, 1992; Oda *et al.*, 1992; Sheu *et al.*, 1992; Hollstein *et al.*, 1993; Yap *et al.*, 1993) as well as in the presence and absence of tumour HBV DNA (Scorsone *et al.*, 1992; Li *et al.*, 1993). An association between HBxAg and *p53* both *in vitro* and *in vivo* has been described (Feitelson *et al.*, 1993).

(b) Activation of cellular oncogenes

The search for activated oncogenes in DNA from HCCs using the NIH3T3 cell transformation assay has not been successful in most cases. A transforming DNA, *lca* (liver cancer), was characterized in a very small number of tumours (2/4) (Ochiya *et al.*, 1986). This new oncogene is expressed at a proliferative stage in fetal liver; its expression in liver cancer has not been associated with gross rearrangement of the gene (Shiozawa *et al.*, 1988). Another transforming gene, *hst*-1, was identified by this method in a tumour from an HBsAg-seronegative patient (Yuasa & Sudo, 1987); and co-amplification of integrated HBV sequences and *hst*-1 was reported in another case (Hatada *et al.*, 1988). Conflicting results have been obtained concerning the *ras* genes in the NIH3T3 cell transformation assay. Direct sequencing of the c-Ha-*ras*, c-Ki-*ras* and N-*ras* genes has shown a very low incidence of point mutations in liver tumours (Tsuda *et al.*, 1989; Tada *et al.*, 1990; Ogata *et al.*, 1991).

Increased expression of c-*myc* protooncogene has been described in a majority of human HCCs but also occurs in cirrhosis (Gu *et al.*, 1986; Himeno *et al.*, 1988). In rare cases, it was associated with genetic amplification of the c-*myc* locus (Trowbridge *et al.*, 1988).

4.3 Other observations relevant to possible mechanisms of action of HBV in carcinogenesis

4.3.1 *Cell division and tissue regeneration in response to HBV infection*

Increased incidences of HCC have been reported in association with liver diseases other than that caused by HBV infection, in which cirrhosis occurs with accompanying regenerative nodules (e.g. alcoholic cirrhosis, haemochromatosis, HCV-induced cirrhosis), suggesting that the active cell division associated with cirrhosis may contribute in an important way to the development of HCC (Colombo *et al.*, 1989; Simonetti *et al.*, 1992). Although cirrhosis is not essential to HCC (see above), the necrosis and inflammation associated with both chronic active hepatitis and cirrhosis may be important. This would explain the absence of tumours in chronically HBV-infected chimpanzees (see 3.1.1(*a*)) in which inflammatory changes are usually limited to the portal spaces and cell necrosis is normally absent or minimal (Shouval *et al.*, 1980). In support of this view is the high incidence of HCC observed in mutant LEC rats in which fulminant hepatitis occurs four months after birth, followed by chronic hepatitis and HCC in association with low levels of ceruloplasmin and heavy hepatic copper deposits (Ono *et al.*, 1991). The changes that occur in the lineages of transgenic mice in which HBsAg accumulates and induces cell necrosis and regeneration, described above, constitute yet another observation in support of this hypothesis (Chisari *et al.*, 1989).

4.3.2 *Immune response*

In patients with chronic HBV infection, it is now clear that immunological mechanisms are involved in the lysis of infected hepatocytes. At least in acute HBV infection, CD8 cytotoxic T lymphocytes that recognize hepatocytes which express HBV core peptides in association with major histocompatibility class I proteins have been demonstrated (Penna *et al.*, 1991). In chronic HBV infection, however, cytotoxic T cells are difficult to demonstrate. It is suggested that the secretion of processed nucleocapsid proteins, such as HBeAg, are involved in inducing tolerance of T cells that can react to HBe and HBc proteins (Thomas *et al.*, 1988). During the course of chronic infection, e antigen/antibody seroconversion may occur at a rate of approximately 5–10% of cases per year. This results in elimination of hepatocytes, indicating that HBV replication perhaps occurs by immune recognition of HBe by anti-HBe. In some patients, e-negative virus then emerges, and viraemia and inflammatory liver disease continue (Carman *et al.*, 1993). These patients progress to cirrhosis, and it has been argued that the associated cycles of liver-cell necrosis and regeneration regulated by growth factors contribute to the multi-step process that leads to the development of HCC in patients with chronic hepatitis with or without cirrhosis. The immunological selection pressure operating against the hepatocytes that support productive HBV infection (expressing nucleocapsid proteins) will favour selective regeneration of uninfected hepatocytes and of hepatocytes containing only integrated HBV sequences, not expressing c and e but perhaps expressing HBsAg (Fowler *et al.*, 1986). These cells are under a strong regenerative stimulus, and it is proposed that it is these cells that give rise to regenerative nodules and HCC (Shafritz *et al.*, 1981; Shafritz, 1982; Thomas *et al.*, 1982).

4.3.3 Hepatocellular carcinoma-associated tumour markers

The best-studied marker of HCC is α-fetoprotein, which is used to diagnose the tumour (Abelev, 1974). Whether there is a specific relationship between HBV and expression of this protein is uncertain (Chan *et al.*, 1980; Trichopoulos *et al.*, 1980b; Kew & Macerollo, 1988).

4.3.4 Role of aflatoxins and possible modification of the effect of HBV

Little information is available as to whether there is a biological interaction between HBV and aflatoxin, although it is established that aflatoxin is mutagenic, and both factors can induce liver injury resulting in increased cell proliferation. One hypothesis is that HBV infection and the associated hepatitis may alter carcinogen metabolism, and some evidence has been provided in humans and woodchucks to support this idea (De Flora *et al.*, 1985, 1989). Aflatoxin B_1 is immunosuppressive (Pier & McLoughlin, 1985; Richard, 1991), but its influence on the immune response to HBV infection has not been investigated.

5. Summary of Data Reported and Evaluation

5.1 Exposure data

Hepatitis B virus (HBV) is a small DNA virus made up of an outer envelope, bearing hepatitis B surface antigen (HBsAg), and an internal nucleocapsid. The nucleocapsid contains the hepatitis B core antigen (HBcAg), DNA polymerase/reverse transcriptase and the viral DNA genome. The viral genome is a circular, partially double-stranded DNA molecule about 3.2 kilobases long. It has four open reading frames, which encode for the different viral antigens, including hepatitis B e antigen (HBeAg) and hepatitis B x antigen (HBxAg), and replicates asymmetrically by reverse transcription of an RNA intermediate. Naturally occurring HBV mutants have been identified, but their pathobiological significance has not been defined. HBV belongs to a group of hepatotropic DNA viruses (hepadnaviruses) which include the hepatitis viruses of the woodchuck (*Marmota monax*), Beechey ground squirrel (*Spermophilus beecheyi*) and domestic duck (*Anas domesticus*). These viruses are highly species specific; they infect primarily hepatocytes.

Current serological methods of detection are highly sensitive and specific and are based on the detection of viral antigens, antibodies to viral antigens and viral DNA. The presence of HBsAg or HBV DNA indicates current HBV infection. The presence of HBeAg indicates a high level of viral replication. Seroconversion to anti-HBe is usually associated with reductions in replication and in disease activity. The presence of immunoglobulin M class anti-HBc indicates acute HBV infection; the immunoglobulin G class anti-HBc appears after acute HBV infection and persists during chronic HBV infection.

Transmission of infection in areas of high prevalence is predominantly between children; mother-to-child (perinatal) transmission plays a particularly important role in Asia. The modes of transmission in childhood are unclear. In areas of intermediate and low endemicity, the pattern of perinatal, childhood and adult infection is mixed. In adults, sexual transmission is a major mode of transmission, although intravenous use of drugs plays an important role in some populations. In many cases in areas of low endemicity, the mode of transmission is unknown.

The course and clinical manifestations of HBV infection are highly variable and depend on age at infection, gender, the immune competence of the host and, possibly, viral factors. Infection perinatally and in early childhood is the major risk factor for chronicity, which frequently leads to progressive liver disease and cirrhosis.

The prevalence of chronic HBV infection varies markedly around the world. High rates of infection, defined as prevalences $\geq 8\%$, occur in China, Southeast Asia, the Pacific Basin, sub-Saharan Africa and the Amazon Basin. In western Europe, North America, Australia and New Zealand, the prevalences of chronic infection are low ($< 2\%$), and infection occurs predominantly in adults. Intermediate prevalences of infection, between 2 and 7%, occur elsewhere in the world.

The incidence of infection is reduced by vaccination with plasma-derived or recombinant vaccines, which are highly immunogenic and confer long-lasting protection against acute hepatitis and chronic infection. The efficacy of vaccines against chronic infection is in excess of 85% in regions where child and adult infection predominate and greater than 70% in regions where perinatal infection plays an important role. The efficacy of vaccination in preventing perinatal infection is improved by the addition of hepatitis B immunoglobulin administration soon after birth.

5.2 Human carcinogenicity data

In 15 cohort studies, carrier status for HBV was determined by the presence of HBsAg in serum. In all studies, the risk for hepatocellular carcinoma increased in association with HBsAg seropositivity, with estimates of relative risk ranging from 5.3 to 148.

Many case–control studies have been reported on the association between hepatocellular carcinoma and chronic infection with HBV, as determined by HBsAg seropositivity. Most of the studies were conducted in Asia and in Africa, but some have been reported from Europe and North America. The studies were of variable quality, but the majority showed a strong association, with relative risks between 5 and 30.

Potential confounding by aflatoxin, infection with hepatitis C virus, cigarette smoking and alcohol drinking appears to have been excluded in studies in which those factors were evaluated.

Serological patterns of HBV markers other than HBsAg, such as anti-HBc and anti-HBs, have been examined in many studies, but variability in methods of determination and reporting of results precluded evaluation of their association with hepatocellular carcinoma.

In general, cohort studies have not reported increased risks for cancers other than hepatocellular carcinoma. No consistent evidence of increased risk was found in case–control studies of other cancers (including cholangiocarcinoma of the liver).

5.3 Animal carcinogenicity data

Hepatitis B virus

Studies over the past two decades have shown that chimpanzees can be infected with HBV and can become carriers, exhibiting mild hepatitis. Progressive liver disease, including hepatocellular carcinoma, is not known to develop in HBV-infected chimpanzees, although reporting of long-term studies of infected animals is sparse and inadequate. A single report suggested that Asian macaques are susceptible to HBV infection and to progressive liver lesions; a possible hepatocellular carcinoma developed in an HBV-infected macaque.

In three studies in transgenic mice on the expression of integrated HBV genes (pre-S, S and/or X genes) in hepatocytes, increased numbers of liver tumours were associated with a high level of expression of the large surface antigen and X proteins. The relevance of the finding that hepatocellular carcinomas are produced in these transgenic mice for evaluating the carcinogenicity of HBV is unclear.

Other hepadnaviruses

Woodchucks are susceptible to infection with the related hepadnaviruses, woodchuck and ground squirrel hepatitis viruses (WHV and GSHV), both of which lead to chronic hepatitis but not to cirrhosis. In one study of naturally infected, captive adults, one study of experimentally infected adults and newborns and one study of experimentally infected newborns, infection with WHV was associated with development of hepatocellular carcinoma in up to 85% of woodchucks with chronic infection. Uninfected animals did not develop hepatocellular carcinoma. Newborn woodchucks experimentally infected with GSHV also developed hepatocellular carcinoma. Beechey ground squirrels are susceptible to infection with GSHV, with the development of mild chronic hepatitis but not cirrhosis. In one study of Beechey ground squirrels captured in the wild, 11/24 (45%) animals naturally infected with GSHV developed hepatocellular carcinoma, while 2/26 (8%) uninfected animals developed the tumour. One study showed that captive Richardson ground squirrels may be infected with a similar but poorly characterized hepadnavirus, but the association of viral infection and hepatocellular carcinoma in this species has not been firmly demonstrated. Domestic ducks are susceptible to infection with a hepadnavirus, duck hepatitis B virus (DHBV). Hepatocellular carcinoma has been observed in free-ranging ducks infected with DHBV, but in three studies of experimentally infected animals and one study of congenitally infected ducks, no increase in the incidence of hepatocellular carcinoma was observed.

5.4 Other relevant data

The mechanisms whereby HBV may induce hepatocellular carcinoma are uncertain. HBV does not contain a known oncogene. HBV DNA is integrated into host DNA in the great majority of hepatocellular carcinomas in HBV carriers, and chromosomal translocations associated with integrated HBV sequences have been reported. In only three cases of hepatocellular carcinoma have HBV DNA sequences been shown to be integrated into any known host gene. This molecular event is, however, common in woodchucks: in about 50% of hepatocellular carcinomas arising in animals infected chronically with WHV, viral DNA sequences were integrated in or adjacent to c-*myc* or N-*myc* genes. In humans, sequences of the S and X genes of HBV are almost always present in integrated HBV DNA, and X gene protein has been shown to *trans*-activate both HBV and cellular genes. There is no well documented evidence for overexpression of known oncogenes as a result of HBV DNA integration in human hepatocellular carcinoma. Deletions on multiple chromosomes and mutations of the *p53* tumour suppressor gene occur in hepatocellular carcinoma, but no pattern of these changes has been found to be specific to hepatocellular carcinomas arising in chronically HBV-infected humans.

The great majority of hepatocellular carcinomas that arise in association with chronic HBV infection occur in conjunction with cirrhosis or chronic hepatitis. Chronic HBV infection is generally established in early childhood, and several decades of chronic hepatitis usually precede development of the cancer. Studies of HBV integration have demonstrated that many regenerative nodules in cirrhotic liver have independent clonal origins; clonal regeneration reflects the extensive cell turnover that renders host DNA more susceptible to mutagenesis.

5.5 Evaluation[1]

There is *sufficient evidence* in humans for the carcinogenicity of chronic infection with hepatitis B virus.

There is *inadequate evidence* in experimental animals for the carcinogenicity of hepatitis B virus. Some hepadnaviruses closely related to hepatitis B virus produce hepatocellular carcinoma in susceptible species.

Overall evaluation

Chronic infection with hepatitis B virus *is carcinogenic to humans (Group 1)*.

6. References

Abelev, G.I. (1974) Alpha-fetoprotein as a marker of embryo-specific differentiations in normal and tumor tissues. *Transplant. Rev.*, **20**, 3–37

Akahane, Y., Yamanaka, T., Suzuki, H., Sugai, Y., Tsuda, F., Yotsumoto, S., Omi, S., Okamoto, H., Miyakawa, Y. & Mayumi, M. (1990) Chronic active hepatitis with hepatitis B virus DNA and antibody against e antigen in the serum. Disturbed synthesis and secretion of e antigen from hepatocytes due to a point mutation in the precore region. *Gastroenterology*, **99**, 1113–1119

Alberts, S.R., Lanier, A.P., McMahon, B.J., Harpster, A., Bulkow, L.R., Heyward, W.L. & Murray, C. (1991) Clustering of hepatocellular carcinoma in Alaska native families. *Gen. Epidemiol.*, **8**, 127–139

Alexander, G.J.M., Brahm, J., Fagan, E.A., Smith, H.M., Daniels, H.M., Eddleston, A.L.W.F. & Williams, R. (1987) Loss of HBsAg with interferon therapy in chronic hepatitis B virus infection. *Lancet*, **ii**, 66–69

Al-Sarraf, M., Kithier, K., Sardesai, S., Vaitkevicius, V.K. & Poulik, M.D. (1973) The incidence and significance of Australia antigen in cancer patients. *Oncology*, **27**, 128–136

---

[1]For definition of the italicized terms, see Preamble, pp. 30–34.

Alter, M.J., Coleman, P.J., Alexander, W.J., Kramer, E., Miller, J.K., Mandel, E., Hadler, S.C. & Margolis, H.S. (1989) Importance of heterosexual activity in the transmission of hepatitis B and non-A, non-B hepatitis. *J. Am. med. Assoc.*, **262**, 1201–1205

Alter, M.J., Hadler, S.C., Margolis, H.S., Alexander, W.J., Hu, P.Y., Judson, F.N., Mares, A., Miller, J.K. & Moyer, L.A. (1990) The changing epidemiology of hepatitis B in the United States. Need for alternative vaccination strategies. *J. Am. med. Assoc.*, **263**, 1218–1222

Alward, W.L.M., McMahon, B.J., Hall, D.B., Heyward, W.L., Francis, D.P. & Bender, T.R. (1985) The long-term serological course of asymptomatic hepatitis B virus carriers and the development of primary hepatocellular carcinoma. *J. infect. Dis.*, **151**, 604–609

Anthony, P.P. (1984) Hepatocellular carcinoma: an overview. In: Williams, A.O., O'Conor, G.T., de-Thé, G.B. & Johnson, C.A., eds, *Virus-associated Cancers in Africa* (IARC Scientific Publications No. 63), Lyon, IARC, pp. 3–58

Arakawa, M., Kage, M., Sugihara, S., Nakashima, T., Suenaga, M. & Okuda, K. (1986) Emergence of malignant lesions within an adenomatous hyperplastic nodule in a cirrhotic liver. Observations in five cases. *Gastroenterology*, **91**, 198–208

Araki, K., Miyazaki, J.-I., Hino, O., Tomita, N., Chisaka, O., Matsubara, K. & Yamamura, K.-I. (1989) Expression and replication of hepatitis B virus genome in transgenic mice. *Proc. natl Acad. Sci. USA*, **86**, 207–211

Arya, S.C., Ashraf, S.J., Parande, C.M., Tobeiqi, M.S. & Ageel, A.R. (1988) Hepatitis B and delta markers in primary hepatocellular carcinoma patients in the Gizan area of Saudi Arabia. *Acta pathol. microbiol. immunol. Scand.*, **Suppl. 3**, 30–34

Austin, H., Delzell, E., Grufferman, S., Levine, R., Morrison, A.S., Stolley, P.D. & Cole, P. (1986) A case–control study of hepatocellular carcinoma and the hepatitis B virus, cigarette smoking, and alcohol consumption. *Cancer Res.*, **46**, 962–966

Babinet, C., Farza, H., Morello, D., Hadchouel, M. & Pourcel, C. (1985) Specific expression of hepatitis B surface antigen (HBsAg) in transgenic mice. *Science*, **230**, 1160–1163

Balsano, C., Avantaggiati, M.L., Natoli, G., De Marzio, E., Elfassi, E., Will, H. & Levrero, M. (1991) Transactivation of c-*fos* and c-*myc* protooncogenes by both full-length and truncated versions of the HBV-X protein. In: Hollinger, F.B., Lemon, S.M. & Margolis, H.S., eds, *Viral Hepatitis and Liver Disease*, Baltimore, Williams & Wilkins, pp. 572–576

Bancroft, W.H., Mundon, F.K. & Russell, P.K. (1972) Detection of additional antigenic determinants of hepatitis B antigen. *J. Immunol.*, **109**, 842–848

Barin, F., Perrin, J., Chotard, J., Denis, F., N'Doye, R., Mar, I.D., Chiron, J.-P., Coursaget, P., Goudeau, A. & Maupas, P. (1981) Cross-sectional and longitudinal epidemiology of hepatitis B in Senegal. *Prog. med. Virol.*, **27**, 148–162

Barker, L.F., Maynard, J.E., Purcell, R.H., Hoofnagle, J.H., Berquist, K.R., London, W.T., Gerety, R.J. & Krushak, D.H. (1975) Hepatitis B virus infection in chimpanzees: titration of subtypes. *J. infect. Dis.*, **132**, 451–458

Bartenschlager, R., Kuhn, C. & Schaller, H. (1992) Expression of the P-protein of the human hepatitis B virus in a vaccinia virus system and detection of the nucleocapsid-associated P-gene product by radiolabelling at newly introduced phosphorylation sites. *Nucleic Acids Res.*, **20**, 195–202

Bassendine, M.F., Della Seta, L., Salmeron, J., Thomas, H.C. & Sherlock, S. (1983) Incidence of hepatitis B virus infection in alcoholic liver disease, HBsAg negative chronic active liver disease and primary liver cell cancer in Britain. *Liver*, **3**, 65–70

Beasley, R.P. & Hwang, L.-Y. (1991) Overview on the epidemiology of hepatocellular carcinoma. In: Hollinger, F.B., Lemon, S.M. & Margolis, H.S., eds, *Viral Hepatitis and Liver Disease*, Baltimore, Williams & Wilkins, pp. 532–535

Beasley, R.P. & Lin, C.-C. (1978) Hepatoma risk among HBsAg carriers (Abstract). *Am. J. Epidemiol.*, **108**, 247

Beasley, R.P., Trepo, C., Stevens, C.E. & Szmuness, W. (1977) The e antigen and vertical transmission of hepatitis B surface antigen. *Am. J. Epidemiol.*, **105**, 94–98

Beasley, R.P., Hwang, L.-Y., Lin, C.-C. & Chien, C.-S. (1981) Hepatocellular carcinoma and hepatitis B virus. A prospective study of 22 707 men in Taiwan. *Lancet*, **ii**, 1129-1133

Beasley, R.P., Lin, C.-C., Chien, C.-S., Chen, C.-J. & Hwang, L.-Y. (1982) Geographic distribution of HBsAg carriers in China. *Hepatology*, **2**, 553–556

Beasley, R.P., Hwang, L.-Y., Stevens, C.E., Lin, C.-C., Hsieh, F.-J., Wang, K.-Y., Sun, T.-S. & Szmuness, W. (1983) Efficacy of hepatitis B immune globulin for prevention of perinatal transmission of the hepatitis B virus carrier state: final report of a randomized double-blind, placebo-controlled trial. *Hepatology*, **3**, 135–141

Bensabath, G., Hadler, S.C., Pereira Soares, M.C., Fields, H. & Maynard, J.E. (1987) Epidemiologic and serologic studies of acute viral hepatitis in Brazil's Amazon basin. *Pan Am. Health Org. Bull.*, **21**, 16–27

Berger, I. & Shaul, Y. (1987) Integration of hepatitis B virus: analysis of unoccupied sites. *J. Virol.*, **61**, 1180–1186

Bernier, R.H., Sampliner, R., Gerety, R., Tabor, E., Hamilton, F. & Nathanson, N. (1982) Hepatitis B infection in households of chronic carriers of hepatitis B surface antigen. *Am. J. Epidemiol.*, **116**, 199–211

Bhat, R.A., Ulrich, P.P. & Vyas, G.N. (1990) Molecular characterization of a new variant of hepatitis B virus in a persistently infected homosexual man. *Hepatology*, **11**, 271–276

Blum, H.E., Stowring, L., Figus, A., Montgomery, C.K., Haase, A.T. & Vyas, G.N. (1983) Detection of hepatitis B virus DNA in hepatocytes, bile duct epithelium, and vascular elements by in situ hybridization. *Proc. natl Acad. Sci. USA*, **80**, 6685–6688

Blum, H.E., Gerok, W. & Vyas, G.N. (1989a) The molecular biology of hepatitis B virus. *Trends Genet.*, **5**, 154–158

Blum, H.E., Walter, E., Teubner, K., Offensperger, W.-B., Offensperger, S. & Gerok, W. (1989b) Hepatitis B virus in non-hepatocytes. In: Bannasch, P., Keppler, D. & Weber, G., eds, *Liver Cell Carcinoma*, Dordrecht, Kluwer Academic Publishers, pp. 169–183

Blum, H.E., Liang, T.J. & Wands, J.R. (1990) Hepatitis B virus carrier and hepatocellular carcinoma. In: Bianchi, L., Gerok, W., Maier, K.-P. & Deinhardt, F., eds, *Infectious Diseases of the Liver*, Dordrecht, Kluwer Academic Publishers, pp. 261–273

Blum, H.E., Galun, E., Liang, T.J., von Weizsäcker, F. & Wands, J.R. (1991) Naturally occurring missense mutation in the polymerase gene terminating hepatitis B virus replication. *J. Virol.*, **65**, 1836–1842

Blum, H.E., Zhang, Z.-S., Galun, E., von Weizsäcker, F., Garner, B., Liang, T.J. & Wands, J.R. (1992) Hepatitis B virus X protein is not central to the viral life cycle *in vitro*. *J. Virol.*, **66**, 1223–1227

Blumberg, B.S. & London, W.T. (1982) Hepatitis B virus: pathogenesis and prevention of primary cancer of the liver. *Cancer*, **50**, 2657–2665

Blumberg, B.S. & London, W.T. (1985) Hepatitis B virus and the prevention of primary cancer of the liver. *J. natl Cancer Inst.*, **74**, 267–273

Blumberg, B.S., Alter, H.J. & Visnich, S. (1965) A 'new' antigen in leukemia sera. *J. Am. med. Assoc.*, **191**, 101–106

Blumberg, B.S., Millman, I., Venkateswaran, P.S. & Thyagarajan, S.P. (1990) Hepatitis B virus and primary hepatocellular carcinoma: treatment of HBV carriers with *Phyllanthus amarus*. *Vaccine*, **8** (Suppl.), S86–S92

Boender, P.J., Schalm, S.W. & Heijtink, R.A. (1985) Detection of integration during active replication of hepatitis B virus in the liver. *J. med. Virol.*, **16**, 47–54

Bortolotti, F., Cadrobbi, P., Crivellaro, C., Guido, M., Rugge, M., Noventa, F., Calzia, R. & Realdi, G. (1990) Long-term outcome of chronic type B hepatitis in patients who acquire hepatitis B virus infection in childhood. *Gastroenterology*, **99**, 805–810

Bouffard, P., Lamelin, J.-P., Zoulim, F., Lepot, D. & Trepo, C. (1992) Phytohemagglutinin and concanavalin A activate hepatitis B virus in peripheral blood mononuclear cells of patients with chronic hepatitis B infection. *J. med. Virol.*, **37**, 255–262

Bowry, T.R. & Shah, M.V. (1980) A study of hepatitis Bs antigen titres and alpha-foetoprotein levels in primary hepatocellular carcinoma in Kenya. *East Afr. med. J.*, **57**, 382–389

Bowry, T.R., Shah, M.V. & Ahmad, Z. (1981) A controlled study of hepatitis core antibody (HBcAb) in primary hepatocellular carcinoma and liver cirrhosis in Kenya. *East Afr. med. J.*, **58**, 576–582

Bréchot, C. (1987) Hepatitis B virus (HBV) and hepatocellular carcinoma. HBV DNA status and its implications. *J. Hepatol.*, **4**, 269–279

Bréchot, C., Pourcel, C., Louise, A., Rain, B. & Tiollais, P. (1980) Presence of integrated hepatitis B virus DNA sequences in cellular DNA of human hepatocellular carcinoma. *Nature*, **286**, 533–535

Bréchot, C., Hadchouel, M., Scotto, J., Fonck, M., Potet, F., Vyas, G.N. & Tiollais, P. (1981a) State of hepatitis B virus DNA in hepatocytes of patients with hepatitis B surface antigen-positive and -negative liver diseases. *Proc. natl Acad. Sci. USA*, **78**, 3906–3910

Bréchot, C., Hadchouel, M., Scotto, J., Degos, F., Charnay, P., Trépo, C. & Tiollais, P. (1981b) Detection of hepatitis B virus DNA in liver and serum: a direct appraisal of the chronic carrier state. *Lancet*, **ii**, 765–768

Bréchot, C., Pourcel, C., Hadchouel, M., Dejean, A., Louise, A., Scotto, J. & Tiollais, P. (1982) State of hepatitis B virus DNA in liver diseases. *Hepatology*, **2**, 27S–34S

Bréchot, C., Degos, F., Lugassy, C., Thiers, V., Zafrani, S., Franco, D., Bismuth, H., Trépo, C., Benhamou, J.-P., Wands, J., Isselbacher, K., Tiollais, P. & Berthelot, P. (1985) Hepatitis B virus DNA in patients with chronic liver disease and negative tests for hepatitis B surface antigen. *New Engl. J. Med.*, **312**, 270–276

Bréchot, C., Kremsdorf, D., Paterlini, P. & Thiers, V. (1991) Hepatitis B virus DNA in HBsAg-negative patients. Molecular characterization and clinical implications. *J. Hepatol.*, **13** (Suppl. 4), S49–S55

Bressac, B., Galvin, K.M., Liang, T.J., Isselbacher, K.J., Wands, J.R. & Ozturk, M. (1990) Abnormal structure and expression of p53 gene in human hepatocellular carcinoma. *Proc. natl Acad. Sci. USA*, **87**, 1973–1977

Bressac, B., Kew, M., Wands, J. & Ozturk, M. (1991) Selective G to T mutations of p53 gene in hepatocellular carcinoma from southern Africa. *Nature*, **350**, 429–431

Brook, M.G., Karayiannis, P. & Thomas, H.C. (1989) Which patients with chronic hepatitis B virus infection will respond to alpha-interferon therapy? A statistical analysis of predictive factors. *Hepatology*, **10**, 761–763

Bruguera, M., Cremades, M., Salinas, R., Costa, J., Grau, M. & Sans, J. (1992) Impaired response to recombinant hepatitis B vaccine in HIV-infected persons. *J. clin. Gastroenterol.*, **14**, 27–30

Brunetto, M.R., Stemler, M., Bonino, F., Schodel, F., Oliveri, F., Rizzetto, M., Verme, G. & Will, H. (1990) A new hepatitis B virus strain in patients with severe anti-HBe positive chronic hepatitis B. *J. Hepatol.*, **10**, 258-261

Buendia, M.A. (1992) Hepatitis B viruses and hepatocellular carcinoma. *Adv. Cancer Res.*, **59**, 167-226

Buetow, K.H., Murray, J.C., Israel, J.L., London, W.T., Smith, M., Kew, M., Blanquet, V., Bréchot, C., Redeker, A. & Govindarajah, S. (1989) Loss of heterozygosity suggests tumor suppressor gene responsible for primary hepatocellular carcinoma. *Proc. natl Acad. Sci. USA*, **86**, 8852-8856

Buetow, K.H., Sheffield, V.C., Zhu, M., Zhou, T., Shen, F.-M., Hino, O., Smith, M., McMahon, B.J., Lanier, A.P., London, W.T., Redeker, A.G. & Govindarajan, S. (1992) Low frequency of p53 mutations observed in a diverse collection of primary hepatocellular carcinomas. *Proc. natl Acad. Sci. USA*, **89**, 9622-9626

Bunyaratvej, S., Rochanawutanon, M. & Chaimuangraj, S. (1979) Hepatitis B surface antigen in liver tissue and primary liver carcinomas in Thailand. *J. med. Assoc. Thailand*, **62**, 414-421

Burk, R.D., DeLoia, J.A., El Awady, M.K. & Gearhart, J.D. (1988) Tissue preferential expression of the hepatitis B virus (HBV) surface antigen gene in two lines of HBV transgenic mice. *J. Virol.*, **62**, 649-654

Carman, W.F., Jacyna, M.R., Hadziyannis, S., Karayiannis, P., McGarvey, M.J., Makris, A. & Thomas, H.C. (1989) Mutation preventing formation of hepatitis B e antigen in patients with chronic hepatitis B infection. *Lancet*, **ii**, 588-591

Carman, W.F., Zanetti, A.R., Karayiannis, P., Waters, J., Manzillo, G., Tanzi, E., Zuckerman, A.J. & Thomas, H.C. (1990) Vaccine-induced escape mutant of hepatitis B virus. *Lancet*, **336**, 325-329

Carman, W.F., Fagan, E.A., Hadziyannis, S., Karayiannis, P., Tassopoulos, N.C., Williams, R. & Thomas, H.C. (1991a) Association of a precore genomic variant of hepatitis B virus with fulminant hepatitis. *Hepatology*, **14**, 219-222

Carman, W.F., Hadziyannis, S., Karayiannis, P., Fagan, E.A., Tassopoulos, N.C., Williams, R. & Thomas, H.C. (1991b) Association of the precore variant of HBV with acute and fulminant hepatitis B infection. In: Hollinger, F.B., Lemon, S.M. & Margolis, H., eds, *Viral Hepatitis and Liver Disease*, Baltimore, Williams & Wilkins, pp. 216-219

Carman, W., Thomas, H. & Domingo, E. (1993) Viral genetic variation: hepatitis B virus as a clinical example. *Lancet*, **341**, 349-353

Carreño, V., Castillo, I., Molina, J., Porres, J.C. & Bartolomé, J. (1992) Long-term follow-up of hepatitis B chronic carriers who responded to interferon therapy. *J. Hepatol.*, **15**, 102-106

Caselmann, W.H., Eisenburg, J., Hofschneider, P.H. & Koshy, R. (1989) Beta- and gamma-interferon in chronic active hepatitis B. A pilot trial of short-term combination therapy. *Gastroenterology*, **96**, 449-455

Caselmann, W.H., Meyer, M., Kekulé, A.S., Lauer, U., Hofschneider, P.H. & Koshy, R. (1990) A trans-activator function is generated by integration of hepatitis B virus preS/S sequences in human hepatocellular carcinoma DNA. *Proc. natl Acad. Sci. USA*, **87**, 2970-2974

Catterall, A.P., Moyle, G.J., Hopes, E.A., Harrison, T.J., Gazzard, B.G. & Murray-Lyon, I.M. (1992) Dideoxyinosine for chronic hepatitis B infection. *J. med. Virol.*, **37**, 307-309

Chainuvati, T., Viranuvatti, V. & Pongpipat, D. (1975) Relationship of hepatitis B antigen in cirrhosis and hepatoma in Thailand. An etiological significance. *Gastroenterology*, **68**, 1261-1264

Chakraborty, P.R., Ruiz-Opazo, H., Shouval, D. & Shafritz, D.A. (1980) Identification of integrated hepatitis B virus DNA and expression of viral RNA in an HBsAg-producing human hepatocellular carcinoma cell line. *Nature*, **286**, 531-533

Challen, C., Lunec, J., Warren, W., Collier, J. & Bessendine, M.F. (1992) Analysis of the p53 tumor-suppressor gene in hepatocellular carcinomas from Britain. *Hepatology*, **16**, 1362–1366

Chan, S.H., Simons, M.J. & Oon, C.J. (1980) HLA antigen in Chinese patients with hepatocellular carcinomas. *J. natl Cancer Inst.*, **65**, 21–23

Chang, M.-H., Chen, P.-J., Chen, J.-Y., Lai, M.-Y., Hsu, H.-C., Lian, D.-C., Liu, Y.-G. & Chen, D.-S. (1991) Hepatitis B virus integration in hepatitis B virus-related hepatocellular carcinoma in childhood. *Hepatology*, **13**, 316–320

Chau, K.H., Hargie, M.P., Decker, R.H., Mushahwar, I.K. & Overby, L.R. (1983) Serodiagnosis of recent hepatitis B infection by IgM class anti-HBc. *Hepatology*, **3**, 142–149

Chen, D.-S. & Sung, J.L. (1978) Hepatitis B virus infection and chronic liver disease in Taiwan. *Acta hepato-gastroenterol.*, **25**, 423–430

Chen, D.-S., Hsu, N.H.-M., Sung, J.-L., Hsu, T.-C., Hsu, S.-T., Kuo, Y.-T., Lo, K.-J., Shih, Y.-T. & the Hepatitis Steering Committee and the Hepatitis Control Committee (1987) A mass vaccination program in Taiwan against hepatitis B virus infection in infants of hepatitis B surface antigen-carrier mothers. *J. Am. med. Assoc.*, **257**, 2597–2603

Chen, C.-J., Liang, K.-Y., Chang, A.-S., Chang, Y.-C., Lu, S.-N., Liaw, Y.-F., Chang, W.-Y., Sheen, M.-W. & Lin, T.-M. (1991) Effects of hepatitis B virus, alcohol drinking, cigarette smoking and familial tendency on hepatocellular carcinoma. *Hepatology*, **13**, 398–406

Chen, H.-S., Kew, M.C., Hornbuckle, W.E., Tennant, B.C., Cote, P.J., Gerin, J.L., Purcell, R.H. & Miller, R.H. (1992) The precore gene of the woodchuck hepatitis virus genome is not essential for viral replication in the natural host. *J. Virol.*, **66**, 5682–5684

Chen, Y., Robinson, W.S. & Marion, P.L. (1992) Naturally occurring point mutation in the C terminus of the polymerase gene prevents duck hepatitis B virus RNA packaging. *J. Virol.*, **66**, 1282–1287

Chen, H.-S., Kaneko, S., Girones, R., Anderson, R.W., Hornbuckle, W.E., Tennant, B.C., Cote, P.J., Gerin, J.L., Purcell, R.H. & Miller, R.H. (1993) The woodchuck hepatitis virus X gene is important for establishment of virus infection in woodchucks. *J. Virol.*, **67**, 1218–1226

Chien, M.-C., Tong, M.J., Lo, K.-J., Lee, J.-K., Milich, D.R., Vyas, G.N. & Murphy, B.L. (1981) Hepatitis B viral markers in patients with primary hepatocellular carcinoma in Taiwan. *J. natl Cancer Inst.*, **66**, 475–479

Chisari, F.V. (1991) Analysis of hepadnavirus gene expression, biology and pathogenesis in the transgenic mouse. *Curr. Top. Microbiol. Immunol.*, **168**, 85–101

Chisari, F.V., Pinkert, C.A., Milich, D.R., Filippi, P., McLachlan, A., Palmiter, R.D. & Brinster, R.L. (1985) A transgenic mouse model of the chronic hepatitis B surface antigen carrier state. *Science*, **230**, 1157–1160

Chisari, F.V., Filippi, P., McLachlan, A., Milich, D.R., Riggs, M., Lee, S., Palmiter, R.D., Pinkert, C.A. & Brinster, R.L. (1986) Expression of hepatitis B virus large envelope polypeptide inhibits hepatitis B surface antigen secretion in transgenic mice. *J. Virol.*, **60**, 880–887

Chisari, F.V., Filippi, P., Buras, J., McLachlan, A., Popper, H., Pinkert, C.A., Palmiter, R.D. & Brinster, R.L. (1987) Structural and pathological effects of synthesis of hepatitis B virus large envelope polypeptide in transgenic mice. *Proc. natl Acad. Sci. USA*, **84**, 6909–6913

Chisari, F.V., Klopchin, K., Moriyama, T., Pasquinelli, C., Dunsford, H.A., Sell, S., Pinkert, C.A., Brinster, R.L. & Palmiter, R.D. (1989) Molecular pathogenesis of hepatocellular carcinoma in hepatitis B virus transgenic mice. *Cell*, **59**, 1145–1156

Christenson, B. (1986) Epidemiological aspects of the transmission of hepatitis B by HBsAg positive adopted children. *Scand. J. infect. Dis.*, **18**, 105–109

Chuang, W.-L., Chang, W.-Y., Lu, S.-N., Su, W.-P., Lin, Z.-Y., Chen, S.-C., Hsieh, M.-Y., Wang, L.-Y., You, S.-L. & Chen, C.-J. (1992) The role of hepatitis B and C viruses in hepatocellular carcinoma in a hepatitis B endemic area: a case–control study. *Cancer*, **69**, 2052–2054

Chung, W.K., Sun, H.S., Park, D.H., Minuk, G.Y. & Hoofnagle, J.H. (1983) Primary hepatocellular carcinoma and hepatitis B virus infection in Korea. *J. med. Virol.*, **11**, 99–104

Collier, A.C., Corey, L., Murphy, V.L. & Handsfield, H.H. (1988) Antibody to human immunodeficiency virus (HIV) and suboptimal response to hepatitis B vaccination. *Ann. intern. Med.*, **109**, 101–105

Colloredo Mels, G., Paris, B., Bertone, V. & Angeli, G. (1986) Primary hepatocellular carcinoma: epidemiological case–control study in the province of Bergamo. *Min. med.*, **77**, 297–306 (in Italian)

Colombo, M. (1992) Hepatocellular carcinoma. *J. Hepatol.*, **15**, 225–236

Colombo, M., Kuo, G., Choo, Q.L., Donato, M.F., Del Ninno, E., Tommasini, M.A., Dioguardi, N. & Houghton, M. (1989) Prevalence of antibodies to hepatitis C virus in Italian patients with hepatocellular carcinoma. *Lancet*, **ii**, 1006–1008

Colombo, M., de Franchis, R., Del Ninno, E., Sangiovanni, A., De Fazio, C., Tommasini, M., Donato, M.F., Piva, A., Di Carlo, V. & Dioguardi, N. (1991) Hepatocellular carcinoma in Italian patients with cirrhosis. *New Engl. J. Med.*, **325**, 675–680

Cordier, S., Thuy, Le Thi Bich, Verger, P., Bard, D., Dai, Le Cao, Larouze, B., Dazza, M.C., Quinh, Hoang Trong & Abenhaim, L. (1993) Risk factors for hepatocellular carcinoma in Vietnam. *Int. J. Epidemiol.*, **55**, 196–201

Coursaget, P., Maupas, P., Goudeau, A., Chiron, J.-P., Drucker, J., Denis, F. & Diop-Mar, I. (1980) Primary hepatocellular carcinoma in intertropical Africa: relationship between age and hepatitis B virus etiology. *J. natl Cancer Inst.*, **65**, 687–690

Coursaget, P., Maupas, P., Goudeau, A., Chiron, J.-P., Raynaud, B., Drucker, J., Barin F., Denis, F., Diop-Mar, I. & Diop, B. (1981) A case/control study of hepatitis B virus serologic markers in Senegalese patients suffering from primary hepatocellular carcinoma. *Prog. med. Virol.*, **27**, 49–59

Coursaget, P., Chiron, J.P., Barres, J.L., Barin, F., Cottey, P., Tortey, E., Yvonnet, B., Diop, B., MBoup, S., Diop-Mar, I., Kocheleff, P., Perrin, J. & Duflo, B. (1984) Hepatitis B virus serological markers in Africans with liver cirrhosis and hepatocellular carcinoma. In: Williams, A.O., O'Conor, G.T., de-Thé, G.B. & Johnson, C.A., *Virus-associated Cancers in Africa* (IARC Scientific Publications No. 63), Lyon, IARC, pp. 181–198

Coursaget, P., Yvonnet, B., Barres, J.L., Perrin, J., Tortey, E., Diop, B., Kocheleff, P., Duflo, B., M'Boup, S., Diop-Mar, I., Bocande, J.E. & Chiron, J.-P. (1985) Hepatitis B virus and primary liver cancer in intertropical Africa. *Rev. Epidémiol. Santé publ.*, **33**, 267–275 (in French)

Coursaget, P., Yvonnet, B., Chotard, J., Sarr, M., Vincelot, P., N'Doye, R., Diop-Mar, I. & Chiron, J.-P. (1986) Seven-year study of hepatitis B vaccine efficacy in infants from an endemic area (Senegal). *Lancet*, **ii**, 1143–1145

Coursaget, P., Yvonnet, B., Chotard, J., Vincelot, P., Sarr, M., Diouf, C., Chiron, J.-P. & Diop-Mar, I. (1987) Age- and sex-related study of hepatitis B virus chronic carrier state in infants from an endemic area (Senegal). *J. med. Virol.*, **22**, 1–5

Coursaget, P., Buisson, Y., Bourdil, C., Yvonnet, B., Molinié, C., Diop, M.T., Chiron, J.-P., Bao, O. & Diop-Mar, I. (1990) Antibody response to preS1 in hepatitis-B-virus-induced liver disease and after immunization. *Res. Virol.*, **141**, 563-570

Cova, L., Wild, C.P., Mehrotra, R., Turusov, V., Shirai, T., Lambert, V., Jacquet, C., Tomatis, L., Trépo, C. & Montesano, R. (1990) Contribution of aflatoxin B_1 and hepatitis B virus infection in the induction of liver tumors in ducks. *Cancer Res.*, **50**, 2156–2163

Craig, J.R., Klatt, E.C. & Yu, M. (1991) Role of cirrhosis and the development of HCC: evidence from histologic studies and large population studies. In: Tabor, E., Di Bisceglie, A.M. & Purcell, R.H., eds, *Etiology, Pathology, and Treatment of Hepatocellular Carcinoma in North America* (Advances in Applied Biotechnology Series Vol. 13), Houston, TX, Gulf Publishing, pp. 177–190

Craven, D.E., Awdeh, Z.L., Kunches, L.M., Yunis, E.J., Dienstag, J.L., Werner, B.G., Polk, B.F., Snydman, D.R., Platt, R., Crumpacker, C.S., Grady, G.F. & Alper, C.A. (1986) Nonresponsiveness to hepatitis B vaccine in health care workers. Results of revaccination and genetic typings. *Ann. intern. Med.*, **105**, 356–360

Cullen, J.M., Marion, P.L. & Newbold, J.E. (1989) A sequential histologic and immunohistochemical study of duck hepatitis B virus infection in Pekin ducks. *Vet. Pathol.*, **26**, 164–172

Cullen, J.M., Marion, P.L., Sherman, G.J., Hong, X. & Newbold, J.E. (1990) Hepatic neoplasms in aflatoxin B_1-treated, congenital duck hepatitis B virus-infected, and virus-free Pekin ducks. *Cancer Res.*, **50**, 4072–4080

Cullen, J.M., Newbold, J.E. & Sherman, G.J. (1991) Teratoma in a duck infected congenitally with duck hepatitis B virus. *Avian Dis.*, **35**, 61–64

D'Amelio, R., Matricardi, P.M., Biselli, R., Stroffolini, T., Mele, A., Spada, E., Chionne, P., Rapicetta, M., Ferrigno, L. & Pasquini, P. (1992) Changing epidemiology of hepatitis B in Italy: public health implications. *Am. J. Epidemiol.*, **135**, 1012–1018

Davis, G.L. (1989) Interferon treatment of viral hepatitis in immunocompromised patients. *Semin. Liver Dis.*, **9**, 267–272

De Flora, S., Romano, M., Basso, C., Serra, D., Astengo, M. & Picciotto, A. (1985) Metabolic activation of hepatocarcinogens in chronic hepatitis B. *Mutat. Res.*, **144**, 213–219

De Flora, S., Hietanen, E., Bartsch, H., Camoirano, A., Izzotti, A., Bagnasco, M. & Millman, I. (1989) Enhanced metabolic activation of chemical hepatocarcinogens in woodchucks infected with hepatitis B virus. *Carcinogenesis*, **10**, 1099–1106

De Franchis, R., Primignani, M., Vecchi, M., Zannier, P.M., Colombo, M., Colucci, G., Antoniozzi, F. & Tommasini, M. (1982) Serum HBV markers in hepatocellular carcinoma and chronic liver disease. *Ann. Sclavo*, **24**, 37–48 (in Italian)

De Franchis, R., Meucci, G., Vecchi, M., Tatarella, M., Colombo, M., Del Ninno, E., Rumi, M.G., Donato, M.F. & Ronchi, G. (1993) The natural history of asymptomatic hepatitis B surface antigen carriers. *Ann. intern. Med.*, **118**, 191–194

Degos, F. & Degott, C. (1989) Hepatitis in renal transplant recipients. *J. Hepatol.*, **9**, 114–123

Dejean, A. & de-Thé, H. (1990) Hepatitis B virus as an insertional mutagen in a human hepatocellular carcinoma. *Mol. biol. Med.*, **7**, 213–222

Dejean, A., Sonigo, P., Wain-Hobson, S. & Tiollais, P. (1984) Specific hepatitis B virus integration in hepatocellular carcinoma DNA through a viral 11-base-pair direct repeat. *Proc. natl Acad. Sci. USA*, **81**, 5350–5354

Dejean, A., Bougueleret, L., Grzeschik, K.-H. & Tiollais, P. (1986) Hepatitis B virus DNA integration in a sequence homologous to v-*erb*-A and steroid receptor genes in a hepatocellular carcinoma. *Nature*, **322**, 70–72

De Jongh, F.E., Janssen, H.L.A., De Man, R.A., Hop, W.C.J., Schalm, S.W. & Van Blankenstein, M. (1992) Survival and prognostic indicators in hepatitis B surface antigen-positive cirrhosis of the liver. *Gastroenterology*, **103**, 1630–1635

Diamantis, I.D., McGandy, C., Pult, I., Bühler, H., Schmid, M., Gudat, F. & Bianchi, L. (1992) Polymerase chain reaction detects hepatitis B virus DNA in paraffin-embedded liver tissue from patients sero- and histo-negative for active hepatitis B. *Virchows Arch. A. Pathol. Anat.*, **420**, 11-15

Di Bisceglie, A.M., Order, S.E., Klein, J.L., Waggoner, J.G., Sjogren, M.H., Kuo, G., Houghton, M., Choo, Q.-L. & Hoofnagle, J.H. (1991) The role of chronic viral hepatitis in hepatocellular carcinoma in the United States. *Am. J. Gastroenterol.*, **86**, 335-338

Dienstag, J.L., Stevens, C.E., Bhan, A.K. & Szmuness, W. (1982) Hepatitis B vaccine administered to chronic carriers of hepatitis B surface antigen. *Ann. intern. Med.*, **96**, 575-579

Ding, Z.G., Li, R.C., Gong, J., Feng, Y.Z., Cheng, K.L., Li, Y.P., Nong, Y.Z., Li, C.Z., Wei, L.D. & Li, Y.C. (1988) Epidemiological study on relationship between hepatitis B and liver cancer—a prospective study on development of liver cancer and distribution of HBsAg carriers and liver damage in persons in Guangxi. *Chin. J. Epidemiol.*, **9**, 220-223 (in Chinese)

Dodd, R.Y. & Nath, N. (1987) Increased risk for lethal forms of liver disease among HBsAg-positive blood donors in the United States. *J. virol. Methods*, **17**, 81-94

Dragani, T.A., Manenti, G., Farza, H., Della Porta, G., Tiollais, P. & Pourcel, C. (1990) Transgenic mice containing hepatitis B virus sequences are more susceptible to carcinogen-induced hepatocarcinogenesis. *Carcinogenesis*, **11**, 953-956

Dunsford, H.A., Sell, S. & Chisari, F.V. (1990) Hepatocarcinogenesis due to chronic liver cell injury in hepatitis B virus transgenic mice. *Cancer Res.*, **50**, 3400-3407

Dusheiko, G., Xu, J. & Zuckermann, A.J. (1992) Clinical diagnosis of hepatitis B infection: applications of the polymerase chain reaction. In: Becker, Y. & Darai, G., eds, *Frontiers of Virology*, Berlin, Springer Verlag, pp. 67-85

Edman, J.C., Gray, P., Valenzuela, P., Rall, L.B. & Rutter, W.J. (1980) Integration of hepatitis B virus sequences and their expression in a human hepatoma cell. *Nature*, **286**, 535-537

Edmunds, W.J., Medley, G.F., Nokes, D.J., Hall, A.J. & Whittle, H.C. (1993) The influence of age on the development of the hepatitis B carrier state. *Proc. R. Soc. Lond. B. Biol. Sci.*, **253**, 197-201

Ehata, T., Omata, M., Yokosuka, O., Hosoda, K. & Ohto, M. (1992) Variations in codons 84-101 in the core nucleotide sequence correlate with hepatocellular injury in chronic hepatitis B virus infection. *J. clin. Invest.*, **89**, 332-338

Elfassi, E., Haseltine, W.A. & Dienstag, J.L. (1986) Detection of hepatitis B virus X product using an open reading frame *Escherichia coli* expression vector. *Proc. natl Acad. Sci. USA*, **83**, 2219-2222

Fakunle, Y.M., Abdurrahman, M.B. & Whittle, H.C. (1980) Hepatitis-B virus infection in children and adults in northern Nigeria: a preliminary survey. *Trans. R. Soc. trop. Med. Hyg.*, **75**, 626-629

Farza, H., Hadchouel, M., Scotto, J., Tiollais, P., Babinet, C. & Pourcel, C. (1988) Replication and gene expression of hepatitis B virus in a transgenic mouse that contains the complete viral genome. *J. Virol.*, **62**, 4144-4152

Fattovich, G., Rugge, M., Brollo, L., Pontisso, P., Noventa, F., Guido, M., Alberti, A. & Realdi, G. (1986) Clinical, virologic and histologic outcome following seroconversion from HBeAg to anti-HBe in chronic hepatitis type B. *Hepatology*, **6**, 167-172

Fattovich, G., Brollo, L., Alberti, A., Realdi, G., Pontisso, P., Giustina, G. & Ruol, A. (1990) Spontaneous reactivation of hepatitis B virus infection in patients with chronic type B hepatitis. *Liver*, **10**, 141-146

Fattovich, G., Brollo, L., Giustina, G., Noventa, F., Pontisso, P., Alberti, A., Realdi, G. & Ruol, A. (1991) Natural history and prognostic factors for chronic hepatitis type B. *Gut*, **32**, 294-298

Fattovich, G., Farci, P., Rugge, M., Brollo, L., Mandas, A., Pontisso, P., Giustina, G., Lai, M.E., Belussi, F., Busatto, G., Balestrieri, A., Ruol, A. & Alberti, A. (1992) A randomized controlled trial of lymphoblastoid interferon-alpha in patients with chronic hepatitis B lacking HBeAg. *Hepatology*, **15**, 584–589

Feitelson, M.A. (1992) Hepatitis B virus infection and primary hepatocellular carcinoma. *Clin. Microbiol. Rev.*, **5**, 275–301

Feitelson, M.A., Millman, I. & Blumberg, B.S. (1986a) Tree squirrel hepatitis B virus: antigenic and structural characterization. *Proc. natl Acad. Sci. USA*, **83**, 2994–2997

Feitelson, M.A., Millman, I., Halbherr, T., Simmons, H. & Blumberg, B.S. (1986b) A newly identified hepatitis B type virus in tree squirrels. *Proc. natl Acad. Sci. USA*, **83**, 2233–2237

Feitelson, M.A., Zhu, M., Duan, L.-X. & London, W.T. (1993) Hepatitis B x antigen and p53 are associated *in vitro* and in liver tissues from patients with primary hepatocellular carcinoma. *Oncogene*, **8**, 1109–1117

Féray, C., Zigneno, A.L., Samuel, D., Bismuth, A., Reynes, A., Tiollais, P., Bismuth, H. & Bréchot, C. (1990) Persistent hepatitis B virus infection of mononuclear blood cells without concomitant liver infection. *Transplantation*, **49**, 1155–1158

Ferrari, C., Penna, A., Giuberti, T., Tong, M.J., Ribera, E., Fiaccadori, F. & Chisari, F.V. (1987) Intrahepatic, nucleocapsid antigen-specific T cells in chronic active hepatitis B. *J. Immunol.*, **139**, 2050–2058

Ferrari, C., Penna, A., Bertoletti, A., Cavalli, A., Valli, A., Missale, G., Pilli, M., Marchelli, S., Giuberti, T. & Fiaccadori, F. (1992) Immune pathogenesis of hepatitis B. *Arch. Virol.*, **Suppl. 4**, 11–18

Ferrell, L., Wright, T., Lake, J., Roberts, J. & Ascher, N. (1992) Incidence and diagnostic features of macroregenerative nodules *vs.* small hepatocellular carcinoma in cirrhotic liver. *Hepatology*, **16**, 1372–1381

Filippazzo, M.G., Aragona, E., Cottone, M., Dardanoni, G., Lanzarone, F., Marenghini, A., Patti, C., Sciarrino, E., Simonetti, R., Tinè, F. & Pagliaro, L. (1985) Assessment of some risk factors for hepatocellular carcinoma: a case control study. *Stat. Med.*, **4**, 345–351

Fortuin, M., Chotard, J., Jack, A.D., Maine, N.P., Mendy, M., Hall, A.J., Inskip, H.M., George, M.O. & Whittle, H.C. (1993) Efficacy of hepatitis B vaccine in the Gambian expanded programme on immunization. *Lancet*, **341**, 1129–1131

Foster, O., Ajdukiewicz, A., Ryder, R., Whittle, H. & Zuckerman, A.J. (1984) Hepatitis B virus transmission in West Africa: a role for tropical ulcer? (Letter to the Editor). *Lancet*, **i**, 576-577

Fourel, G., Trépo, C., Bougueleret, L., Henglein, B., Ponzetto, A., Tiollais, P. & Buendia, M.-A. (1990) Frequent activation of N-*myc* genes by hepadnavirus insertion in woodchuck liver tumours. *Nature*, **347**, 294–298

Fowler, M.J.F., Thomas, H.C. & Monjardino, J. (1986) Cloning and analysis of integrated hepatitis B virus DNA of the *adr* subtype derived from a human primary liver cell carcinoma. *J. gen. Virol.*, **67**, 771-775

Fox, E., Abbatte, E.A., Said, S, Constantine, N.T., Wassef, H.H. & Woody, J.N. (1988) Viral hepatitis markers in Djibouti: an epidemiological survey. *Trans. R. Soc. trop. Med. Hyg.*, **82**, 750–752

Francis, D.P., Hadler, S.C., Thompson, S.E., Maynard, J.E., Ostrow, D.G., Altman, N., Braff, E.H., O'Malley, P., Hawkins, D., Judson, F.N., Penley, K., Nylund, T., Christie, G., Meyers, F., Moore, J.N., Jr, Gardner, A., Doto, I.L., Miller, J.H., Reynolds, G.H., Murphy, B.L., Schable, C.A., Clark, B.T., Curran, J.W. & Redeker, A.G. (1982) The prevention of hepatitis B with vaccine. Report of the Centers for Disease Control Multi-center Efficacy Trial among homosexual men. *Ann. intern. Med.*, **97**, 362–366

Freiman, J.S., Jilbert, A.R., Dixon, R.J., Holmes, M., Gowans, E.J., Burrell, C.J., Wills, E.J. & Cossart, Y.E. (1988) Experimental duck hepatitis B virus infection: pathology and evolution of hepatic and extrahepatic infection. *Hepatology*, **8**, 507–513

Freytag von Loringhoven, A., Koch, S., Hofschneider, P.H. & Koshy, R. (1985) Co-transcribed 3′ host sequences augment expression of integrated hepatitis B virus DNA. *EMBO J.*, **4**, 249–255

Fried, M.W., Korenman, J.C., Di Bisceglie, A.M., Park, Y., Waggoner, J.G., Mitsuya, H., Hartman, N.R., Yarchoan, R., Broder, S. & Hoofnagle, J.H. (1992) A pilot study of 2′,3′-dideoxyinosine for the treatment of chronic hepatitis B. *Hepatology*, **16**, 861–864

Friede, A., Harris, J.R., Kobayashi, J.M., Shaw, F.E., Jr, Shoemaker-Nawas, P.C. & Kane, M.A. (1988) Transmission of hepatitis B virus from adopted Asian children to their American families. *Am. J. public Health*, **78**, 26–29

Fujii, H., Moriyama, K., Sakamoto, N., Kondo, T., Yasuda, K., Hiraizumi, Y., Yamazaki, M., Sakaki, Y., Okochi, K. & Nakajima, E. (1992) Gly^{145} to Arg substitution in HBs antigen of immune escape mutant of hepatitis B virus. *Biochem. biophys. Res. Commun.*, **184**, 1152–1157

Fujimori, M., Tokino, T., Hino, O., Kitagawa, T., Imamura, T., Okamoto, E., Mitsunobu, M., Ishikawa, T., Nakagama, H., Harada, H., Yagura, M., Matsubara, K. & Nakamura, Y. (1991) Allelotype study of primary hepatocellular carcinoma. *Cancer Res.*, **51**, 89–93

Fukao, A. (1985) An epidemiological study on relationship between hepatitis B virus and hepatocellular carcinoma. *Jpn. J. Gastroenterol.*, **82**, 232–238 (in Japanese)

Ganem, D. & Varmus, H.E. (1987) The molecular biology of the hepatitis B virus. *Ann. Rev. Biochem.*, **56**, 651–693

Garcia, G., Smith, C.I., Weissberg, J.I., Eisenberg, M., Bissett, J., Nair, P.V., Mastre, B., Rosno, S., Roskamp, D., Waterman, K., Pollard, R.B., Tong, M.J., Brown, B.W., Jr, Robinson, W.S., Gregory, P.B. & Merigan, T.C. (1987) Adenine arabinoside monophosphate (vidarabine phosphate) in combination with human leukocyte interferon in the treatment of chronic hepatitis B. *Ann. intern. Med.*, **107**, 278–285

Gashau, W. & Mohammed, I. (1991) Hepatitis B viral markers in Nigerian patients with primary liver cancer. *Trop. geogr. Med.*, **43**, 64–67

Ge, X., Huang, G.-Y., Jie, C., Wang, S.-S., Huang, D.-C., Wei, L., Jiang, Y.-Z. & Li, R.-J. (1991) Studies on experimental infection of *Macaca assamensis* with human hepatitis B virus. In: Hollinger, F.B., Lemon, S.M. & Margolis, H.S., eds, *Viral Hepatitis and Liver Disease*, Baltimore, Williams & Wilkins, pp. 301–303

Gerin, J.L., Cote, P.J., Korba, B.E. & Tennant, B.C. (1989) Hepadnavirus-induced liver cancer in woodchucks. *Cancer Detect. Prev.*, **14**, 227–229

Girones, R. & Miller, R.H. (1989) Mutation rate of the hepadnavirus genome. *Virology*, **170**, 595–597

Gombe, C.M. (1984) HBsAg: marker of the relationship between hepatitis B virus and primary liver cancer: situation at Brazzaville in 1984. In: Williams, A.O., O'Conor, G.T., de-Thé, G.B. & Johnson, C.A., eds, *Virus-associated Cancers in Africa* (IARC Scientific Publications No. 63), Lyon, IARC, pp. 221–226 (in French)

Goudeau, A., Maupas, P., Dubois, F., Coursaget, P. & Bougnoux, P. (1981) Hepatitis B infection in alcoholic liver disease and primary hepatocellular carcinoma in France. *Prog. med. Virol.*, **27**, 26–34

Gu, J.-R., Hu, L.-F., Cheng, Y.-C. & Wan, D.-F. (1986) Oncogenes in human primary hepatic cancer. *J. cell. Physiol.*, **Suppl. 4**, 13–20

Guan, R., Yap, I., Wong, L., Tan, L.H., Oon, C.J. & Wee, A. (1989) Evidence of viral replication in HBsAg positive patients with hepatocellular carcinoma: measurement of serum hepatitis B virus deoxyribonucleic acid (HBV-DNA). *Ann. Acad. Med.*, **18**, 8–11

Günther, S., Meisel, H., Reip, A., Miska, S., Krüger, D.H. & Will, H. (1992) Frequent and rapid emergence of mutated pre-C sequences in HBV from e-antigen positive carriers who seroconvert to anti-HBe during interferon treatment. *Virology*, **187**, 271–279

Gyorkey, F., Melnick, J.L., Mirkovic, R., Cabral, G.A., Gyorkey, P. & Hollinger, F.B. (1977) Experimental carcinoma of liver in macaque monkeys exposed to diethylnitrosamine and hepatitis B virus. *J. natl Cancer Inst.*, **59**, 1451–1457

Hadler, S.C., Francis, D.P., Maynard, J.E., Thompson, S.E., Judson, F.N., Echenberg, D.F., Ostrow, D.G., O'Malley, P.M., Penley, K.A., Altman, N.L., Braff, E., Shipman, G.F., Coleman, P.J. & Mandel, E.J. (1986) Long-term immunogenicity and efficacy of hepatitis B vaccine in homosexual men. *New Engl. J. Med.*, **315**, 209–214

Hadziyannis, S.J., Merikas, G.E. & Afroudakis, A.P. (1970) Hepatitis-associated antigen in chronic liver disease (Letter to the Editor). *Lancet*, **i**, 100

Halevy, J., Achiron, A., Spiegel, D., Nili, M., Luboshits, J., Yerushalmi, Y. & Theodor, E. (1990) Recombinant alpha-interferon may be efficacious in acute hepatitis B. *Am. J. Gastroenterol.*, **85**, 210–212

Hall, A.J., Winter, P.D. & Wright, R. (1985) Mortality of hepatitis B positive blood donors in England and Wales. *Lancet*, **i**, 91–93

Halliday, M.L., Kang, L.-Y., Rankin, J.G., Coates, R.A., Corey, P.N.J., Hu, Z.-H., Zhou, T.-K., Yuan, G.-J. & Yao, F.-L. (1992) An efficacy trial of a mammalian cell-derived recombinant DNA hepatitis B vaccine in infants born to mothers positive for HBsAg, in Shanghai, China. *Int. J. Epidemiol.*, **21**, 564–573

Halpern, M.S., England, J.M., Deery, D.T., Petcu, D.J., Mason, W.S. & Molnar-Kimber, K.L. (1983) Viral nucleic acid synthesis and antigen accumulation in pancreas and kidney of Pekin ducks infected with duck hepatitis B virus. *Proc. natl Acad. Sci. USA*, **80**, 4865–4869

Halpern, M.S., Egan, J., Mason, W.S. & England, J.M. (1984) Viral antigen in endocrine cells of the pancreatic islets and adrenal cortex of Pekin ducks infected with duck hepatitis B virus. *Virus Res.*, **1**, 213–223

Han, K.-H., Hollinger, F.B., Noonan, C.A. & Yoffe, B. (1992) Simultaneous detection of HBV-specific antigens and DNA in paraffin-embedded liver tissue by immunohistochemistry and in situ hybridization using a digoxigenin-labeled probe. *J. virol. Methods*, **37**, 89–98

Hansen, L.J., Tennant, B.C., Seeger, C. & Ganem, D. (1993) Differential activation of *myc* gene family members in hepatic carcinogenesis by closely related hepatitis B viruses. *Mol. cell. Biol.*, **13**, 659–667

Harrison, T.J., Hopes, E.A., Oon, C.J., Zanetti, A.R. & Zuckerman, A.J. (1991) Independent emergence of a vaccine-induced escape mutant of hepatitis B virus. *J. Hepatol.*, **13** (Suppl. 4), S105–S107

Haruna, Y., Hayashi, N., Katamaya, K., Yuki, N., Kasahara, A., Sasaki, Y., Fusamoto, H. & Kamada, T. (1991) Expression of X protein and hepatitis B virus replication in chronic hepatitis. *Hepatology*, **13**, 417–421

Hasegawa, K., Huang, J., Wands, J.R., Obata, H. & Liang, T.J. (1991) Association of hepatitis B viral precore mutations with fulminant hepatitis B in Japan. *Virology*, **185**, 460–463

Hatada, I., Tokino, T., Ochiya, T. & Matsubara, K. (1988) Co-amplification of integrated hepatitis B virus DNA and transforming gene *hst-1* in a hepatocellular carcinoma. *Oncogene*, **3**, 537–540

Heyward, W.L., Lanier, A.P., McMahon, B.J., Fitzgerald, M.A., Kilkenny, S. & Paprocki, T.R. (1985) Early detection of primary hepatocellular carcinoma. Screening for primary hepatocellular carcinoma among persons infected with hepatitis B virus. *J. Am. med. Assoc.*, **254**, 3052–3054

Hilger, C., Velhagen, I., Zentgraf, H. & Schröder, C.H. (1991) Diversity of hepatitis B virus X gene-related transcripts in hepatocellular carcinoma: a novel polyadenylation site on viral DNA. *J. Virol.*, **65**, 4284–4291

Hilleman, M.R., Buynak, E.B., Roehm, R.R., Tytell, A.A., Bertland, A.U. & Lampson, G.P. (1975) Purified and inactivated human hepatitis B vaccine: progress report. *Am. J. med. Sci.*, **270**, 401–404

Himeno, Y., Fukuda, Y., Hatanaka, M. & Imura, H. (1988) Expression of oncogenes in human liver disease. *Liver*, **8**, 208–212

Hino, O., Kitagawa, T., Koike, K., Kobayashi, M., Hara, M., Mori, W., Nakashima, T., Hattori, N. & Sugano, H. (1984) Detection of hepatitis B virus DNA in hepatocellular carcinomas in Japan. *Hepatology*, **4**, 90–95

Hino, O., Kitagawa, T. & Sugano, H. (1985) Relationship between serum and histochemical markers for hepatitis B virus and rate of viral integration in hepatocellular carcinomas in Japan. *Int. J. Cancer*, **35**, 5–10

Hino, O., Shows, T.B. & Rogler, C.E. (1986) Hepatitis B virus integration site in hepatocellular carcinoma at chromosome 17;18 translocation. *Proc. natl Acad. Sci. USA*, **83**, 8338–8342

Hino, O., Ohtake, K. & Rogler, C.E. (1989) Features of two hepatitis B virus (HBV) DNA integrations suggest mechanisms of HBV integration. *J. Virol.*, **63**, 2638–2643

Hino, O., Tabata, S. & Hotta, Y. (1991) Evidence for increased in vitro recombination with insertion of human hepatitis B virus DNA. *Proc. natl Acad. Sci. USA*, **88**, 9248–9252

Ho, J.C.I., Wu, P.-C. & Mak, T.-K. (1981) Liver cell dysplasia in association with hepatocellular carcinoma, cirrhosis and hepatitis B surface antigen in Hong Kong. *Int. J. Cancer*, **28**, 571–574

Hohenberger, P. (1985) Pancreas as target organ of hepatitis virus—immunohistological demonstration of HBsAg in pancreatic carcinoma and in chronic pancreatitis. *Leber Magen Darm*, **15**, 58–63 (in German)

Höhne, M., Schaefer, S., Seifer, M., Feitelson, M.A., Paul, D. & Gerlich, W.H. (1990) Malignant transformation of immortalized transgenic hepatocytes after transfection with hepatitis B virus DNA. *EMBO J.*, **9**, 1137–1145

Hollstein, M.C., Sidransky, D., Vogelstein, B. & Harris, C.C. (1991) p53 Mutations in human cancers. *Science*, **253**, 49–53

Hollstein, M.C., Wild, C.P., Bleicher, F., Chutimataewin, S., Harris, C.C., Srivatanakul, P. & Montesano, R. (1993) p53 Mutations and aflatoxin B1 exposure in hepatocellular carcinoma patients from Thailand. *Int. J. Cancer*, **53**, 51–55

Holman, C.D.J., Quadros, C.F., Bucens, M.R. & Reid, P.M. (1987) Occurrence and distribution of hepatitis B infection in the aboriginal population of western Australia. *Aust. N.Z. J. Med.*, **17**, 518–525

Hoofnagle, J.H., Peters, M., Mullen, K.D., Jones, D.B., Rustgi, V., Di Bisceglie, A., Hallahan, C., Park, Y., Meschievitz, C. & Jones, E.A. (1988) Randomized, controlled trial of recombinant human alpha-interferon in patients with chronic hepatitis B. *Gastroenterology*, **95**, 1318–1325

Horiike, N., Michitaka, K., Onji, M., Murota, T. & Ohta, Y. (1989) HBV-DNA hybridization in hepatocellular carcinoma associated with alcohol in Japan. *J. med. Virol.*, **28**, 189–192

Horiike, N., Blumberg, B.S. & Feitelson, M.A. (1991) Characteristics of hepatitis B X antigen, antibodies to X antigen, and antibodies to the viral polymerase during hepatitis B virus infection. *J. infect. Dis.*, **164**, 1104–1112

Hosono, S., Lee, C.-S., Chou, M.-J., Yang, C.-S. & Shih, C. (1991) Molecular analysis of the p53 alleles in primary hepatocellular carcinomas and cell lines. *Oncogene*, **6**, 237–243

Howe, A.Y.M., Elliott, J.F. & Tyrrell, D.L.J. (1992) Duck hepatitis B virus polymerase produced by in vitro transcription and translation possesses DNA polymerase and reverse transcriptase activities. *Biochem. biophys. Res. Commun.*, **189**, 1170–1176

Hsia, C.C., Evarts, R.P., Nakatsukasa, H., Marsden, E.R. & Thorgeirsson, S.S. (1992) Occurrence of oval-type cells in hepatitis B virus-associated human hepatocarcinogenesis. *Hepatology*, **16**, 1327–1333

Hsieh, C.-C., Tzonou, A., Zavitsanos, X., Kaklamani, E., Lan, S.-J. & Trichopoulos, D. (1992) Age at first establishment of chronic hepatitis B virus infection and hepatocellular carcinoma risk: a birth order study. *Am. J. Epidemiol.*, **136**, 1115–1121

Hsing, A.W., Guo, W., Chen, J., Li, J.-Y., Stone, B.J., Blot, W.J. & Fraumeni, J.F., Jr (1991) Correlates of liver cancer mortality in China. *Int. J. Epidemiol.*, **20**, 54–59

Hsu, T.-Y., Möröy, T., Etiemble, J., Louise, A., Trépo, C., Tiollais, P. & Buendia, M.-A. (1988) Activation of c-*myc* by woodchuck hepatitis virus insertion in hepatocellular carcinoma. *Cell*, **55**, 627–635

Hsu, T.-Y., Fourel, G., Etiemble, J., Tiollais, P. & Buendia, M.-A. (1990) Integration of hepatitis virus DNA near c-*myc* in woodchuck hepatocellular carcinoma. *Gastroenterol. Jpn.*, **25**, 43–48

Hsu, H.-C., Chiou, T.-J., Chen, J.-Y., Lee, C.-S., Lee, P.-H. & Peng, S.-Y. (1991) Clonality and clonal evolution of hepatocellular carcinoma with multiple nodules. *Hepatology*, **13**, 923–928

Hsu, I.C., Metcalf, R.A., Sun, T., Welsh, J.A., Wang, N.J. & Harris, C.C. (1991) Mutational hotspot in the p53 gene in human hepatocellular carcinomas. *Nature*, **350**, 427–428

IARC (1987) *IARC Monographs on the Evaluation of Carcinogenic Risks to Humans*, Suppl. 7, *Overall Evaluations of Carcinogenicity: An Updating of* IARC Monographs *Volumes 1 to 42*, Lyon, pp. 297–308

IARC (1988) *IARC Monographs on the Evaluation of Carcinogenic Risks to Humans*, Vol. 44, *Alcohol Drinking*, Lyon

IARC (1993) *IARC Monographs on the Evaluation of Carcinogenic Risks to Humans*, Vol. 56, *Some Naturally Occurring Substances: Food Items and Constituents, Heterocyclic Aromatic Amines and Mycotoxins*, Lyon, pp. 245–395

IARC (undated) *Hepatitis B and Liver Cancer. The Gambia Hepatitis Intervention Study*, Lyon

Iijima, T., Saitoh, N., Nobutomo, K., Nambu, M. & Sakuma, K. (1984) A prospective cohort study of hepatitis B surface antigen carriers in a working population. *Gann*, **75**, 571–573

Iizuka, H., Ohmura, K., Ishijima, A., Satoh, K., Tanaka, J., Tsuda, F., Okamoto, H., Miyakawa, Y. & Mayumi, M. (1992) Correlation between anti-HBc titers and HBV DNA in blood units without detectable HBsAg. *Vox sang.*, **63**, 107–111

Imai, M., Hoshi, Y., Okamoto, H., Matsui, T., Tsurimoto, T., Matsubara, K., Miyakawa, Y. & Mayumi, M. (1987) Free and integrated forms of hepatitis B virus DNA in human hepatocellular carcinoma cells (PLC/342) propagated in nude mice. *J. Virol.*, **61**, 3555–3560

Imazeki, F., Yaginuma, K., Omata, M., Okuda, K., Kobayashi, M. & Koike, K. (1988) Integrated structures of duck hepatitis B virus DNA in hepatocellular carcinoma. *J. Virol.*, **62**, 861–865

Inaba, Y., Maruchi, N., Matsuda, M., Yoshihara, N. & Yamamoto, S.-I. (1984) A case-control study on liver cancer with special emphasis on the possible aetiological role of schistosomiasis. *Int. J. Epidemiol.*, **13**, 408-412

Inskip, H.M., Hall, A.J., Chotard, J., Loik, F. & Whittle, H. (1991) Hepatitis B vaccine in the Gambian Expanded Programme on Immunization: factors influencing antibody response. *Int. J. Epidemiol.*, **20**, 764-769

Itoh, Y., Takai, E., Ohnuma, H., Kitajima, K., Tsuda, F., Machida, A., Mishiro, S., Nakamura, T., Miyakawa, Y. & Mayumi, M. (1986) A synthetic peptide vaccine involving the product of the pre-S(2) region of hepatitis B virus DNA: protective efficacy in chimpanzees. *Proc. natl Acad. Sci. USA*, **83**, 9174-9178

Jackowska, T., Kalinowska, B., Rokicka-Milewska, R., Derulska, D., Sopyl/o, B. & Makowska, K. (1990) Hepatitis B virus infection in children with leukaemias and lymphomas. *Wiad. Lek.*, **43**, 645-651 (in Polish)

Janssen, H.L.A., Berk, L., Schalm, S.W., Heijtink, R.A., Hess, G., Rossol, S., Meyer zum Buschenfelde, K.-H., Chamuleau, R.A.F.M., Jansen, P.L.M., Reesink, H.W., Meyer, B., Beglinger, C., den Ouden-Muller, J.W., de Jong, M. & Mulder, C.J.J. (1992) Antiviral effect of prolonged intermittent lymphoblastoid alpha interferon treatment in chronic hepatitis B. *Gut*, **33**, 1094-1098

Jilg, W., Schmidt, M., Weinel, B., Küttler, T., Brass, H., Bommer, J., Müller, R., Schulte, B., Schwarzbeck, A. & Deinhardt, F. (1986) Immunogenicity of recombinant hepatitis B vaccine in dialysis patients. *J. Hepatol.*, **3**, 190-195

Johnson, P.J. (1991) Epidemiology of hepatocellular carcinoma in the West. *Pathol. Biol.*, **39**, 896-897

Joubert, J.J., Jupp, P.G., Prozesky, O.W. & Lourens, J.G.H. (1985) Infection of wild populations of the tampan, *Ornithodoros moubata* Murray, with hepatitis B virus in the Kavango, northern Namibia. *South Afr. J. Sci.*, **81**, 167-168

Junge, U. & Deinhardt, F. (1985) The acute manifestations of hepatitis B virus infection. In: Gerety, R.J., ed., *Hepatitis B*, New York, Academic Press, pp. 93-118

Kaklamani, E., Trichopoulos, D., Tzonou, A., Zavitsanos, X., Koumantaki, Y., Hatzakis, A., Hsieh, C.C. & Hatziyannis, S. (1991) Hepatitis B and C viruses and their interaction in the origin of hepatocellular carcinoma. *J. Am. med. Assoc.*, **265**, 1974-1976

Kashala, L.O., Conne, B., Kapanci, Y., Frei, P.C., Lambert, P.H., Kalengayi, M.R., Essex, M. (1992) Hepatitis B virus, alpha-fetoprotein synthesis, and hepatocellular carcinoma in Zaire. *Liver*, **12**, 330-340

Kato, I., Tominaga, S. & Ikari, A. (1992) The risk and predictive factors for developing liver cancer among patients with decompensated liver cirrhosis. *Jpn. J. Clin. Oncol.*, **22**, 278-285

Kay, A., Mandart, E., Trépo, C. & Galibert, F. (1985) The HBV HBx gene expressed in *E. coli* is recognised by sera from hepatitis patients. *EMBO J.*, **4**, 1287-1292

Kekulé, A.S., Lauer, U., Meyer, M., Caselmann, W.H., Hofschneider, P.H. & Koshy, R. (1990) The preS2/S region of integrated hepatitis B virus DNA encodes a transcriptional transactivator. *Nature*, **343**, 457-461

Kekulé, A.S., Lauer, U., Weiss, L., Luber, B. & Hofschneider, P.H. (1993) Hepatitis B virus transactivator HBx uses a tumour promotor signalling pathway (Letter to the Editor). *Nature*, **361**, 742-745

Kent, G.P., Brondum, J., Keenlyside, R.A., LaFazia, L.M. & Denman Scott, H. (1988) A large outbreak of acupuncture-associated hepatitis B. *Am. J. Epidemiol.*, **127**, 591-598

Kew, M.C. & Macerollo, P. (1988) Effect of age on the etiologic role of the hepatitis B virus in hepatocellular carcinoma in blacks. *Gastroenterology*, **94**, 439–442

Kew, M.C., Geddes, E.W., Macnab, G.M. & Bersohn I. (1974) Hepatitis-B antigen and cirrhosis in Bantu patients with primary liver cancer. *Cancer*, **34**, 539–541

Kew, M.C., Desmyter, J., Bradburne, A.F. & Macnab, G.M. (1979) Hepatitis B virus infection in southern African blacks with hepatocellular cancer. *J. natl Cancer Inst.*, **62**, 517–520

Kew, M.C., Desmyter, J., De Groote, G., Frösner, G., Roggendorf, M. & Deinhardt, F. (1981) Hepatocellular cancer in southern African blacks: HBeAg, anti-HBe, IgM-anti-HBc and other markers of hepatitis B. *Prog. med. Virol.*, **27**, 41–48

Kew, M.C., Kassianides, C., Hodkinson, J., Coppin, A. & Paterson, A.C. (1986a) Hepatocellular carcinoma in urban born blacks: frequency and relation to hepatitis B virus infection. *Br. med. J.*, **293**, 1339–1341

Kew, M.C., Fujita, Y., Takahashi, H., Coppins, A. & Wands, J.R. (1986b) Comparison between polyclonal and first and second generation monoclonal radioimmunoassays in the detection of hepatitis B surface antigen in patients with hepatocellular carcinoma. *Hepatology*, **6**, 636–639

Kim, C.-M., Koike, K., Saito, I., Miyamura, T. & Jay, G. (1991) HBx gene of hepatitis B virus induces liver cancer in transgenic mice. *Nature*, **351**, 317–320

Kim, S.H., Hong, S.P., Kim, S.K., Lee, W.S. & Rho, H.M. (1992) Replication of a mutant hepatitis B virus with a fused X–C reading frame in hepatoma cells. *J. gen. Virol.*, **73**, 2421–2424

Kingsley, L.A., Rinaldo, C.R., Jr, Lyter, D.W., Valdiserri, R.O., Belle, S.H. & Ho, M. (1990) Sexual transmission efficiency of hepatitis B virus and human immunodeficiency virus among homosexual men. *J. Am. med. Assoc.*, **264**, 230–234

Koch, S., Freytag von Loringhoven, A., Hofschneider, P.H. & Koshy, R. (1984) Amplification and rearrangement in hepatoma cell DNA associated with integrated hepatitis B virus DNA. *EMBO J.*, **3**, 2185–2189

Kojima, M., Shimizu, M., Tsuchimochi, T., Koyasu, M., Tanaka, S., Iizuka, H., Tanaka, T., Okamoto, H., Tsuda, F., Miyakawa, Y. & Mayumi, M. (1991) Posttransfusion fulminant hepatitis B associated with precore-defective HBV mutants. *Vox sang.*, **60**, 34–39

Korba, B.E., Wells, F.V., Baldwin, B., Cote, P.J., Tennant, B.C., Popper, H. & Gerin, J.L. (1989) Hepatocellular carcinoma in woodchuck hepatitis virus-infected woodchucks: presence of viral DNA in tumor tissue from chronic carriers and animals serologically recovered from acute infections. *Hepatology*, **9**, 461–470

Kosaka, Y., Takase, K., Kojima, M., Shimizu, M., Inoue, K., Yoshiba, M., Tanaka, S., Akahane, Y., Okamoto, H., Tsuda, F., Miyakawa, Y. & Mayumi, M. (1991) Fulminant hepatitis B: induction by hepatitis B virus mutants defective in the precore region and incapable of encoding e antigen. *Gastroenterology*, **100**, 1087–1094

Koshy, R. & Wells, J. (1991) Deregulation of cellular gene expression by HBV *trans*-activators in hepatocarcinogenesis. *Adv. appl. Biotechnol. Ser.*, **13**, 159–170

Koshy, R., Koch, S., Freytag von Loringhoven, A., Kahmann, R., Murray, K. & Hofschneider, P.H. (1983) Integration of hepatitis B virus DNA: evidence for integration in the single-stranded gap. *Cell*, **34**, 215–223

Kremsdorf, D., Thiers, V., Garreau, F., Nakajima, E., Chappey, C., Schellekens, H., Wands, J.R., Sninsky, J., Tiollais, P. & Bréchot, C. (1991) Nucleotide sequence analysis of hepatitis B virus genomes isolated from serologically negative patients. In: Hollinger, F.B., Lemon, S.M. & Margolis, H., eds, *Viral Hepatitis and Liver Disease*, Baltimore, Williams & Wilkins, pp. 222–226

Kress, S., Jahn, U.-R., Buchmann, A., Bannasch, P. & Schwarz, M. (1992) p53 Mutations in human hepatocellular carcinomas in Germany. *Cancer Res.*, **52**, 3220–3223

Krogsgaard, K., Kryger, P., Aldershvile, J., Andersson, P., Bréchot, C. & the Copenhagen Hepatitis Acuta Programme (1985) Hepatitis B virus DNA in serum from patients with acute hepatitis B. *Hepatology*, **5**, 10–13

Krugman, S., Giles, J.P. & Hammond, J. (1970) Hepatitis virus: effect of heat on the infectivity and antigenicity of the MS-1 and MS-2 strain. *J. infect. Dis.*, **122**, 432–436

Krugman, S., Overby, L.R., Mushahwar, I.K., Ling, C.-M., Frösner, G.G. & Deinhardt, F. (1979) Viral hepatitis, type B. Studies on natural history and prevention re-examined. *New Engl. J. Med.*, **300**, 101–106

Kruskall, M.S., Alper, C.A., Awdeh, Z., Yunis, E.J. & Marcus-Bagley, D. (1992) The immune response to hepatitis B vaccine in humans: inheritance patterns in families. *J. exp. Med.*, **175**, 495–502

Kubo, Y., Okuda, K., Hashimoto, M., Nagasaki, Y., Ebata, H., Nakajima, Y., Musha, H., Sakuma, K. & Ohtake, H. (1977) Antibody to hepatitis B core antigen in patients with hepatocellular carcinoma. *Gastroenterology*, **72**, 1217–1220

Lai, M.-Y., Chen, P.-J., Yang, P.-M., Sheu, J.-C., Sung, J.-L. & Chen, D.-S. (1990) Identification and characterization of intrahepatic hepatitis B virus DNA in HBsAg-seronegative patients with chronic liver disease and hepatocellular carcinoma in Taiwan. *Hepatology*, **12**, 575–581

Lai, M.E., Melis, A., Mazzoleni, A.P., Farci, P. & Balestrieri, A. (1991) Sequence analysis of hepatitis B virus genome of a new mutant of ayw subtype isolated in Sardinia. *Nucleic Acids Res.*, **19**, 5078

Lam, K.C., Yu, M.C., Leung, J.W.C. & Henderson, B.E. (1982) Hepatitis B virus and cigarette smoking: risk factors for hepatocellular carcinoma in Hong Kong. *Cancer Res.*, **42**, 5246–5248

Lampertico, P., Malter, J.S., Colombo, M. & Gerber, M.A. (1990) Detection of hepatitis B virus DNA in formalin-fixed, paraffin-embedded liver tissue by the polymerase chain reaction. *Am. J. Pathol.*, **137**, 253–258

Larouzé, B., London, W.T., Saimot, G., Werner, B.G., Lustbader, E.D., Payet, M. & Blumberg, B.S. (1976) Host responses to hepatitis-B infection in patients with primary hepatic carcinoma and their families: a case/control study in Senegal, West Africa. *Lancet*, **ii**, 534–538

Lauer, U., Weiss, L., Hofschneider, P.H. & Kekulé, A.S. (1992) The hepatitis B virus pre-S/S^t transactivator is generated by 3′ truncations within a defined region of the S gene. *J. Virol.*, **66**, 5284–5289

Laukamm-Josten, U., von Laer, G., Feldmeier, H., Bienzle, U., Uy, A., Thomssen, R. & Guggenmoos-Holzmann, I. (1987) Active immunization against hepatitis B: immunogenicity of a recombinant DNA vaccine in females, heterosexual and homosexual males. *Postgrad. med. J.*, **63** (Suppl. 2), 143–146

Leandro, G. & Duca, P. (1993) The role of hepatitis B and C viruses in hepatocellular carcinoma in a hepatitis B endemic area: a case–control study (Letter to the Editor). *Cancer*, **71**, 510–511

Leandro, G., Colloredo, G., Cozzolongo, R. & Elba, S. (1990) Hepatocellular carcinoma in cirrhotic patients: role of hepatitis B virus. *Ital. J. Gastroenterol.*, **22**, 66–69

Le Bouvier, G.L. (1971) The heterogeneity of Australia antigen. *J. infect. Dis.*, **123**, 671–675

Lee, A.K.Y. (1975) Hepatitis B antigen and auto-antibodies in chronic liver diseases in Hong Kong. *Aust. N.Z. J. Med.*, **5**, 235–239

Lee, T.-H., Finegold, M.J., Shen, R.-F., DeMayo, J.L., Woo, S.L.C. & Butel, J.S. (1990) Hepatitis B virus transactivator X protein is not tumorigenic in transgenic mice. *J. Virol.*, **64**, 5939–5947

Levrero, M., Jean-Jean, O., Balsano, C., Will, H. & Perricaudet, M. (1990) Hepatitis B virus (HBV) X gene expression in human cells and anti-HBx antibodies detection in chronic HBV infection. *Virology*, **174**, 299–304

Levrero, M., Stemler, M., Pasquinelli, C., Alberti, A., Jean-Jean, O., Franco, A., Balsano, C., Diop, D., Bréchot, C., Melegari, M., Villa, E., Barnaba, V., Perricaudet, M. & Will, H. (1991) Significance of anti-HBx antibodies in hepatitis B virus infection. *Hepatology*, **13**, 143–149

Li, D., Cao, Y., He, L., Wang, N.J. & Gu, J.-R. (1993) Aberrations of p53 gene in human hepatocellular carcinoma from China (Accelerated paper). *Carcinogenesis*, **14**, 169–173

Liang, T.J., Isselbacher, K.J. & Wands, J.R. (1989) Rapid identification of low level hepatitis B-related viral genome in serum (Rapid publication). *J. clin. Invest.*, **84**, 1367–1371

Liang, T.J., Hasegawa, K., Rimon, N., Wands, J.R. & Ben-Porath, E. (1991a) A hepatitis B virus mutant associated with an epidemic of fulminant hepatitis. *New Engl. J. Med.*, **324**, 1705–1709

Liang, T.J., Baruch, Y., Ben-Porath, E., Enat, R., Bassan, L., Brown, N.V., Rimon, N., Blum, H.E. & Wands, J.R. (1991b) Hepatitis B virus infection in patients with idiopathic liver disease. *Hepatology*, **6**, 1044–1051

Liaw, Y.-F., Tai, D.-I., Chu, C.-M., Lin, D.-Y., Sheen, I.-Y., Chen, T.-J. & Pao, C.C. (1986) Early detection of hepatocellular carcinoma in patients with chronic type B hepatitis. A prospective study. *Gastroenterology*, **90**, 263–267

Lin, T.-M., Tsu, W.T. & Chen, C.J. (1986) Mortality of hepatoma and cirrhosis of liver in Taiwan. *Br. J. Cancer*, **54**, 969–976

Lin, T.-M., Chen, C.-J., Lu, S.-N., Chang, A.-S., Chang, Y.-C., Hsu, S.-T., Liu, J.-Y., Liaw, Y.-F. & Chang, W.-Y. (1991) Hepatitis B virus e antigen and primary hepatocellular carcinoma. *Anticancer Res.*, **11**, 2063–2066

Lingao, A.L. (1989) The relationship of hepatocellular carcinoma and liver cirrhosis to hepatitis B virus infection in the Philippines. *Gastroenterol. Jpn.*, **24**, 425–433

Lingao, A.L., Domingo, E.O. & Nishioka, K. (1981) Hepatitis B virus profile of hepatocellular carcinoma in the Philippines. *Cancer*, **48**, 1590–1595

Lok, A.S.F., Lai, C.-L. & Wu, P.-C. (1986) Interferon therapy of chronic hepatitis B virus infection in Chinese. *J. Hepatol.*, **3** (Suppl. 2), S209–S215

Lok, A.S.F., Lai, C.-L., Wu, P.-C., Leung, E.K.Y. & Lam, T.-S. (1987) Spontaneous hepatitis B e antigen to antibody seroconversion and reversion in Chinese patients with chronic hepatitis B virus infection. *Gastroenterology*, **92**, 1839–1843

Lok, A.S.F., Liang, R.H.S., Chiu, E.K.W., Wong, K.-L., Chan, T.-K. & Todd, D. (1991) Reactivation of hepatitis B virus replication in patients receiving cytotoxic therapy. *Gastroenterology*, **100**, 182–188

Lok, A.S.F., Wu, P.-C., Lai, C.-L., Lau, J.Y.N., Leung, E.K.Y., Wong, L.S.K., Ma, O.C.K., Lauder, I.J., Ng, C.P.L. & Chung, H.-T. (1992) A controlled trial of interferon with or without prednisone priming for chronic hepatitis B. *Gastroenterology*, **102**, 2091–2097

Loncarevic, I.F., Zentgraf, H. & Schröder, C.H. (1990) Sequence of a replication competent hepatitis B virus genome with a pre-X open reading frame. *Nucleic Acids Res.*, **18**, 4940

London, W.T. (1979) Sex differences in response to hepatitis B virus. Introduction. *Arth. Rheum.*, **22**, 1258–1260

London, W.T. (1981) Primary hepatocellular carcinoma—etiology, pathogenesis, and prevention. *Hum. Pathol.*, **12**, 1085–1097

Lu, C.Q., Chung, H., Liu, H., Ping, H. & Tsa, C. (1988) A study of correlation between primary hepatocellular carcinoma and hepatitis B. *Chin. J. Pathol.*, **9**, 5–7 (in Chinese)

Lu, S.N., Lin, T.M., Chen, C.J., Chen, J.S., Liaw, Y.F., Chang, W.Y. & Hsu, S.T. (1988) A case–control study of primary hepatocellular carcinoma in Taiwan. *Cancer*, **62**, 2051–2055

Luo, S., Ye, F.-S., Mo, Z.-C., Su, Y.-X., He, J.-S., Zhou, C.-Q., Tong, M.J., Henderson, B.E. & Yu, M.C. (1988) Prevalence of hepatitis B viral markers in hepatitis B endemic areas of China. *Chin. med. J.*, **101**, 654–658

Maddrey, W.C. & Van Thiel, D.H. (1988) Liver transplantation: an overview. *Hepatology*, **8**, 948–959

Marion, P.L. (1991) Ground squirrel hepatitis virus. In: McLachlan, A., ed., *Molecular Biology of the Hepatitis B Virus*, Boca Raton, FL, CRC Press, pp. 39–51

Marion, P.L. & Cullen, J.M. (1992) Animal models of human disease: hepatitis B virus infection. *Comp. Pathol. Bull.*, **24**, 3–4

Marion, P.L., Oshiro, L.S., Regnery, D.C., Scullard, G.H. & Robinson, W.S. (1980) A virus in Beechey ground squirrels that is related to hepatitis B virus of humans. *Proc. natl Acad. Sci. USA*, **77**, 2941–2945

Marion, P.L., Knight, S.S., Salazar, F.H., Popper, H. & Robinson, W.S. (1983) Ground squirrel hepatitis virus infection. *Hepatology*, **3**, 519–527

Marion, P.L., Knight, S.S., Ho, B.-K., Guo, Y.-Y., Robinson, W.S. & Popper, H. (1984) Liver disease associated with duck hepatitis B virus infection of domestic ducks. *Proc. natl Acad. Sci. USA*, **81**, 898–902

Marion, P.L., Van Davelaar, M.J., Knight, S.S., Salazar, F.H., Garcia, G., Popper, H. & Robinson, W.S. (1986) Hepatocellular carcinoma in ground squirrels persistently infected with ground squirrel hepatitis virus. *Proc. natl Acad. Sci. USA*, **83**, 4543–4546

Marion, P.L., Popper, H., Azcarraga, R.R., Steevens, C., Van Davelaar, M.J., Garcia, G. & Robinson, W.S. (1987) Ground squirrel hepatitis virus and hepatocellular carcinoma. In: Koike, K., Robinson, W. & Will, H., eds, *Hepadna Viruses* (UCLA Symposia on Molecular and Cellular Biology Vol. 70), New York, Alan R. Liss, pp. 337–348

Marshall, C.J. (1991) Tumor suppressor genes. *Cell*, **64**, 313–326

Martin, P., Munoz, S.J. & Friedman L.S. (1992) Liver transplantation for viral hepatitis: current status. *Am. J. Gastroenterol.*, **87**, 409–418

Mason, W.S. & Taylor, J.M. (1989) Experimental systems for the study of hepadnavirus and hepatitis delta virus infections. *Hepatology*, **9**, 635–645

Mason, W.S., Seal, G. & Summers, J. (1980) Virus of Pekin ducks with structural and biological relatedness to human hepatitis B virus. *J. Virol.*, **36**, 829–836

Mason, A., Yoffe, B., Noonan, C., Mearns, M., Campbell, C., Kelley, A. & Perrillo, R.P. (1992) Hepatitis B virus DNA in peripheral-blood mononuclear cells in chronic hepatitis B after HBsAg clearance. *Hepatology*, **16**, 36–41

Matsubara, K. & Tokino, T. (1990) Integration of hepatitis B virus DNA and its implications for hepatocarcinogenesis. *Mol. biol. Med.*, **7**, 243–260

Maupas, P. & Melnick, J.L. (1981) Hepatitis B infection and primary liver cancer. *Prog. med. Virol.*, **27**, 1–5

Maupas, P., Coursaget, P., Goudeau, A., Drucker, J., Sankale, M., Linhard, J. & Diebolt, G. (1977) Hepatitis B virus and primary liver carcinoma: evidences for a filiation hepatitis B, cirrhosis and primary liver cancer. *Ann. Microbiol. (Inst. Pasteur)*, **128A**, 245–253

Maupas, P., Chiron, J.-P., Barin, F., Coursaget, P., Goudeau, A., Perrin, J., Denis, F. & Diop-Mar, I. (1981) Efficacy of hepatitis B vaccine in prevention of early HBsAg carrier state in children. Controlled trial in an endemic area (Senegal). *Lancet*, **i**, 289–292

Maynard, J.E., Kane, M.A. & Hadler, S.C. (1989) Global control of hepatitis B through vaccination: role of hepatitis B vaccine in the Expanded Programme on Immunization. *Rev. infect. Dis.*, **11** (Suppl. 3), S574–S578

McLean, A.A., Guess, H.A. & Scolnick, E.M. (1985) Suboptimal response to hepatitis B vaccine given by injection into the buttock. *Morb. Mortal. Wkly Rep.*, **34**, 105–108, 113

McMahon, B.J., Alward, W.L.M., Hall, D.B., Heyward, W.L., Bender, T.R., Francis, D.P. & Maynard, J.E. (1985) Acute hepatitis B virus infection: relation of age to the clinical expression of the disease and subsequent development of the carrier state. *J. infect. Dis.*, **151**, 599–603

McMahon, B.J., Rhoades, E.R., Heyward, W.L., Tower, E., Ritter, D., Lanier, A.P., Wainwright, R.B. & Helminiak, C. (1987) A comprehensive programme to reduce the incidence of hepatitis B virus infection and its sequelae in Alaskan natives. *Lancet*, **ii**, 1134–1136

McMahon, B.J., Alberts, S.R., Wainwright, R.B., Bulkow, L. & Lanier, A.P. (1990a) Hepatitis B-related sequelae. Prospective study in 1400 hepatitis B surface antigen-positive Alaska native carriers. *Arch. intern. Med.*, **150**, 1051–1054

McMahon, B.J., Lanier, A.P., Wainwright, R.B. & Kilkenny S.J. (1990b) Hepatocellular carcinoma in Alaska Eskimos: epidemiology, clinical features, and early detection. *Prog. Liver Dis.*, **9**, 643–655

McMahon, B.J., Parkinson, A.J., Helminiak, C., Wainwright, R.B., Bulkow, L., Kellerman-Douglas, A., Schoenberg, S. & Ritter, D. (1992) Response to hepatitis B vaccine of persons positive for antibody to hepatitis B core antigen. *Gastroenterology*, **103**, 590–594

McMahon, G., Ehrlich, P.H., Moustafa, Z.A., McCarthy, L.A., Dottavio, D., Tolpin, M.D., Nadler, P.I. & Östberg, L. (1992) Genetic alterations of the gene encoding the major HBsAg: DNA and immunological analysis of recurrent HBsAg derived from monoclonal antibody-treated liver transplant patients. *Hepatology*, **15**, 757–766

McNair, A.N.B., Main, J. & Thomas, H.C. (1992) Interactions of the human immunodeficiency virus and the hepatotropic viruses. *Semin. Liver Dis.*, **12**, 188–196

McQuillan, G.M., Townsend, T.R., Fields, H.A., Carroll, M., Leahy, M. & Polk, B.F. (1989) Seroepidemiology of hepatitis B virus infection in the United States. *Am. J. Med.*, **87** (Suppl. 3A), 5S–10S

McSweeney, P.A., Carter, J.M., Green, G.J. & Romeril, K.R. (1988) Fatal aplastic anemia associated with hepatitis B viral infection. *Am. J. Med.*, **85**, 255–256

Melegari, M., Jung, M.-C., Schneider, R., Santantonio, T., Bagnulo, S., Luchena, N., Pastore, G., Pape, G., Scaglioni, P.P., Villa, E. & Will, H. (1991) Conserved core protein sequences in hepatitis B virus infected patients without anti-HBc. *J. Hepatol.*, **13**, 187–191

Meyers, M.L., Vitvitski Trépo, L., Nath, N. & Snisky, J.J. (1986) Hepatitis B virus polypeptide X: expression in *Escherichia coli* and identification of specific antibodies in sera from hepatitis B virus-infected humans. *J. Virol.*, **57**, 101–109

Michon, J., Prince, A.M., Szmuness, W., Demaille, J., Diebolt, G., Linhard, J., Quenum, C. & Sankale, M. (1975) Primary liver cancer and hepatitis B infection in Senegal. Comparison between cancer patients and two controls. *Biomedicine*, **23**, 263–266 (in French)

Mikhailov, M.I., Papernova, N.Y., Zinovyeva, L.I., Durnov, L.A. & Makhonova, L.A. (1986) Hepatitis B markers in infant cancer patients. *Vopr. Onkol.*, **32**, 70–74 (in Russian)

Milich, D.R., Hughes, J.L., Houghten, R., McLachlan, A. & Jones, J.E. (1989) Functional identification of agretopic and epitopic residues within an HBcAg T cell determinant. *J. Immunol.*, **143**, 3141–3147

Miller, R.H. & Robinson, W.S. (1986) Common evolutionary origin of hepatitis B virus and retroviruses. *Proc. natl Acad. Sci. USA*, **83**, 2531–2535

Millman, I., Southam, L., Halbherr, T., Simmons, H. & Kang, C.M. (1984) Woodchuck hepatitis virus: experimental infection and natural occurrence. *Hepatology*, **4**, 817–823

Milne, A., Allwood, G.K., Moyes, C.D., Pearce, N.E. & Lucas, C.R. (1985) Prevalence of hepatitis B infections in a multiracial New Zealand community. *N.Z. med. J.*, **98**, 529–532

Minuk, G.Y., Shaffer, E.A., Hoar, D.I. & Kelly, J. (1986) Ground squirrel hepatitis virus (GSHV) infection and hepatocellular carcinoma in the Canadian Richardson ground squirrel (*Spermophilus richardsonii*). *Liver*, **6**, 350–356

Mitamura, K., Hoyer, B.H., Ponzetto, A., Nelson, J., Purcell, R.H. & Gerin, J.L. (1982) Woodchuck hepatitis virus DNA in woodchuck liver tissues. *Hepatology*, **2**, 47S–50S

Mitsuda, T., Mori, T., Ookawa, N., Aihara, Y., Kosuge, K., Yokota, S., Ibe, M., Shimizu, H., Yoshida, N. & Matsuyama, S. (1989) Demonstration of mother-to-infant transmission of hepatitis B virus by means of polymerase chain reaction. *Lancet*, **ii**, 886–888

Mitsui, T., Iwano, K., Suzuki, S., Yamazaki, C., Masuko, K., Tsuda, F., Aihara, S., Akahane, Y., Miyakawa, Y. & Mayumi, M. (1989) Combined hepatitis B immune globulin and vaccine for postexposure prophylaxis of accidental hepatitis B virus infection in hemodialysis staff members: comparison with immune globulin without vaccine in historical controls. *Hepatology*, **10**, 324–327

Miyaki, M., Sato, C., Gotanda, T., Matsui, T., Mishiro, S., Imai, M. & Mayumi, M. (1986) Integration of region X of hepatitis B virus genome in human primary hepatocellular carcinomas propagated in nude mice. *J. gen. Virol.*, **67**, 1449–1454

Mizusawa, H., Taira, M., Yaginuma, K., Kobayashi, M., Yoshida, E. & Koike, K. (1985) Inversely repeating integrated hepatitis B virus DNA and cellular flanking sequences in the human hepatoma-derived cell line huSP. *Proc. natl Acad. Sci. USA*, **82**, 208–212

Mohamed, A.E., Kew, M.C & Groeneveld, H.T. (1992) Alcohol consumption as a risk factor for hepatocellular carcinoma in urban southern African blacks. *Int. J. Cancer*, **51**, 537–541

Mondelli, M., Vergani, G.M., Alberti, A., Vergani, D., Portmann, B., Eddleston, A.L.W.F. & Williams, R. (1982) Specificity of T lymphocytes cytotoxicity to autologous hepatocytes in chronic hepatitis B virus infection: evidence that T cells are directed against HBV core antigen expressed on hepatocytes. *J. Immunol.*, **129**, 2773–2778

Moriarty, A.M., Alexander, H., Lerner, R.A. & Thornton, G.B. (1985) Antibodies to peptides detect new hepatitis B antigen: serological correlation with hepatocellular carcinoma. *Science*, **227**, 429–433

Möröy, T., Marchio, A., Etiemble, J., Trépo, C., Tiollais, P. & Buendia, M.-A. (1986) Rearrangement and enhanced expression of c-*myc* in hepatocellular carcinoma of hepatitis virus infected woodchucks. *Nature*, **324**, 276–279

Muchmore, E., Socha, W.W. & Krawczynski, C. (1990) HCC in chimpanzees. In: Sung, J.L., ed., *Viral Hepatitis and Hepatocellular Carcinoma*, Hong Kong, Excerpta Medica, pp. 698–702

Murakami, Y., Hayashi, K., Hirohashi, S. & Sekiya, T. (1991) Aberrations of the tumor suppressor p53 and retinoblastoma genes in human hepatocellular carcinomas. *Cancer Res.*, **51**, 5520–5525

Mutchnick, M.G., Appelman, H.D., Chung, H.T., Aragona, E., Gupta, T.P., Cummings, G.D., Waggoner, J.G., Hoofnagle, J.H. & Shafritz, D.A. (1991) Thymosin treatment of chronic hepatitis B: a placebo-controlled pilot trial. *Hepatology*, **14**, 409–415

Nagaya, T., Nakamura, T., Tokino, T., Tsurimoto, T., Imai, M., Mayumi, T., Kamino, K., Yamamura, K. & Matsubara, K. (1987) The mode of hepatitis B virus DNA integration in chromosomes of human hepatocellular carcinoma. *Genes Dev.*, **1**, 773–782

Nakamura, T., Tokino, T., Nagaya, T. & Matsubara, K. (1988) Microdeletion associated with the integration process of hepatitis B virus DNA. *Nucleic Acids Res.*, **16**, 4865–4873

Naoumov, N.V., Schneider, R., Grötzinger, T., Jung, M.C., Miska, S., Pape, G.R. & Will, H. (1992) Precore mutant hepatitis B virus infection and liver disease. *Gastroenterology*, **102**, 538–543

Nasidi, A., Harry, T.O., Vyazov, S.O., Manube, G.M.R., Azzan, B.B. & Ananiev, V.A. (1986) Prevalence of hepatitis B infection markers in representative areas of Nigeria. *Int. J. Epidemiol.*, **15**, 274–276

Nayak, N.C. & Sachdeva, R. (1975) Localization of hepatitis B surface antigen in conventional paraffin sections of the liver. *Am. J. Pathol.*, **81**, 479–492

Nayak, N.C., Dhar, A., Sachdeva, R., Mittal, A., Seth, H.N., Sudarsanam, D., Reddy, B., Wagholikar, U.L. & Reddy, C.R.R.M. (1977) Association of human hepatocellular carcinoma and cirrhosis with hepatitis B virus surface and core antigens in the liver. *Int. J. Cancer*, **20**, 643–654

Neurath, A.R., Kent, S.B.H., Strick, N. & Parker, K. (1986) Identification and chemical synthesis of a host cell receptor binding site on hepatitis B virus. *Cell*, **46**, 429–436

Neurath, A.R., Strick, N., Sproul, P., Ralph, H.E. & Valinsky, J. (1990) Detection of receptors for hepatitis B virus on cells of extrahepatic origin. *Virology*, **176**, 448–457

Nielsen, J.O., Dietrichson, O., Elling, P. & Christoffersen, P. (1971) Incidence and meaning of persistence of Australia antigen in patients with acute viral hepatitis: development of chronic hepatitis. *New Engl. J. Med.*, **285**, 1157–1160

Nishida, N., Fukuda, Y., Kokuryu, H., Sadamoto, T., Isowa, G., Honda, K., Yamaoka, Y., Ikenaga, M., Imura, H. & Ishizaki, K. (1992) Accumulation of allelic loss on arms of chromosomes 13q, 16q and 17p in the advanced stages of human hepatocellular carcinoma. *Int. J. Cancer*, **51**, 862–868

Nishida, N., Fukuda, Y., Kokuryu, H., Toguchida, J., Yandell, D.W., Ikenega, M., Imura, H. & Ishizaki, K. (1993) Role and mutational heterogeneity of the p53 gene in hepatocellular carcinoma. *Cancer Res.*, **53**, 368–372

Nishioka, K., Levin, A.G. & Simons, M.J. (1975) Hepatitis B antigen, antigen subtypes and hepatitis B antibody in normal subjects and patients with liver disease. Results of a collaborative study. *Bull. World Health Organ.*, **52**, 293–300

Nomura, A., Stemmermann, G.N. & Wasnich, R.D. (1982) Presence of hepatitis B surface antigen before primary hepatocellular carcinoma. *J. Am. med. Assoc.*, **247**, 2247–2249

Ochiya, T., Fujiyama, A., Fukushige, S., Hatada, I. & Matsubara, K. (1986) Molecular cloning of an oncogene from a human hepatocellular carcinoma. *Proc. natl Acad. Sci. USA*, **83**, 4993–4997

Oda, T., Tsuda, H., Scarpa, A., Sakamoto, M. & Hirohashi, S. (1992) p53 Gene mutation spectrum in hepatocellular carcinoma. *Cancer Res.*, **52**, 6358–6364

Ogata, N., Kamimura, T. & Asakura, H. (1991) Point-mutation, allelic loss and increased methylation of c-Ha-*ras* gene in human hepatocellular carcinoma. *Hepatology*, **13**, 31–37

Ogston, C.W., Jonak, G.J., Rogler, C.E., Astrin, S.M. & Summers, J. (1982) Cloning and structural analysis of integrated woodchuck hepatitis virus sequences from hepatocellular carcinomas of woodchucks. *Cell*, **29**, 385–394

Ohaki, Y., Misugi, K., Sasaki, Y. & Tsunoda, A. (1983) Hepatitis B surface antigen positive hepatocellular carcinoma in children. Report of a case and review of the literature. *Cancer*, **51**, 822–828

Okamoto, H., Imai, M., Tsuda, F., Tanaka, T., Miyakawa, Y. & Mayumi, M. (1987) Point mutation in the *S* gene of hepatitis B virus for a d/y or w/r subtypic change in two blood donors carrying a surface antigen of compound subtype adyr or adwr. *J. Virol.*, **61**, 3030–3034

Okamoto, H., Yano, K., Nozaki, Y., Matsui, A., Miyazaki, H., Yamamoto, K., Tsuda, F., Machida, A. & Mishiro, S. (1992) Mutations within the S gene of hepatitis B virus transmitted from mothers to babies immunized with hepatitis B immune globulin and vaccine. *Pediatr. Res.*, **32**, 264–268

Okochi, K. & Murakami, S. (1968) Observations on Australia antigen in Japanese. *Vox sang.*, **15**, 374–385

Okuda, K., Kasai, Y., Sugawara, K., Mizumoto, R., Tsuzuki, T., Ichida, F., Sasaki, H., Endo, Y., Hattori, N., Nakashima, T., Mori, W., Tobe, T., Maetani, S., Matsumoto, Y., Suzuki, N. & Hiarkawa, A. (1980) Primary liver cancers in Japan. *Cancer*, **45**, 2663–2669

Omata, M. (1990) Significance of extrahepatic replication of hepatitis B virus. *Hepatology*, **12**, 364–366

Omata, M., Ashcavai, M., Liew, C.-T. & Peters, R.L. (1979) Hepatocellular carcinoma in the USA, etiologic considerations. Localization of hepatitis B antigens. *Gastroenterology*, **76**, 279–287

Omata, M., Uchiumi, K., Ito, Y., Yokosuka, O., Mori, J., Terao, K., Ye, W.-F., O'Connell, A., London, W.T. & Okuda, K. (1983) Duck hepatitis B virus and liver diseases. *Gastroenterology*, **85**, 260–267

Omata, M., Yokosuka, O., Imazeki, F., Matsuyama, Y., Uchiumi, K., Ito, Y., Mori, J. & Okuda, K. (1984) Transmission of duck hepatitis B virus from Chinese carrier ducks to Japanese ducklings: a study of viral DNA in serum and tissue. *Hepatology*, **4**, 603–607

Omata, M., Zhou, Y.-Z., Uchiumi, K., Hirota, K., Ito, Y., Yokosuka, O. & Okuda, K. (1987) Hepatitis B virus DNA, antigen, and liver pathology in ducks: an animal model of human liver disease. In: Koike, K., Robinson, W. & Will, H., eds, *Hepadna Viruses* (UCLA Symposia on Molecular and Cellular Biology Vol. 70), New York, Alan R. Liss, pp. 349–356

Ono, T., Abe, S. & Yoshida, M.C. (1991) Hereditary low level of plasma ceruloplasmin in LEC rats associated with spontaneous development of hepatitis and liver cancer. *Jpn. J. Cancer Res.*, **82**, 486–489

Oshima, A., Tsukuma, H., Hiyama, T., Fujimoto, I., Yamano, H. & Tanaka, M. (1984) Follow-up study of HBsAg-positive blood donors with special reference to effect of drinking and smoking on development of liver cancer. *Int. J. Cancer*, **34**, 775–779

Osmond, D.H., Charlebois, E., Sheppard, H.W., Page, K., Winkelstein, W., Moss, A.R. & Reingold, A. (1993) Comparison of risk factors for hepatitis C and hepatitis B virus infection in homosexual men. *J. infect. Dis.*, **167**, 66–71

Otu, A.A. (1987) Hepatocellular carcinoma, hepatic cirrhosis, and hepatitis B virus infection in Nigeria. *Cancer*, **60**, 2581–2585

Ou, J.-H. & Rutter, W.J. (1985) Hybrid hepatitis B virus–host transcripts in a human hepatoma cell. *Proc. natl Acad. Sci. USA*, **82**, 83–87

Ozturk, M., Bressac, B., Puisieux, A., Kew, M., Volkmann, M., Bozcall, S., Mura, J.M., de la Monte, S., Carlson, R., Blum, H., Wands, J., Takahashi, H., von Weizsäcker, F., Galun, E., Siddhartha, K., Carr, B.L., Schröder, C.H., Erken, E., Varinii, S., Rustgi, V.K., Prat, J., Toda, G., Koch, H.K., Liang, X.H., Tang, Z.-Y., Shouval, D., Lee, H.-S., Vyas, G.N. & Sarosi, I. (1991) p53 Mutation in hepatocellular carcinoma after aflatoxin exposure. *Lancet*, **338**, 1356–1359

Pagliaro, L., Saracci, R., Bardelli, D., Filippazzo, G. & a group of the Italian Association for the Study of the Liver (AISF) (1982) Chronic liver disease, alcohol consumption and HBsAg antigen in Italy: a multiregional case–control study. *Ital. J. Gastroenterol.*, **14**, 90–95

Pagliaro, L., Simonetti, R.G., Craxì, A., Spanò, C., Filippazzo, M.G., Palazzo, U., Patti, S., Giannuoli, G., Marraffa, A., Colombo, M., Tommasini, M., Bellentani, S., Villa, E., Manenti, F., Caporaso, N., Coltorti, M., Del Vecchio-Blanco, C., Farsi, P., Smedile, A. & Verme, G. (1983) Alcohol and HBV infection as risk factors for hepatocellular carcinoma in Italy: a multicentric, controlled study. *Hepato-gastroenterology*, **30**, 48–50

Parkin, D.M., Srivatanakul, P., Khlat, M., Chenvidhya, D., Chotiwan, P., Insiripong, S., L'Abbé, K.A. & Wild, C.P. (1991) Liver cancer in Thailand. I. A case-control study of cholangiocarcinoma. *Int. J. Cancer*, **48**, 323-328

Paronetto, F. & Tennant, B.C. (1990) Woodchuck hepatitis virus infection: a model of human hepatic diseases and hepatocellular carcinoma. *Prog. Liver Dis.*, **9**, 463-483

Pasquinelli, C., Garreau, F., Bougueleret, L., Cariani, E., Grzeschik, K.H., Thiers, V., Croissant, O., Hadchouel, M., Tiollais, P. & Bréchot, C. (1988) Rearrangement of a common cellular DNA domain on chromosome 4 in human primary liver tumors. *J. Virol.*, **62**, 629-632

Pastore, G., Santantonio, T., Milella, M., Monno, L., Mariano, N., Moschetta, R. & Pollice, L. (1992) Anti-HBe-positive chronic hepatitis B with HBV-DNA in the serum response to a 6-month course of lymphoblastoid interferon. *J. Hepatol.*, **14**, 221-225

Paterlini, P., Driss, F., Nalpas, B., Pisi, E., Franco, D., Berthelot, P. & Bréchot, C. (1993) Persistence of hepatitis B and hepatitis C viral genomes in primary liver cancers from HBsAg-negative patients: a study of a low-endemic area. *Hepatology*, **17**, 20-29

Payet, M., Camain, R. & Pene, P. (1956) Primary liver cancer. Critical study of 240 cases. *Rev. int. Hepatol.*, **6**, 1-20 (in French)

Pedreira, J.D., Vargas, V., Vilaseca, J., Esteban, R., Hernández-Sánchez, J.M., Guardia, J. & Bacardí, R. (1980) Primary liver carcinoma and markers of virus of type B hepatitis. *Med. clín. (Barcelona)*, **75**, 58-60 (in Spanish)

Penna, A., Chisari, F.V., Bertoletti, A., Missale, G., Fowler, P., Giuberti, T., Fiaccadori, F. & Ferrari, C. (1991) Cytotoxic T lymphocytes recognize an HLA-A2-restricted epitope within the hepatitis B virus nucleocapsid antigen. *J. exp. Med.*, **174**, 1565-1570

Penner, E., Maida, E., Mamoli, B. & Gangl, A. (1982) Serum and cerebrospinal fluid immune complexes containing hepatitis B surface antigen in Guillain-Barré syndrome. *Gastroenterology*, **82**, 576-580

Perrillo, R.P., Chau, K.H., Overby, L.R. & Decker, R.H. (1983) Anti-hepatitis B core immunoglobulin M in the serologic evaluation of hepatitis B virus infection and simultaneous infection with type B, delta agent and non-A, non-B viruses. *Gastroenterology*, **85**, 163-167

Perrillo, R.P., Schiff, E.R., Davis, G.L., Bodenheimer, H.C., Jr, Lindsay, K., Payne, J., Dienstag, J.L., O'Brien, C., Tamburro, C., Jacobson, I.M., Sampliner, R., Feit, D., Lefkowitch, J., Kuhns, M., Meschievitz, C., Sanghvi, B., Albrecht, J., Gibas, A. and the Hepatitis Interventional Therapy Group (1990) A randomized, controlled trial of interferon alfa-2a alone and after prednisone withdrawal for the treatment of chronic active hepatitis B. *New Engl. J. Med.*, **323**, 295-301

Peters, R.L. (1975) Viral hepatitis: a pathologic spectrum. *Am. J. med. Sci.*, **270**, 17-31

Peters, R.L., Afroudakis, A.P. & Tatter, D. (1977) The changing incidence of association of hepatitis B with hepatocellular carcinoma in California. *Am. J. clin. Pathol.*, **68**, 1-7

Pier, A.C. & McLoughlin, M.E. (1985) Mycotoxic suppression of immunity. In: Lacey, J., ed., *Trichothecenes and Other Mycotoxins*, New York, John Wiley & Sons, pp. 507-519

Pirovino, M., Heer, M., Joller-Jemelka, H.P., Altorfer, J., Akovbiantz, A. & Schmid, M. (1983) Hepatocellular carcinoma and hepatitis B virus infection. Analysis of 75 cases from Switzerland. *Liver*, **3**, 398-402

Planes, N., De Somoza, N. & Morgenfeld, M.C. (1976) Surface antigen of hepatitis B in malignant lymphoma. *Sangre*, **21**, 492-498 (in Spanish)

Polakoff, S. (1990) Acute viral hepatitis B, reported to the public health laboratory service. *J. Infect.*, **20**, 163-168

Pontisso, P., Locasciulli, A., Schiavon, E., Cattoretti, G., Schirò, R., Stenico, D. & Alberti, A. (1987) Detection of hepatitis B virus DNA sequences in bone marrow of children with leukemia. *Cancer*, **59**, 292–296

Popper, H. (1977) Pathologic aspects of cirrhosis. A review. *Am. J. Pathol.*, **87**, 228–264

Popper, H., Shih, J.W.-K., Gerin, J.L., Wong, D.C., Hoyer, B.H., London, W.T., Sly, D.L. & Purcell, R.H. (1981) Woodchuck hepatitis and hepatocellular carcinoma: correlation of histologic with virologic observations. *Hepatology*, **1**, 91–98

Popper, H., Roth, L., Purcell, R.H., Tennant, B.C. & Gerin, J.L. (1987) Hepatocarcinogenicity of the woodchuck hepatitis virus. *Proc. natl Acad. Sci. USA*, **84**, 866–870

Prince, A.M. (1970) Prevalence of serum-hepatitis-related-antigen (SH) in different geographic regions. *Am. J. trop. Med. Hyg.*, **19**, 872–879

Prince, A.M. & Alcabes, P. (1982) The risk of development of hepatocellular carcinoma in hepatitis B virus carriers in New York. A preliminary estimate using death-records matching. *Hepatology*, **2**, 15S–20S

Prince, A.M., Leblanc, L., Krohn, K., Masseyeff, R. & Alpert, M.E. (1970) SH antigen and chronic liver disease (Letter to the Editor). *Lancet*, **ii**, 717–718

Prince, A.M., Metselaar, D., Kafuko, G.W., Mukwaya, L.G., Ling, C.M. & Overby, L.R. (1972) Hepatitis B antigen in wild-caught mosquitoes in Africa. *Lancet*, **ii**, 247–250

Prince, A.M., Szmuness, W., Michon, J., Demaille, J., Diebolt, G., Linhard, J., Quenum, C. & Sankale, M. (1975) A case/control study of the association between primary liver cancer and hepatitis B infection in Senegal. *Int. J. Cancer*, **16**, 376–383

Quade, K., Saldanha, J., Thomas, H. & Monjardino, J. (1992) Integration of hepatitis B virus DNA through a mutational hot spot within the cohesive region in a case of hepatocellular carcinoma. *J. gen. Virol.*, **73**, 179–182

Redeker, A.G. (1975) Viral hepatitis: clinical aspects. *Am. J. med. Sci.*, **270**, 9–16

Repp, R., Keller, C., Borkhardt, A., Csecke, A., Schaefer, S., Gerlich, W.H. & Lampert, F. (1992) Detection of a hepatitis B virus variant with a truncated X gene and enhancer II. *Arch. Virol.*, **125**, 299–304

Reys, L.L., Purcell, R.H., Holland, P.V. & Alter, H.J. (1977) The relationship between hepatitis B virus infection and hepatic cell carcinoma in Mozambique. *Trop. geogr. Med.*, **29**, 251–256

Richard, J.L. (1991) Mycotoxins as immunomodulators in animal systems. In: Bray, G.A. & Ryan, D., eds, *Mycotoxins, Cancer and Health*, Baton Rouge, LA, Louisiana State University Press, pp. 197–220

Röckelein, G. & Hecken-Emmel, M. (1988) Risk factors of hepatocellular carcinoma in Germany: hepatitis B or liver cirrhosis? *Hepato-gastroenterology*, **35**, 151–157

Rogler, C.E. (1991) Cellular and molecular mechanisms of hepatocarcinogenesis associated with hepadnavirus infection. *Curr. Top. Microbiol. Immunol.*, **168**, 103–140

Rogler, C.E. & Summers, J. (1984) Cloning and structural analysis of integrated woodchuck hepatitis virus sequences from a chronically infected liver. *J. Virol.*, **50**, 832–837

Rogler, C.E., Sherman, M., Su, C.Y., Shafritz, D.A., Summers, J., Shows, T.B., Henderson, A. & Kew, M. (1985) Deletion in chromosome 11p associated with a hepatitis B integration site in hepatocellular carcinoma. *Science*, **230**, 319–322

Rosenblum, L., Darrow, W., Witte, J., Cohen, J., French, J., Gil, P.S., Potterat, J., Sikes, K., Reich, R. & Hadler, S. (1992) Sexual practices in the transmission of hepatitis B virus and prevalence of delta virus infection in female prostitutes in the United States. *J. Am. med. Assoc.*, **267**, 2477–2481

Ross, R.K., Yuan, J.-M., Yu, M.C., Wogan, G.N., Qian, G.-S., Tu, J.-T., Groopman, J.D., Gao, Y.-T. & Henderson, B.E. (1992) Urinary aflatoxin biomarkers and risk of hepatocellular carcinoma. *Lancet*, **339**, 943–946

Rossner, M.T. (1992) Review: hepatitis B virus X-gene product: a promiscuous transcriptional activator. *J. med. Virol.*, **36**, 101–117

Roth, L., King, J.M., Hornbuckle, W.E., Harvey, H.J. & Tennant, B.C. (1985) Chronic hepatitis and hepatocellular carcinoma associated with persistent woodchuck hepatitis virus infection. *Vet. Pathol.*, **22**, 338–343

Ruiz-Moreno, M., Rúa, M.J., Moraleda, G., Guardia, L., Moreno, A. & Carreño, V. (1992) Treatment with interferon gamma versus interferons alfa and gamma in children with chronic hepatitis B. *Pediatrics*, **90**, 254–258

Ryder, R.W., Whittle, H.C., Sanneh, A.B.K., Ajdukiewicz, A.B., Tulloch, S. & Yvonnet, B. (1992) Persistent hepatitis B virus infection and hepatoma in the Gambia, West Africa. A case–control study of 140 adults and their 603 family contacts. *Am. J. Epidemiol.*, **136**, 1122–1131

Sakamoto, M., Hirohashi, S., Tsuda, H., Shimosato, Y., Makuuchi, M. & Hosoda, Y. (1989) Multicentric independent development of hepatocellular carcinoma revealed by analysis of hepatitis B virus integration pattern. *Am. J. surg. Pathol.*, **13**, 1064–1067

Sakuma, K., Saitoh, N., Kasai, M., Jitsukawa, H., Yoshino, I., Yamaguchi, M., Nobutomo, K., Yamumi, M., Tsuda, F., Komazawa, T., Nakamura, T., Yoshida, Y. & Okuda, K. (1988) Relative risks of death due to liver disease among Japanese male adults having various statuses for hepatitis B s and e antigen/antibody in serum: a prospective study. *Hepatology*, **8**, 1642–1646

Santantonio, T., Jung, M.-C., Miska, S., Pastore, G., Pape, G.R. & Will, H. (1991a) High prevalence and heterogeneity of HBV preC mutants in anti-HBe-positive carriers with chronic liver disease in southern Italy. *J. Hepatol.*, **13** (Suppl. 4), S78–S81

Santantonio, T., Jung, M.-C., Schneider, R., Pastore, G., Pape, G.R. & Will, H. (1991b) Selection for a pre-C stop codon mutation during interferon treatment. *J. Hepatol.*, **13**, 368–371

Schek, N., Fischer, M. & Schaller, H. (1991) The hepadnaviral X protein. In: McLachlan, A., ed., *The Hepadnaviral X Protein*, Boca Raton, FL, CRC Press, pp. 181–192

Scheuer, P.J. (1991) Classification of chronic viral hepatitis: a need for reassessment. *J. Hepatol.*, **13**, 372–374

Scheuer, P.J. & Thaler, H. (1977) Acute and chronic hepatitis revisited. Review by an international group. *Lancet*, **ii**, 914–919

Schödel, F., Sprengel, R., Weimer, T., Fernholz, D., Schneider, R. & Will, H. (1989) Animal hepatitis B viruses. In: Klein, G., ed., *Advances in Viral Oncology*, Vol. 8, New York, Raven Press, pp. 73–102

Schödel, F., Weimer, T., Fernholz, D., Schneider, R., Sprengel, R., Wildner, G. & Will, H. (1991) The biology of avian hepatitis B viruses. In: McLachlan, A., ed., *Molecular Biology of the Hepatitis B Virus*, Boca Raton, FL, CRC Press, pp. 53–80

Scorsone, K.A., Zhou, Y.-Z., Butel, J.S. & Slagle, B.L. (1992) p53 Mutations cluster at codon 249 in hepatitis B virus-positive hepatocellular carcinomas from China. *Cancer Res.*, **52**, 1635–1638

Sebti, M.F. (1984) Acute viral hepatitis and markers of HB virus in chronic liver diseases and in primary liver cancers. In: Williams, A.O., O'Conor, G.T., de-Thé, G.B. & Johnson, C.A., eds, *Virus-associated Cancers in Africa* (IARC Scientific Publications No. 63), Lyon, IARC, pp. 227–236 (in French)

Seeger, C., Ganem, D. & Varmus H.E. (1986) Biochemical and genetic evidence for the hepatitis B virus replication strategy. *Science*, **232**, 477–484

Seeger, C., Baldwin, B., Hornbuckle, W.E., Yeager, A.E., Tennant, B.C., Cote, P., Ferrell, L., Ganem, D. & Varmus, H.E. (1991) Woodchuck hepatitis virus is a more efficient oncogenic agent than ground squirrel hepatitis virus in a common host. *J. Virol.*, **65**, 1673–1679

Seelig, R., Renz, M. & Seelig, H.P. (1992) PCR (polymerase chain reaction) in the diagnosis of viral hepatitis. *Ann. Med.*, **24**, 225–230

Seifer, M., Heermann, K.H. & Gerlich, W.H. (1990) Expression pattern of the hepatitis B virus genome in transfected mouse fibroblasts. *Virology*, **179**, 287–299

Seifer, M., Höhne, M., Schaefer, S. & Gerlich, W.H. (1991) In vitro tumorigenicity of hepatitis B virus DNA and HBx protein. *J. Hepatol.*, **13** (Suppl. 4), S61–S65

Sell, S., Hunt, J.M., Dunsford, H.A. & Chisari, F.V. (1991) Synergy between hepatitis B virus expression and chemical hepatocarcinogens in transgenic mice. *Cancer Res.*, **51**, 1278–1285

Shafritz, D.A. (1982) Hepatitis B virus DNA molecules in the liver of HBsAg carriers: mechanistic considerations in the pathogenesis of hepatocellular carcinoma. *Hepatology*, **2**, 35S–41S

Shafritz, D.A., Shouval, D., Sherman, H.I., Hadziyannis, S.J. & Kew, M.C. (1981) Integration of hepatitis B virus DNA into the genome of liver cells in chronic liver disease and hepatocellular carcinoma. Studies in percutaneous liver biopsies and post-mortem tissue specimens. *New Engl. J. Med.*, **305**, 1067–1073

Shaul, Y., Garcia, P.D., Schonberg, S. & Rutter, W.J. (1986) Integration of hepatitis B virus DNA in chromosome-specific satellite sequences. *J. Virol.*, **59**, 731–734

Sherker, A.H. & Marion, P.L. (1991) Hepadnaviruses and hepatocellular carcinoma. *Ann. Rev. Microbiol.*, **45**, 475–508

Sherlock, S. (1989) Classifying chronic hepatitis. *Lancet*, **ii**, 1168–1170

Sherlock, S., Fox, R.A., Niazi, S.P. & Scheurer, P.J. (1970) Chronic liver disease and primary liver-cell cancer with hepatitis-associated (Australia) antigen in serum. *Lancet*, **i**, 1243–1247

Sheu, J.-C., Huang, G.-T., Lee, P.-H., Chung, J.-C, Chou, H.-C., Lai, M.-Y., Wang, J.-T., Lee, H.-S., Shih, L.-N., Yang, P.-M., Wang, T.-H. & Chen, D.-S. (1992) Mutation of p53 gene in hepatocellular carcinoma in Taiwan. *Cancer Res.*, **52**, 6098–6100

Shih, C., Burke, K., Chou, M.-J., Zeldis, J.B., Yang, C.-S., Lee, C.-S., Isselbacher, K.J., Wands, J.R. & Goodman, H.M. (1987) Tight clustering of human hepatitis B virus integration sites in hepatomas near a triple-stranded region. *J. Virol.*, **61**, 3491–3498

Shikata, T., Uzawa, T., Yoshiwara, N., Akatsaka, T. & Yamasaki, S. (1974) Staining method of Australia antigen in paraffin section. Detection of cytoplasmic inclusion bodies. *Jpn. J. exp. Med.*, **44**, 25–36

Shimoda, T., Uchida, T., Miyata, H., Abe, K., Ariga, H., Shikata, T. & Fujii, Y. (1980) A 6-year-old boy having hepatocelllar carcinoma associated with hepatitis B surface antigenemia. *Am. J. clin. Pathol.*, **74**, 827–831

Shiozawa, M., Ochiya, T., Hatada, I., Imamura, T., Okudaira, Y., Hiraoka, H. & Matsubara, K. (1988) The *lca* as an onco-fetal gene: its expression in human fetal liver. *Oncogene*, **2**, 523–526

Shirakata, Y., Kawada, M., Fujiki, Y., Sano, H., Oda, M., Yaginuma, K., Kobayashi, M. & Koike, K. (1989) The X gene of hepatitis B virus induced growth stimulation and tumorigenic transformation of mouse NIH3T3 cells. *Jpn. J. Cancer Res.*, **80**, 617–621

Shouval, D., Chakraborty, P.R., Ruiz-Opazo, N., Baum, S., Spigland, I., Muchmore, E., Gerber, M.A., Thung, S.N., Popper, H. & Shafritz, D.A. (1980) Chronic hepatitis in champanzee carriers of hepatitis B virus: morphologic, immunologic, and viral DNA studies. *Proc. natl Acad. Sci. USA*, **77**, 6147–6151

Shusterman, N. & London, W.T. (1984) Hepatitis B and immune-complex disease. *New Engl. J. Med.*, **310**, 43–46

Simon, D., Knowles, B.B. & Weith, A. (1991) Abnormalities of chromosome 1 and loss of heterozygosity on 1p in primary hepatomas. *Oncogene*, **6**, 765–770

Simonetti, R.G., Cammà, C., Fiorello, F., Cottone, M., Rapicetta, M., Marino, L., Fiorentino, G., Craxì, A., Ciccaglione, A., Giuseppetti, R., Stroffolini, T. & Pagliaro, L. (1992) Hepatitis C virus infection as a risk factor for hepatocellular carcinoma in patients with cirrhosis. A case–control study. *Ann. intern. Med.*, **116**, 97–102

Simons, M.J., Yap, E.H., Yu, M., Seah, C.S., Chew, B.K., Fung, W.P., Tan, A.Y.O. & Shanmugaratnam, K. (1971) Australia antigen in Singapore Chinese patients with hepatocellular carcinoma. *Lancet*, **i**, 1149–1151

Simons, M.J., Yap, E.H., Yu, M. & Shanmugaratnam, K. (1972) Australia antigen in Singapore Chinese patients with hepatocellular carcinoma and comparison groups: influence of technique sensitivity on differential frequencies. *Int. J. Cancer*, **10**, 320–325

Sjøgren, M.H., Lemon, S.M., Chung, W.K., Sun, H.S. & Hoofnagle, J.H. (1984) IgM antibody to hepatitis B core antigen in Korean patients with hepatocellular carcinoma. *Hepatology*, **4**, 615–618

Sjøgren, M.H., Dusheiko, G.M., Kew, M.C. & Song, E. (1988) Hepatitis B virus infection and hepatocellular carcinoma: correlation between IgM antibody to hepatitis B core antigen, hepatitis B e antigen, and hepatitis B DNA. *Am. J. trop. Med. Hyg.*, **39**, 582–585

Slagle, B.L., Zhou, Y.-Z. & Butel, J.S. (1991) Hepatitis B virus integration event in human chromosome 17p near the p53 gene identifies the region of the chromosome commonly deleted in virus-positive hepatocellular carcinomas. *Cancer Res.*, **51**, 49–54

Slagle, B.L., Lee, T.-H. & Butel, J.S. (1992) Hepatitis B virus and hepatocellular carcinoma. *Prog. med. Virol.*, **39**, 167–203

Smith, J.B. & Blumberg, B.S. (1969) Viral hepatitis, postnecrotic cirrhosis, and hepatocellular carcinoma (Letter to the Editor). *Lancet*, **ii**, 953

Snyder, R.L. (1968) Hepatomas of captive woodchucks (Abstract No. 68). *Am. J. Pathol.*, **52**, 32a–33a

Soběslavský, O. (1980) Prevalence of markers of hepatitis B virus infection in various countries: a WHO collaborative study. *Bull. World Health Organ.*, **58**, 621–628

Sokal, E.M., Ulla, L. & Otte, J.B. (1992) Hepatitis B vaccine response before and after transplantation in 55 extrahepatic biliary atresia children. *Dig. Dis. Sci.*, **37**, 1250–1252

Sprengel, R., Kaleta, E.F. & Will, H. (1988) Isolation and characterization of a hepatitis B virus endemic in herons. *J. Virol.*, **62**, 3832-3839

Srivatanakul, P., Parkin, D.M., Khlat, M., Chenvidhya, D., Chotiwan, P., Insiripong, S., L'Abbé, K.A. & Wild, C.P. (1991) Liver cancer in Thailand. II. A case–control study of hepatocellular carcinoma. *Int. J. Cancer*, **48**, 329–332

Stevens, C.E., Toy, P.T., Tong, M.J., Taylor, P.E., Vyas, G.N., Nair, P.V., Gudavalli, M. & Krugman, S. (1985) Perinatal hepatitis B virus transmission in the United States. Prevention by passive–active immunization. *J. Am. med. Assoc.*, **253**, 1740–1745

Stevens, C.E., Taylor, P.E., Tong, M.J., Toy, P.T., Vyas, G.N., Nair, P.V., Weissman, J.Y. & Krugman, S. (1987) Yeast-recombinant hepatitis B vaccine. Efficacy with hepatitis B immune globulin in prevention of perinatal hepatitis B virus transmission. *J. Am. med. Assoc.*, **257**, 2612–2616

Stevens, C.E., Toy, P.T., Taylor, P.E., Lee, T. & Yip, H.-Y. (1992) Prospects for control of hepatitis B virus infection: implications of childhood vaccination and long-term protection. *Pediatrics*, **90**, 170–173

Stroffolini, T., Chiaramonte, M., Tiribelli, C., Villa, E., Simonetti, R.G., Rapicetta, M., Stazi, M.A., Bertin, T., Crocè, S.L., Trande, P., Magliocco, A. & Chionne, P. (1992) Hepatitis C virus infection, HBsAg carrier state and hepatocellular carcinoma: relative risk and population attributable risk from a case-control study in Italy. *J. Hepatol.*, **16**, 360–363

Struve, J. (1992) Hepatitis B virus infection among Swedish adults: aspects on seroepidemiology, transmission and vaccine response. *Scand. J. infect. Dis.*, **Suppl. 82**, 1–57

Sugimura, H., Fukazawa, T., Saitoh, M., Nakamura, K.-I., Shimada, H. & Ohtsubo, K. (1991) The histopathology of the liver in older patients with hepatitis B surface antigenaemia. *Virchow's Arch. A Pathol. Anat.*, **419**, 409–415

Summers, J. (1981) Three recently described animal virus models for human hepatitis B virus. *Hepatology*, **1**, 179–183

Summers, J. & Mason, W.S. (1982) Replication of the genome of a hepatitis B-like virus by reverse transcription of an RNA intermediate. *Cell*, **29**, 403–415

Summers, J., Smolec, J.M. & Snyder, R. (1978) A virus similar to human hepatitis B virus associated with hepatitis and hepatoma in woodchucks. *Proc. natl Acad. Sci. USA*, **75**, 4533–4537

Sun, T.-T., Chu, Y.-R., Ni, Z.-Q., Lu, J.-H., Huang, F., Ni, Z.-P., Pei, X.-F., Yu, Z.-I. & Liu, G.-T. (1986) A pilot study on universal immunization of newborn infants in an area of hepatitis B virus and primary hepatocellular carcinoma prevalence with a low dose of hepatitis B vaccine. *J. Cell. Physiol.*, **Suppl. 4**, 83–90

Sun, Z.(T), Zhu, Y., Stjernsward, J., Hilleman, M., Collins, R., Zhen, Y., Hsia, C.C., Lu, J., Huang, F., Ni, Z., Ni, T., Liu, G.T., Yu, Z., Liu, Y., Chen, J.M. & Peto, R. (1991) Design and compliance of HBV vaccination trial on newborns to prevent hepatocellular carcinoma and 5-year results of its pilot study. *Cancer Detect. Prev.*, **15**, 313–318

Sureau, C., Eichberg, J.W., Hubbard, G.B., Romet-Lemonne, J.L. & Essex, M. (1988) A molecular cloned hepatitis B virus produced *in vitro* is infectious in a chimpanzee. *J. Virol.*, **62**, 3064–3067

Suwangool, P. (1979) Orcein staining for detection of hepatitis B surface antigen in cirrhosis and hepatic carcinoma in Thailand. *J. med. Assoc. Thai*, **62**, 422–428

Szmuness, W. (1975) Recent advances in the study of the epidemiology of hepatitis B. *Am. J. Pathol.*, **81**, 629–649

Szmuness, W. (1978) Hepatocellular carcinoma and the hepatitis B virus: evidence for a causal association. *Prog. med. Virol.*, **24**, 40–69

Szmuness, W., Much, M.I., Prince, A.M., Hoofnagle, J.H., Cherubin, C.E., Harley, E.J. & Block, G.H. (1975a) On the role of sexual behavior in the spread of hepatitis B infection. *Ann. intern. Med.*, **83**, 489–495

Szmuness, W., Harley, E.J. & Prince, A.M. (1975b) Intrafamilial spread of asymptomatic hepatitis B. *Am. J. med. Sci.*, **270**, 293–304

Szmuness, W., Harley, E.J., Ikram, H. & Stevens, C.E. (1978a) Sociodemographic aspects of the epidemiology of hepatitis B. In: Vyas, G.N., Cohen, S.N. & Schmidt, R., eds, *Viral Hepatitis*, Philadelphia, Franklin Institute Press, pp. 297–320

Szmuness, W., Stevens, C.E., Ikram, H., Much, M.I., Harley, E.J. & Hollinger, B. (1978b) Prevalence of hepatitis B virus infection and hepatocellular carcinoma in Chinese-Americans. *J. infect. Dis.*, **137**, 822–829

Szmuness, W., Stevens, C.E., Harley, E.J., Zang, E.A., Oleszko, W.R., William, D.C., Sadovsky, R., Morrison, J.M. & Kellner, A. (1980) Hepatitis B vaccine. Demonstration of efficacy in a controlled clinical trial in a high-risk population in the United States. *New Engl. J. Med.*, **303**, 833–841

Tabor, E. (1987) Guillain–Barré syndrome and other neurologic syndromes in hepatitis A, B and non-A, non-B. *J. med. Virol.*, **21**, 207–216

Tabor, E. (1989) Hepatocellular carcinoma: possible etiologies in patients without serologic evidence of hepatitis B virus infection. *J. med. Virol.*, **27**, 1–6

Tabor, E., Gerety, R.J., Vogel, C.L., Bayley, A.C., Anthony, P.P., Chan, C.H. & Barker, L.F. (1977) Hepatitis B virus infection and primary hepatocellular carcinoma. *J. natl Cancer Inst.*, **58**, 1197–1200

Tabor, E., Bayley, A.C., Cairns, J., Pelleu, L. & Gerety, R.J. (1985) Horizontal transmission of hepatitis B virus among children and adults in five rural villages in Zambia. *J. med. Virol.*, **15**, 113–120

Tada, M., Omata, M. & Ohto, M. (1990) Analysis of *ras* gene mutations in human hepatic malignant tumors by polymerase chain reaction and direct sequencing. *Cancer Res.*, **50**, 1121–1124

Tagawa, M., Omata, M., Yokosuka, D., Uchiumi, K., Imazeki, F. & Okuda, K. (1985) Early events in duck hepatitis B virus infection. Sequential appearance of viral deoxyribonucleic acid in liver, pancreas, kidney and spleen. *Gastroenterology*, **89**, 1224–1229

Takada, S. & Koike, K. (1990) Trans-activation function of a 3′ truncated X gene–cell fusion product from integrated hepatitis B virus DNA in chronic hepatitis tissues. *Proc. natl Acad. Sci. USA*, **87**, 5628–5632

Takayama, T., Makuuchi, M., Hirohashi, S., Sakamoto, M., Okazaki, N., Takayasu, K., Kosuge, T., Motoo, Y., Yamazaki, S. & Hasegawa, H. (1990) Malignant transformation of adenomatous hyperplasia to hepatocellular carcinoma. *Lancet*, **336**, 1150–1153

Takeda, K., Akahane, Y., Suzuki, H., Okamoto, H., Tsuda, F., Miyakawa, Y. & Mayumi, M. (1990) Defects in the precore region of the HBV genome in patients with chronic hepatitis B after sustained seroconversion from HBeAg to anti-HBe induced spontaneously or with interferon therapy. *Hepatology*, **12**, 1284–1289

Tan, A.Y.O., Law, C.H. & Lee, Y.S. (1977) Hepatitis B antigen in the liver cells in cirrhosis and hepatocellular carcinoma. *Pathology*, **9**, 57–64

Tanaka, K. & Mori, W. (1985) Hepatitis B surface antigen in hepatocellular carcinoma. *Jpn. J. Cancer Res. (Gann)*, **76**, 603–607

Tanaka, T., Miyamoto, H., Hino, O., Kitagawa, T., Koike, M., Iizuka, T., Sakamoto, H. & Ooshima, A. (1986) Primary hepatocellular carcinoma with hepatitis B virus–DNA integration in a 4-year-old boy. *Hum. Pathol.*, **17**, 202–204

Tanaka, K., Hirohata, T. & Takeshita, S. (1988) Blood transfusion, alcohol consumption, cigarette smoking in causation of hepatocellular carcinoma: a case–control study in Fukuoka, Japan. *Jpn. J. Cancer Res. (Gann)*, **79**, 1075–1082

Tanaka, Y., Esumi, M. & Shikata, T. (1988) Frequent integration of hepatitis B virus DNA in non-cancerous liver tissue from hepatocellular carcinoma patients. *J. med. Virol.*, **26**, 7–14

Tanaka, K., Hirohata, T., Takeshita, S., Hirohata, I., Koga, S., Sugimachi, K., Kanematsu, T., Ohryohji, F. & Ishibashi, H. (1992) Hepatitis B virus, cigarette smoking and alcohol consumption in the development of hepatocellular carcinoma: a case–control study in Fukuoka, Japan. *Int. J. Cancer*, **51**, 509–514

Taylor, P.E. & Stevens, C.E. (1988) Persistence of antibody to hepatitis B surface antigen after vaccination with hepatitis B vaccine. In: Zuckerman, A.J., ed., *Viral Hepatitis and Liver Disease*, New York, Alan R. Liss, pp. 995–997

Taylor, P.E., Stevens, C.E., de Cordoba, S.R. & Rubinstein, P. (1988) Hepatitis B virus and human immunodeficiency virus: possible interactions. In: Zuckerman, A.J., ed., *Viral Hepatitis and Liver Disease*, New York, Alan R. Liss, pp. 198–200

Tennant, B.C., Hornbuckle, W.E., Baldwin, B.H., King, J.M., Cote, P., Popper, H., Purcell, R.H. & Gerin, J.L. (1988) Influence of age on the response to experimental woodchuck hepatitis virus infection. In: Zuckerman, A.J., ed., *Viral Hepatitis and Liver Disease*, New York, Alan R. Liss, pp. 462–464

Tennant, B.C., Hornbuckle, W.E., Yeager, A.E., Baldwin, B.H., Sherman, W.K., Anderson, W.I., Steinberg, H., Cote, P.J., Korba, B.E. & Gerin, J.L. (1990) Effects of aflatoxin B_1 on experimental woodchuck hepatitis virus infection and hepatocellular carcinoma. In: Hollinger, F.B., Lemon, S.M. & Margolis, H., ed., *Viral Hepatitis and Liver Disease*, Baltimore, Williams & Wilkins, pp. 599–600

Tennant, B.C., Mrosovsky, N., McLean, K., Cote, P.J., Korba, B.E., Engle, R.E., Gerin, J.L., Wright, J., Michener, G.R., Uhl, E. & King, J.M. (1991) Hepatocellular carcinoma in Richardson's ground squirrels (*Spermophilus richardsonii*): evidence for association with hepatitis B-like virus infection. *Hepatology*, **13**, 1215–1221

Terazawa, S., Kojima, M., Yamanaka, T., Yotsumoto, S., Okamoto, H., Tsuda, F., Miyakawa, Y. & Mayumi, M. (1990) Hepatitis B virus mutants with precore-region defects in two babies with fulminant hepatitis and their mothers positive for antibody to hepatitis B e antigen. *Pediatr. Res.*, **29**, 5–9

de-Thé, H., Marchio, A., Tiollais, P. & Dejean, A. (1987) A novel steroid thyroid hormone receptor-related gene inappropriately expressed in human hepatocellular carcinoma. *Nature*, **330**, 667–670

The Gambia Hepatitis Study Group (1987) The Gambia Hepatitis Intervention Study. *Cancer Res.*, **47**, 5782–5787

Thomas, H.C., Montano, L., Goodall, A., de Koning, R., Oladapo, J. & Wiedman, K.H. (1982) Immunological mechanisms in chronic hepatitis B virus infection. *Hepatology*, **2**, 116S–121S

Thomas, H.C., Jacyna, M., Waters, J. & Main, J. (1988) Virus–host interaction in chronic hepatitis B virus infection. *Semin. Liver Dis.*, **8**, 342–349

Thyagarajan, S.P., Subramanian, S., Thirunalasundari, T., Venkateswaran, P.S. & Blumberg, B.S. (1988) Effect of *Phyllanthus amarus* on chronic carriers of hepatitis B virus. *Lancet*, **ii**, 764–766

Tiollais, P. & Buendia, M.-A. (1991) Hepatitis B virus. *Sci. Am.*, **April**, 48–54

Tiollais, P., Pourcel, C. & Dejean, A. (1985) The hepatitis B virus. *Nature*, **317**, 489–495

Todo, S., Demetris, A.J., Van Thiel, D., Teperman, L., Fung, J.J. & Starzl, T.E. (1991) Orthotopic liver transplantation for patients with hepatitis B virus-related liver disease. *Hepatology*, **13**, 619–626

Toh, H., Hayashida, H. & Miyata, T. (1983) Sequence homology between retroviral reverse transcriptase and putative polymerases of hepatitis B virus and cauliflower mosaic virus. *Nature*, **305**, 827–829

Tokino, T. & Matsubara, K. (1991) Chromosomal sites for hepatitis B virus integration in human hepatocellular carcinoma. *J. Virol.*, **65**, 6761–6764

Tokino, T., Fukushige, S., Nakamura, T., Nagaya, T., Murotsu, T., Shiga, K., Aoki, N. & Matsubara, K. (1987) Chromosomal translocation and inverted duplication associated with integrated hepatitis B virus in hepatocellular carcinomas. *J. Virol.*, **61**, 3848–3854

Tokudome, S., Ikeda, M., Matsushita, K., Maeda, Y. & Yoshinari, M. (1987) Hepatocellular carcinoma among female Japanese hepatitis B virus carriers. *Hepato-gastroenterology*, **34**, 246–248

Tokudome, S., Ikeda, M., Matsushita, K., Maeda, Y. & Yoshinari, M. (1988) Hepatocellular carcinoma among HBsAg positive blood donors in Fukuoka, Japan. *Eur. J. Cancer clin. Oncol.*, **24**, 235–239

Tong, M.J. & Govindarajan, S. (1988) Primary hepatocellular carcinoma following perinatal transmission of hepatitis B. *West. J. Med.*, **148**, 205–208

Tong, M.J., Sun, S.-C., Schaeffer, B.T., Chang, N.-K., Lo, K.-J. & Peters, R.L. (1971) Hepatitis-associated antigen and hepatocellular carcinoma in Taiwan. *Ann. intern. Med.*, **75**, 687–691

Tong, M.J., Weiner, J.M., Ashcavel, M.W. & Vyas, G.N. (1979) Evidence for clustering of hepatitis B virus infection in families of patients with primary hepatocellular carcinoma. *Cancer*, **44**, 2338–2342

Tong, S., Li, J., Vitvitski, L. & Trépo, C. (1990) Active hepatitis B virus replication in the presence of anti-HBe is associated with viral variants containing an inactive pre-C region. *Virology*, **176**, 596–603

Toukan, A.U. (1987) Hepatitis B virus infection in urban residents of Jordan with particular reference to socioeconomic factors. *Trop. Gastroenterol.*, **8**, 161–166

Toukan, A.U., Sharaiha, Z.K., Abu-El-Rub, O.A., Hmoud, M.K., Dahbour, S.S., Abu-Hassan, H., Yacoub, S.M., Hadler, S.C., Margolis, H.S., Coleman, P.J. & Maynard, J.E. (1990) The epidemiology of hepatitis B virus among family members in the Middle East. *Am. J. Epidemiol.*, **132**, 220–232

Transy, C., Fourel, G., Robinson, W.S., Tiollais, P., Marion, P.L. & Buendia, M.-A. (1992) Frequent amplification of c-*myc* in ground squirrel liver tumors associated with past or ongoing infection with a hepadnavirus. *Proc. natl Acad. Sci. USA*, **89**, 3874–3878

Trichopoulos, D., Tabor, E., Gerety, R.J., Xirouchaki, E., Sparros, L., Muñoz, N. & Linsell, C.A. (1978) Hepatitis B and primary hepatocellular carcinoma in a European population. *Lancet*, **ii**, 1217–1219

Trichopoulos, D., MacMahon, B., Sparros, L. & Merikas, G. (1980a) Smoking and hepatitis B-negative primary hepatocellular carcinoma. *J. natl Cancer Inst.*, **65**, 111–114

Trichopoulos, D., Sizaret, P., Tabor, E., Gerety, R.J., Martel, N., Muñoz, N. & Theodoropoulos, G. (1980b) Alphafetoprotein levels of liver cancer patients and controls in a European population. *Cancer*, **46**, 736–740

Trichopoulos, D., Day, N.E., Kaklamani, E., Tzonou, A., Muñoz, N., Zavitsanos, X., Koumantaki, Y. & Trichopoulou, A. (1987) Hepatitis B virus, tobacco smoking and ethanol consumption in the etiology of hepatocellular carcinoma. *Int. J. Cancer*, **39**, 45–49

Trowbridge, R., Fagan, E.A., Davison, F., Eddleston, A.L.W.F., Williams, R., Linskens, M.H.K. & Farzaneh, F. (1988) Amplification of the c-*myc* gene locus in a human hepatic tumour containing integrated hepatitis B virus DNA. In: Zuckerman, A.J., ed., *Viral Hepatitis and Liver Disease*, New York, Alan R. Liss, pp. 764–768

Tsai, S.L., Chen, P.J., Lai, M.Y., Yang, P.M., Sung, J.L., Huang, J.H., Hwang, L.H., Chang, T.H. & Chen, D.S. (1992) Acute exacerbations of chronic type B hepatitis are accompanied by increased T cell responses to hepatitis B core and e antigens. Implications for hepatitis B e antigen seroconversion. *J. clin. Invest.*, **89**, 87–96

Tsega, E. (1977) Hepatocellular carcinoma in Ethiopia. A prospective clinical study of 100 patients. *East Afr. med. J.*, **54**, 281–292

Tsega, E., Gold, P., Shuster, J., Whittemore, B. & Lester, F.T. (1976) Hepatitis B antigen, alpha-fetoglobulins and primary hepatocellular carcinoma in Ethiopia. *J. trop. Med. Hyg.*, **79**, 230–234

Tsuda, H., Hirohashi, S., Shimosato, Y., Terada, M. & Hasegawa, H. (1988) Clonal origin of atypical adenomatous hyperplasia of the liver and clonal identity with hepatocellular carcinoma. *Gastroenterology*, **95**, 1664–1666

Tsuda, H., Hirohashi, S., Shimosato, Y., Ino, Y., Yoshida, T. & Terada, M. (1989) Low incidence of point mutation of c-Ki-*ras* and N-*ras* oncogenes in human hepatocellular carcinoma. *Jpn. J. Cancer Res.*, **80**, 196–199

Tsuda, H., Zhang, W., Shimosato, Y., Yokota, J., Terada, M., Sugimura, T., Miyamura, T. & Hirohashi, S. (1990) Allele loss on chromosome 16 associated with progression of human hepatocellular carcinoma. *Proc. natl Acad. Sci. USA*, **87**, 6791–6794

Tsukuma, H., Hiyama, T., Oshima, A., Sobue, T., Fujimoto, I., Kasugai, H., Kojima, J., Sasaki, Y., Imaoka, S., Horiuchi, N. & Okuda, S. (1990) A case–control study of hepatocellular carcinoma in Osaka, Japan. *Int. J. Cancer*, **45**, 231–236

Tswana, S.A. & Moyo, S.R. (1992) The interrelationship between HBV-markers and HIV antibodies in patients with hepatocellular carcinoma. *J. med. Virol.*, **37**, 161–164

Tu, J.-T., Gao, R.-N., Zhang, D.-H. & Gu, B.-C. (1985) Hepatitis B virus and primary liver cancer on Chongming Island, People's Republic of China. *Natl Cancer Inst. Monogr.*, **69**, 213–215

Turbitt, M.L., Patrick, R.S., Goudie, R.B. & Buchanan, W.M. (1977) Incidence in south-west Scotland of hepatitis B surface antigen in the liver of patients with hepatocellular carcinoma. *J. clin. Pathol.*, **30**, 1124–1128

Twu, J.-S., Lai, M.-Y., Chen, D.-S. & Robinson, W.S. (1993) Activation of proto-oncogene c-*jun* by the X protein of hepatitis B virus. *Virology*, **192**, 346–350

Tygstrup, N., Andersen P.K., Juhl, E. & a Trial Group of the European Association for the Study of the Liver (1986) Steroids in chronic B-hepatitis. A randomized, double-blind, multinational trial on the effect of low-dose, long-term treatment on survival. *Liver*, **6**, 227–232

Tzonou, A., Trichopoulos, D., Kaklamani, E., Zavitsanos, X., Koumantaki, Y. & Hsieh, C.-C. (1991) Epidemiologic assessment of interactions of hepatitis-C virus with seromarkers of hepatitis-B and -D viruses, cirrhosis and tobacco smoking in hepatocellular carcinoma. *Int. J. Cancer*, **49**, 377–380

Uchida, T., Suzuki, K., Esumi, M., Arii, M. & Shikata, T. (1988) Influence of aflatoxin B_1 intoxication on duck livers with duck hepatitis B virus infection. *Cancer Res.*, **48**, 1559–1565

Ulrich, P.P., Bhat, R.A., Seto, B., Mack, D., Sninsky, J. & Vyas, G.N. (1989) Enzymatic amplification of hepatitis B virus DNA in serum compared with infectivity testing in chimpanzees. *J. infect. Dis.*, **160**, 37–43

Vall Mayans, M., Calvet, X., Bruix, J., Bruguera, M., Costa, J., Estève, J., Bosch, F.X., Bru, C. & Rodés, J. (1990) Risk factors for hepatocellular carcinoma in Catalonia, Spain. *Int. J. Cancer*, **46**, 378–381

Van Den Heever, A., Pretorius, F.J., Falkson, G. & Simson, I.W. (1978) Hepatitis B surface antigen and primary liver cancer. *South Afr. med. J.*, **24**, 359–361

Vento, S. & Eddleston, A.L.W.F. (1987) Immunological aspects of chronic active hepatitis. *Clin. exp. Immunol.*, **68**, 225–232

Vento, S., Di Perri, G., Luzzati, R., Cruciani, M., Garofano, T., Mengoli, C., Concia, E. & Bassetti, D. (1989) Clinical reactivation of hepatitis B in anti-HBs-positive patients with AIDS (Letter to the Editor). *Lancet*, **i**, 332–333

Vijayakumar, T., Sasidharan, V.K., Ankathil, R., Remani, P., Kumari, T.V. & Vasudevan, D.M. (1984) Incidence of hepatitis B surface antigen (HBsAg) in oral cancer and carcinoma of uterine cervix. *Indian J. Cancer*, **21**, 7–10

Villarrubia, V.G., Valladolid, J.M., Elorza, F.L., Sada, G., Vilchez, J.G., Jimenez, M. & Herrerias, J.M. (1992) Therapeutic response of chronic active hepatitis B (CAHB) to a new immunomodulator: AM3. Immunohematological effects. *Immunopharmacol. Immunotoxicol.*, **14**, 141–164

Viola, M.V., Prince, A.M. & Alpert, E. (1972) Hepatitis-associated antigen in patients with cancer. *Yale J. Biol. Med.*, **45**, 64–69

Vitvitski, L., Meyers, M.L., Sninsky, J.J., Berthillon, P., Chevalier, P., Sells, M.A., Acs, G. & Trépo, C. (1988) Expression of the X gene product of hepatitis B virus and WHV in infected livers and transfected 3T3 cells: evidence for cross-reactivity and correlation with core/e gene expression. In: Zuckerman, A.J., ed., *Viral Hepatitis and Liver Disease*, New York, Alan R. Liss, pp. 341–344

Vogel, C.L., Anthony, P.P., Mody, N. & Barker, L.F. (1970) Hepatitis-associated antigen in Ugandan patients with hepatocellular carcinoma. *Lancet*, **ii**, 621–624

Vogel, C.L., Anthony, P.P., Sadikali, F., Barker, L.F. & Peterson, M.R. (1972) Hepatitis-associated antigen and antibody in hepatocellular carcinoma: results of a continuing study. *J. natl Cancer Inst.*, **48**, 1583–1588

Wain-Hobson, S. (1984) Molecular biology of the hepadnaviruses. In: Chisari, F.V., ed., *Advances in Hepatitis Research*, New York, Masson, pp. 49–53

Wainwright, R.B., McMahon, B.J., Bulkow, L.R., Hall, D.B., Fitzgerald, M.A., Harpster, A.P., Hadler, S.C., Lanier, A.P. & Heyward, W.L. (1989) Duration of immunogenicity and efficacy of hepatitis B vaccine in a Yupik Eskimo population. *J. Am. med. Assoc.*, **261**, 2362–2366

Wang, H.-P. & Rogler, C.E. (1988) Deletions in human chromosome arms 11p and 13q in primary hepatocellular carcinomas. *Cytogenet. Cell Genet.*, **48**, 72–78

Wang, H.-P. & Rogler, C.E. (1991) Topoisomerase I-mediated integration of hepadnavirus DNA *in vitro*. *J. Virol.*, **65**, 2381–2392

Wang, G.-H. & Seeger, C. (1992) The reverse transcriptase of hepatitis B virus acts as a protein primer for viral DNA synthesis. *Cell*, **71**, 663–670

Wang, N., Sun, Z., Pang, Q., Zhu, Y. & Xia, Q. (1980) Liver cancer, liver disease background and virus-like particles in serum among ducks from high incidence area of human hepatocellular carcinoma. *Chin. J. Oncol.*, **2**, 176–178 (in Chinese)

Wang, J., Chenivesse, X., Henglein, B. & Bréchot, C. (1990) Hepatitis B virus integration in a cyclin A gene in a hepatocellular carcinoma. *Nature*, **343**, 555–557

Wang, W., London, W.T., Lega, L. & Feitelson, M.A. (1991) HBxAg in the liver from carrier patients with chronic hepatitis and cirrhosis. *Hepatology*, **14**, 29–37

Wang, J., Zindy, F., Chenivesse, X., Lamas, E., Henglein, B. & Bréchot, C. (1992) Modification of cyclin A expression by hepatitis B virus DNA integration in a hepatocellular carcinoma. *Oncogene*, **7**, 1653–1656

Waters, J.A., Kennedy, M., Voet, P., Hauser, P., Petre, J., Carman, W. & Thomas, H.C. (1992) Loss of the common 'a' determinant of hepatitis B surface antigen by a vaccine-induced escape mutant. *J. clin. Invest.*, **90**, 2543–2547

Wei, Y., Fourel, G., Ponzetto, A., Silvestro, M., Tiollais, P. & Buendia, M.-A. (1992) Hepadnavirus integration: mechanisms of activation of the N-*myc*2 retrotransposon in woodchuck liver tumors. *J. Virol.*, **66**, 5265–5276

Whittle, H.C., Bradley, A.K., McLauchlan, K., Ajdukiewicz, A.B., Howard, C.R., Zuckerman, A.J. & McGregor, I.A. (1983) Hepatitis B virus infection in two Gambian villages. *Lancet*, **i**, 1203–1206

Whittle, H.C., Lamb, W.H. & Ryder, R.W. (1987) Trials of intradermal hepatitis B vaccines in Gambian children. *Ann. trop. Paediatr.*, **7**, 6–9

Whittle, H.C., Inskip, H., Bradley, A.K., McLaughlan, K., Shenton, F., Lamb, W., Eccles, J., Baker, B.A. & Hall, A.J. (1990) The pattern of childhood hepatitis B infection in two Gambian villages. *J. infect. Dis.*, **161**, 1112–1115

Whittle, H.C., Inskip, H., Hall, A.J., Mendy, M., Downes, R. & Hoare, S. (1991) Vaccination against hepatitis B and protection against chronic viral carriage in the Gambia. *Lancet*, **337**, 747–750

Will, H., Reiser, W., Weimer, T., Pfaff, E., Büscher, M., Sprengel, R., Cattaneo, R. & Schaller, H. (1987) Replication strategy of human hepatitis B virus. *J. Virol.*, **61**, 904–911

Wills, W., Larouzé, B., London, W.T., Millman, I., Werner, B.G., Ogston, W., Pourtaghva, M., Diallo, S. & Blumberg, B.S. (1977) Hepatitis B virus in bedbugs (*Cimex hemipterus*) from Senegal. *Lancet*, **ii**, 217–220

Wollersheim, M., Debelka, U. & Hofschneider, P.H. (1988) A transactivating function encoded in the hepatitis B virus X gene is conserved in the integrated state. *Oncogene*, **3**, 545–552

Wong, V.C.W., Ip, H.M.H., Reesink, H.W., Nco Lelie, P., Reerink-Brongers, E.E., Yeung, C.Y. & Ma, H.K. (1984) Prevention of the HBsAg carrier state in newborn infants of mothers who are chronic carriers of HBsAg and HbeAg by administration of hepatitis B vaccine and hepatitis B immunoglobulin. *Lancet*, **i**, 921–926

Wright, R., McCollum, R.W. & Klatskin, G. (1969) Australia antigen in acute and chronic liver disease. *Lancet*, **ii**, 117–121

Wright, H.I., Gavaler, J.S. & Van Thiel, D.H. (1992) Preliminary experience with alpha-2b-interferon therapy of viral hepatitis in liver allograft recipients. *Transplantation*, **53**, 121–124

Xu, J., Brown, D., Harrison, T., Lin, Y. & Dusheiko, G. (1992) Absence of hepatitis B virus precore mutants in patients with chronic hepatitis B responding to interferon-alpha. *Hepatology*, **15**, 1002–1006

Yaginuma, K., Kobayashi, M., Yoshida, E. & Koike, K. (1985) Hepatitis B virus integration in hepatocellular carcinoma DNA: duplication of cellular flanking sequences at the integration site. *Proc. natl Acad. Sci. USA*, **82**, 4458–4462

Yaginuma, K., Kobayashi, H., Kobayashi, M., Morishima, T., Matsuyama, K. & Koike, K. (1987) Multiple integration site of hepatitis B virus DNA in hepatocellular carcinoma and chronic active hepatitis tissues from children. *J. Virol.*, **61**, 1808–1813

Yap, E.P.H., Cooper, K., Maharaj, B. & McGee, J.O'D. (1993) p53 Codon 249 scr hot-spot mutation in HBV-negative hepatocellular carcinoma (Letter to the Editor). *Lancet*, **341**, 251

Yarrish, R.L., Werner, B.G. & Blumberg, B.S. (1980) Association of hepatitis B virus infection with hepatocellular carcinoma in American patients. *Int. J. Cancer*, **26**, 711–715

Yasui, H., Hino, O., Ohtake, K., Machinami, R. & Kitagawa, T. (1992) Clonal growth of hepatitis B virus-integrated hepatocytes in cirrhotic liver nodules. *Cancer Res.*, **52**, 6810–6814

Yeh, F.-S., Mo, C.-C., Luo, S., Henderson, B.E., Tong, M.J. & Yu, M.C. (1985a) A serological case-control study of primary hepatocellular carcinoma in Guangxi, China. *Cancer Res.*, **45**, 872–873

Yeh, F.-S., Mo, C.-C. & Yen, R.-C. (1985b) Risk factors for hepatocellular carcinoma in Guangxi, People's Republic of China. *Natl Cancer Inst. Monogr.*, **69**, 47–48

Yeh, F.-S., Yu, M.C., Mo, C.-C., Luo, S., Tong, M.J. & Henderson, B.E. (1989) Hepatitis B virus, aflatoxins, and hepatocellular carcinoma in southern Guangxi, China. *Cancer Res.*, **49**, 2506–2509

Yoffe, B., Burns, D.K., Bhatt, H.S. & Combes, B. (1990) Extrahepatic hepatitis B virus DNA sequences in patients with acute hepatitis B infection. *Hepatology*, **12**, 187–192

Yokosuka, O., Omata, M., Zhou, Y.-Z., Imazeki, F. & Okuda, K. (1985) Duck hepatitis B virus DNA in liver and serum of Chinese ducks: integration of viral DNA in a hepatocellular carcinoma. *Proc. natl Acad. Sci. USA*, **82**, 5180–5184

Yoshizawa, K., Itoh, Y., Akahane, Y. & Tsuda, F. (1977) A direct immunofluorescence method for the detection of hepatitis B core antigen in formalin-fixed and gelatin-embedded liver specimens. *J. clin. Pathol.*, **30**, 776–778

Yu, M.C., Tong, M.J., Coursaget, P., Ross, R.K., Govindarajan, S. & Henderson, B.E. (1990) Prevalence of hepatitis B and C viral markers in black and white patients with hepatocellular carcinoma in the United States. *J. natl Cancer Inst.*, **82**, 1038–1041

Yuasa, Y. & Sudo, K. (1987) Transforming genes in human hepatomas detected by a tumorigenicity assay. *Jpn. J. Cancer Res. (Gann)*, **78**, 1036–1040

Zerial, M., Salinas, J., Filipski, J. & Bernardi, G. (1986) Genomic localization of hepatitis B virus in a human hepatoma cell line. *Nucleic Acids Res.*, **14**, 8373–8386

Zhang, X.-K., Egan, J.O., Huang, D.-P., Sun, Z.-L., Chien, V.K.Y. & Chiu, J.-F. (1992) Hepatitis B virus DNA integration and expression of an erb B-like gene in human hepatocellular carcinoma. *Biochem. biophys. Res. Commun.*, **188**, 344–351

Zhou, Y.-Z., Butel, J.S., Li, P.-J., Finegold, M.J. & Melnick, J.L. (1987) Integrated state of subgenomic fragments of hepatitis B virus DNA in hepatocellular carcinoma from mainland China. *J. natl Cancer Inst.*, **79**, 223–231

Zhou, Y.-Z., Slagle, B.L., Donehower, L.A., vanTuinen, P., Ledbetter, D.H. & Butel, J.S. (1988) Structural analysis of a hepatitis B virus genome integrated into chromosome 17p of a human hepatocellular carcinoma. *J. Virol.*, **62**, 4224–4231

HEPATITIS C VIRUS

1. Exposure Data

1.1 Structure and biology of hepatitis C virus (HCV)

1.1.1 *Structure of the virus*

The etiological agent of most cases of post-transfusion hepatitis and a variable proportion of sporadic non-A, non-B hepatitis was discovered in 1989, by recombinant cDNA immunoscreening of serum from a chimpanzee chronically infected with a contaminated human factor VIII concentrate (Choo *et al.*, 1989). The agent was termed hepatitis C virus (HCV). It is a positive-strand RNA virus distantly related to the pestiviruses and flaviviruses on the basis of similar biophysical characteristics, genome organization, hydrophobicity plots and consensus sequences (Miller & Purcell, 1990; Han *et al.*, 1991; Koonin, 1991).

1.1.2 *Structure of HCV genome and gene products*

The genomic organization and characterization of HCV have been described (Choo *et al.*, 1991; Han *et al.*, 1991; Cha *et al.*, 1992). The viral genome is a positive-strand RNA molecule about 9.4 kilobases long (Fig. 1), which is translated into a viral polyprotein. The prototype HCV nucleotide sequence is called HCV-1 (Choo *et al.*, 1991). The single large open reading frame encodes a polyprotein precursor of about 3010 amino acids, which contains co-linearly structural and nonstructural proteins. Putative boundaries are assigned that separate the 5′ untranslated region, the core protein, the glycoprotein envelope 1 (E1), the nonstructural protein 1/envelope 2 (NS1/E2), the nonstructural proteins 2–5 (NS2, NS3, NS4 and NS5) and the 3′ untranslated region.

1.1.3 *Replication and gene expression of HCV*

HCV RNA is transcribed into minus-strand RNA, the putative replication intermediate. HCV does not appear to produce DNA replicative intermediates, and integrated viral sequences have not been found in the host genome (Choo *et al.*, 1989). Viral proteins or viral particles have not been identified in serum from HCV-infected individuals; however, viral antigens have recently been detected in infected hepatocytes by immunohistochemical analysis (Hiramatsu *et al.*, 1992; Krawczynski *et al.*, 1992). Apart from a study using a human T-cell line (Shimizu, Y.K. *et al.*, 1992), infection of cells with HCV *in vitro* has not been reported.

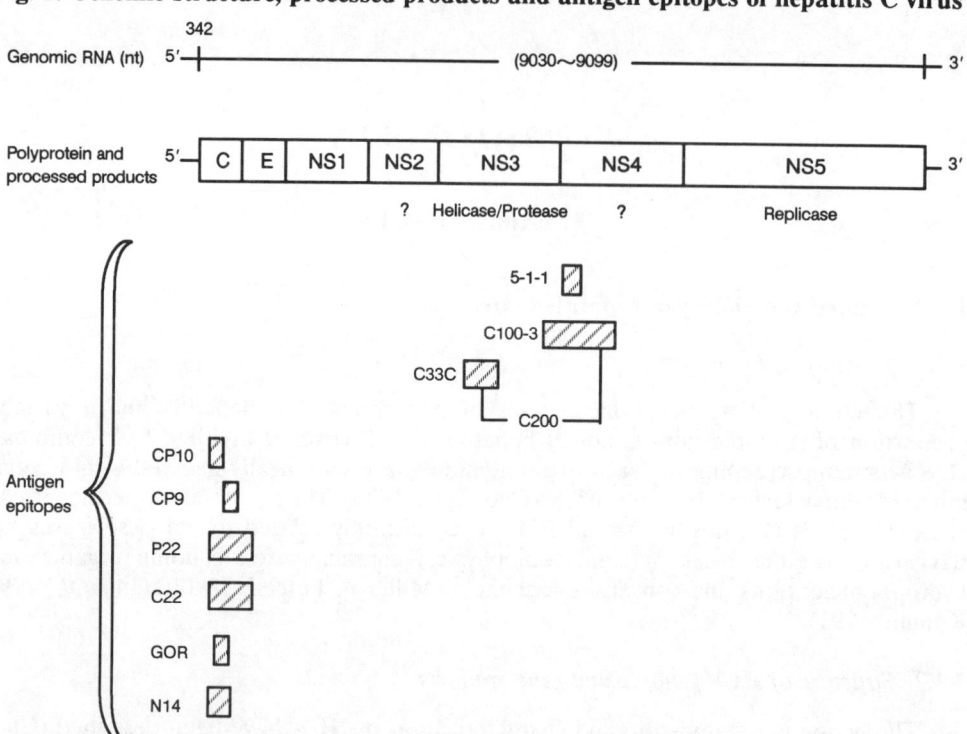

Fig. 1. Genomic structure, processed products and antigen epitopes of hepatitis C virus

Genomic RNA (nt) 5'—|——342——————(9030~9099)——————————|— 3'

Polyprotein and processed products 5'—[C | E | NS1 | NS2 | NS3 | NS4 | NS5]— 3'

? Helicase/Protease ? Replicase

Antigen epitopes:
- 5-1-1
- C100-3
- C33C
- C200
- CP10
- CP9
- P22
- C22
- GOR
- N14

nt, nucleotide; C, core protein; E, envelope; NS, nonstructural protein
From Greenwood & Whittle (1981); Alter, H.J. *et al.* (1989); Kuo *et al.* (1989); McFarlane *et al.* (1990); Mishiro *et al.* (1990); Okamoto *et al.* (1990a); Chiba *et al.* (1991); Houghton *et al.* (1991); Suzuki *et al.* (1991); Watanabe *et al.* (1991a,b); Weiner *et al.* (1991a); Bresters *et al.* (1992); Claeys *et al.* (1992); Kotwal *et al.* (1992a); Matsuura *et al.* (1992); van der Poel *et al.* (1992); Watanabe *et al.* (1993)

It has been possible to identify viral proteins by transcription of RNA from cloned HCV cDNA as well as by transfection of cell lines (Harada *et al.*, 1991; Kumar *et al.*, 1992) *in vitro*, followed by translation of the RNAs *in vitro*. HCV core and envelope proteins, encoded by the NS1/E2 region of the viral genome, have been expressed *in vitro* in *Escherichia coli* (Mita *et al.*, 1992), in insect cells (Matsuura *et al.*, 1992) and in mammalian cells (Matsuura *et al.*, 1992; Spaete *et al.*, 1992). The E2 protein appears to have an amino-terminal hypervariable region that may be the target of immune selection of HCV variants and may be found sequentially in infected individuals (Weiner *et al.*, 1992). The full-length protein NS1/E2 appears to be cell-associated and is not secreted; in contrast, C-terminal truncated proteins were detected extracellularly and may be relevant targets for the host immune response and therefore potential subunit vaccine candidates (Spaete *et al.*, 1992). In the natural course of HCV infection, however, antibodies to the NS1/E2 protein are detected infrequently and do not serve as evidence of viral clearance (Matsuura *et al.*, 1992; Mita *et al.*, 1992).

1.1.4 *HCV animal models*

HCV has been detected in humans and has been successfully transmitted to chimpanzees. At present, the chimpanzee is the only established animal model for non-A, non-B hepatitis (Alter *et al.*, 1978; Tabor *et al.*, 1978; Bradley *et al.*, 1979; Wyke *et al.*, 1979; Yoshizawa *et al.*, 1980) and HCV infection specifically (Shimizu *et al.*, 1990). The natural course of HCV infection has been studied in this animal model (Bradley *et al.* 1990; Abe *et al.*, 1992; Beach *et al.*, 1992; Farci *et al.*, 1992a; Hilfenhaus *et al.*, 1992; Shindo *et al.*, 1992a). Most importantly, studies in champanzees reveal a lack of protective immunity against reinfection with HCV (Farci *et al.*, 1992b; Prince *et al.*, 1992). In contrast to hepatitis B virus (HBV), no naturally occurring HCV-related animal virus has been identified.

1.1.5 *Genotypes of HCV*

After the initial discovery of HCV (Choo *et al.*, 1989), viral isolates from different parts of the world were sequenced, and a huge amount of information on HCV diversity has been published. Complete HCV cDNA sequences have been established for isolates from the USA, including the initial clone HCV-1 (Choo *et al.*, 1991) and the HCV-H virus (Inchauspé *et al.*, 1991), and for isolates from Japan, including HCV-J (Kato *et al.*, 1990), HCV-BK (Takamizawa *et al.*, 1991), HCV-J4 (Okamoto *et al.*, 1990a, 1992a), HCV-J6 (Okamoto *et al.*, 1991) and HCV-J8 (Okamoto, 1992; Okamoto *et al.*, 1992a). Partial HCV cDNA sequences are known for isolates from the USA (Weiner *et al.*, 1991), Japan (Enomoto *et al.*, 1990; Maéno *et al.*, 1990; Okamoto *et al.*, 1990a; Takeuchi *et al.*, 1990a; Hijikata *et al.*, 1991; Tsukiyama-Kohara *et al.*, 1991), Thailand (Mori *et al.*, 1992), China (Chen *et al.*, 1992; Liu *et al.*, 1992; Wang Y. *et al.*, 1992), France (Kremsdorf *et al.* 1991; Li *et al.*, 1991), Germany (Fuchs *et al.*, 1991) and Scotland (Chan, S.-W. *et al.*, 1992).

Comparison of the sequence of the original HCV-1 isolate from the USA (Choo *et al.*, 1989) with a Japanese isolate, HCV-J (Kato *et al.*, 1990), revealed that these HCVs differ both in nucleotide and polypeptide sequence (Kubo *et al.*, 1989; Takeuchi *et al.*, 1990b; Choo *et al.*, 1991). On the basis of nucleotide sequence homology, several genotypes have been identified throughout the world (Enomoto *et al.*, 1990; Houghton *et al.*, 1991; Cha *et al.*, 1992; Chan, S.-W. *et al.*, 1992; Okamoto *et al.*, 1992a,b). On the basis of nucleotide sequence homology of whole sequenced HCV isolates, they were classified into type I (1a), type II (1b), type III (2a) and type IV (2b). Provisionally, type V (3a) and type VI (3b) isolates were reported on the basis of data on partially sequenced genomes.

Apart from the geographic distribution of HCV genotypes mentioned above, recent evidence suggests that HCV exists in infected individuals as different but related genomes, known as quasispecies (Martell *et al.*, 1992; Murakawa *et al.*, 1992; Tanaka, T. *et al.*, 1992; Weiner *et al.*, 1992). Researchers have proposed many classification schemes based primarily on nucleotide sequence homology using different regions of the genome. There is no universally agreed classification.

1.1.6 *Host range and target cells of HCV infection*

The host range of HCV is very narrow, as HCV infects only humans and chimpanzees. The molecular basis of this narrow host range is not known.

In permissive hosts, viral antigens and nucleic acids are found primarily in serum and liver cells. In infected liver tissues, HCV antigens have been detected by immunohistochemical analysis (Hiramatsu *et al.*, 1992; Krawczynski *et al.*, 1992), and RNA has been found in liver and serum by molecular techniques (Fong *et al.*, 1991; Akyol *et al.*, 1992; Bresters *et al.*, 1992; Diamantis *et al.*, 1992; Hosoda *et al.*, 1992; Lamas *et al.*, 1992; Negro *et al.*, 1992; Takehara *et al.*, 1992). HCV RNA has also been detected in peripheral blood mononuclear cells (Qian *et al.*, 1992; Hsieh *et al.*, 1992; Wang, J.-T. *et al.*, 1992; Zignego *et al.*, 1992). Experimental evidence was obtained recently for in-vitro infection and replication of HCV in a human T-cell line (Shimizu, Y.K. *et al.*, 1992).

The biological significance of HCV in cells other than hepatocytes remains largely undefined, however. Blood mononuclear cells may play a critical role in reactivation episodes during chronic HCV infection, after interferon treatment of chronic hepatitis C (Qian *et al.*, 1992) and in reinfection after liver transplantation (Read *et al.*, 1991; Ferrell *et al.*, 1992a; Belli *et al.*, 1993).

1.2 Methods of detection

The detection of infection is based upon assays for viral antibodies and viral nucleic acids. In contrast to HBV infection, no assay system is yet available commercially for detection of HCV antigens in serum or plasma, although they can be detected in serum by research techniques, such as enzyme-linked immunosorbent assay (ELISA) (Takahashi *et al.*, 1992).

1.2.1 *In serum and plasma*

Tests for anti-HCV first became available in 1989. These are known as first-generation assays and had limited sensitivity and specificity; they have been superseded by improved second-generation assays. Neither test distinguishes between current and past HCV infection.

(a) The first-generation anti-HCV assay

In this assay, C100-3 antigen, a recombinant antigen derived from the NS3-NS4 region of the HCV genome (Fig. 1), is used to capture anti-HCV. The labelled anti-HCV is then detected by a second labelled antibody to human immunoglobulin (Kuo *et al.*, 1989). This assay is now available commercially in the ELISA format. In the USA, anti-C100-3 was used to detect anti-HCV in radioimmunoassays in about 90% of blood units implicated in post-transfusion hepatitis (Alter, H.J. *et al.*, 1989).

Screening for anti-C100-3 before blood transfusion reduced the number of cases of post-transfusion non-A, non-B hepatitis in Japan by 60–80% (Japanese Red Cross Non-A, Non-B Hepatitis Research Group, 1991). This test also detected anti-HCV in about 60% of HCV RNA-positive blood donors (Watanabe *et al.*, 1993).

The specificity of the assay is reduced by freezing and thawing serum or plasma and by the presence of high immunoglobulin levels (McFarlane *et al.*, 1990). The latter aspect is particularly important, since in many etiological forms of chronic liver disease immunoglobulin levels are typically elevated, and in individuals living in tropical areas immunoglobulin levels can be very high owing to chronic parasitic infections (Greenwood & Whittle, 1981).

(b) The second-generation anti-HCV assays

In second-generation anti-HCV assays, a recombinant antigen of the non-structural NS3 region, named C33c, and a recombinant antigen of the nucleocapsid (core) region, named C22, were added to the previously used C100-3 antigen for a second-generation ELISA. In another assay, C200 antigen expressed as one polypeptide comprising C100-3 and C33c is used as antigen together with C22 (Bresters et al., 1992; van der Poel et al., 1992). Agglutination tests have also been developed in which gelatin particles coated with second-generation antigens (particle agglutination) and fixed erythrocytes coated with second-generation antigen (passive haemagglutination) have been used to measure anti-HCV. More than 98% of RNA-positive serum samples are detected in second-generation assays for anti-HCV as compared with about 60% in first-generation assays (Watanabe et al., 1993).

Several other systems using other antigens, e.g. NS5, have been described. The second-generation assays are more specific and sensitive than the first-generation assays and to a large degree overcome the limitations mentioned above.

(c) Confirmatory tests

Confirmatory recombinant immunoblot assays (RIBA) and neutralization assays were developed using different viral antigens. The inclusion of additional antigens and a format different from the ELISA improves the specificity of the test. Confirmatory tests give positive results in more than 90% of patients with chronic liver disease or post-transfusion hepatitis tested by ELISA (Suzuki et al., 1991; Watanabe et al., 1991a).

(d) Other anti-HCV assays

Assays have also been based on core and core-related antigens (see Fig. 1), including CP9 (Okamoto et al., 1990b), CP10 (Okamoto et al., 1992c), P22 (Chiba et al., 1991), HCV core (Claeys et al., 1992), HCV-SP (synthetic polypeptide) (Kotwal et al., 1992a), N14 (Watanabe et al., 1993) and GOR (Mishiro et al., 1990; Watanabe et al., 1991b). The relevance of these assays to the natural history of the disease remains to be established.

(e) HCV RNA

HCV infection can also be assessed by detecting HCV RNA by reverse transcription (RT) and the polymerase chain reaction (PCR), which is highly sensitive and has been used for early diagnosis: Quantitative PCR can be used to detect 5–30 molecules of synthetic HCV RNA (Hagiwara et al., 1993). The detection limit of PCR is at present about 10 chimpanzee infectious doses per millilitre of serum (Okamoto et al., 1990c).

Well-controlled procedures for handling samples, extraction and purification of nucleic acids, avoidance of laboratory contamination and use of appropriate negative and positive controls are essential prerequisites for the PCR assay. Selection of primers from the highly conserved 5′ non-coding region is also important for sensitivity and has allowed identification of a broad range of genotypes (Okamoto et al., 1990c).

Testing by PCR has become the 'gold standard' for some workers. The results of these tests correlate well with the risk for transmitting post-transfusion hepatitis, with those of second-generation anti-HCV assays and with liver histology and are useful in monitoring the response of patients to interferon therapy. The test suffers from the risk for contamination, however, and reproducibility between laboratories has been poor (Zaaijer *et al.*, 1993).

1.2.2 *In liver tissues*

(a) *HCV antigen*

HCV antigen can be detected immunohistochemically using fluorescein isothiocyanate-labelled immunoglobulin G fractions from chimpanzee and human sera that are strongly reactive with recombinant structural and non-structural proteins of HCV. In one study, the antigen was localized in the cytoplasm of hepatocytes in all nine chimpanzees with acute hepatitis C, in 5/10 chimpanzees with chronic HCV infection and in 11/12 patients with chronic hepatitis C. Direct immunomorphological evidence for the presence of HCV antigen deposits in hepatocytes using fluorescein isothiocyanate-labelled polyclonal anti-HCV antigen probe was established in absorption experiments using recombinant HCV non-structural proteins. The putative HCV NS3 protein was the most readily detected component of HCV in liver cells (Krawczynski *et al.*, 1992).

(b) *HCV RNA*

HCV RNA can be detected in liver biopsy samples from patients with chronic hepatitis C by RT–PCR and confirmed by Southern blotting. Shieh *et al.* (1991) used primers from both NS3 and core regions and detected the NS3 region more frequently than the core region. HCV RNA was localized by in-situ hybridization in the cytoplasm of hepatocytes in liver biopsy samples obtained from patients with chronic non-A, non-B hepatitis who were seropositive for anti-HCV.

The presence of minus-strand HCV RNA was tested in blood and liver specimens from patients with HCV infection, but it was detected only in the liver. These results suggest that HCV replicates predominantly in liver cells. The detection of minus-strand HCV RNA should be useful for determining HCV replication in tissues other than liver (Takehara *et al.*, 1992).

1.2.3 *Interpretation of serological markers of HCV infection*

Patients infected with HCV may or may not develop clinical and biochemical evidence of acute hepatitis. First-generation assays may give positive results at the time of acute hepatitis or not for months after acute infection, so repeat testing up to 12 months after onset of disease is necessary before HCV infection can be ruled out as a cause of non-A, non-B hepatitis. Even then, given the limited sensitivity and specificity of first-generation assays, the diagnosis cannot be made with certainty. Second-generation assays usually give positive results at the onset of clinical disease, but repeat testing may be necessary even with these tests. After acute infection, approximately 50% of patients become asymptomatic and have normal transaminase levels (Alter *et al.*, 1992); however, anti-HCV remains and RNA is found by PCR in the majority of cases, suggesting persistent infection.

About 50% of patients with clinical evidence of acute HCV infection develop persistent or fluctuating increases in the level of alanine aminotransferase, and most of them have a histological picture of chronic active hepatitis in liver biopsy samples, which may progress to cirrhosis. PCR shows that they also retain anti-HCV and HCV RNA. Thus, the results of tests for both anti-HCV and HCV RNA are usually positive in both individuals with active and those with quiescent HCV infection. Current evidence suggests that few patients resolve HCV infection spontaneously (Alter et al., 1992).

Existing immunoglobulin M–anti-HCV tests, although not commercially available, may prove useful in differentiating acute HCV from exacerbations of chronic disease.

1.3 Epidemiology of infection

Specific tests for hepatitis C became available in 1989 (Kuo et al., 1989), although the existence of a virus distinct from viruses A and B that causes post-transfusion hepatitis had been proposed for years previously (Prince et al., 1974; Anon., 1975). Studies in the USA showed that sporadic cases occurred in addition to those associated with blood transfusion (Alter et al., 1982). The availability of specific tests has begun to clarify the epidemiology. A significant number of false-positive results was obtained using early tests with an ELISA to the C100-3 antigen, particularly in the populations of tropical countries; use of the second-generation tests and confirmation by RIBA has provided more reliable estimates of the prevalence of infection. Table 1 shows the prevalences of specific antibody in various populations and the assays used.

Table 1. Community-based studies of seroprevalence to HCV markers

Region	Assay[a]	Age group (years)	No. of people	% with Ab	Comments	Reference
Cameroon	RIBA	16–70	315	9.8	Rate increased with age; excess in women over men	Mencarini et al. (1991)
Swaziland	RIBA	16–50	194	1.5		Aceti et al. (1992)
Italy	1st-gen. ELISA	20– ≥ 61	812	2.9	Rate increased with age; excess in men over women	Albano et al. (1992)
Italy	RIBA-2	30–69	1484	0.87	Higher prevalence in those 40–59 years old	Rapicetta et al. (1992)
Spain	1st-gen. ELISA	6 mo.–75	497	0.61	Excess in men over women	Dal-Ré et al. (1991)
Peru	RIBA	14–80	2111 (males)	0		Hyams et al. (1992)
Yemen	RIBA	3–80	348	2.6	Rate increased with age	Scott et al. (1992)
Hong Kong	1st-gen. ELISA	0– > 60	382	0.5		Chan, G.C.B. et al. (1992)
Japan	1st-gen. ELISA	> 40	1009	2.3	Rate increased with age; excess in men over women	Ito et al. (1991)
USA	RIBA	≥ 15	2523	18.0		Kelen et al. (1992)

[a]ELISA, enzyme-linked immunosorbent assay; RIBA, recombinant immunoblot assay: sera were initially screened using first- and second-generation ELISA, and reactive sera were further verified with a second-generation immunoblot assay; RIBA-2, second-generation RIBA, with C22, 5.1.1, C100-3 and C33 antigens (sometimes called RIBA 4)

Screening of blood donors has also provided information on prevalence, although the exclusion of high-risk groups and those with a history of hepatitis makes these populations less representative. The results of a sample of donor surveys are shown in Table 2. Surveys have also been carried out of pregnant women (Table 3).

Table 2. Prevalence of HCV antibodies among blood donors in various regions

Country or region	Assay[a]	Age group (years)	No. of people	% with Ab	Reference
Niger	2nd-gen.	mean, 30	1068 men	0.56	Develoux et al. (1992) (abstract)
United Kingdom	RIBA-2	NR	31 936	0.08	Goodrick et al. (1992)
Germany	1st-gen.	18–65	116 700	0.72	Caspari et al. (1991)
Saudi Arabia	RIBA (5-1-1, C100-3)	NR	4580 Saudis 1694 Middle East 1824 Far East 2548 European/American	0.33 1.42 0.27 0.27	Bernvil et al. (1991)
Kuwait	1st-gen.	NR	505	3.0	Al-Nakib et al. (1992)
Thailand	1st-gen.	10–70	390	2.6	Boonmar et al. (1990)
Hong Kong	1st-gen.	NR	4291	1.24	Lin et al. (1992)
China	RIBA-2	18–50	503	1.6	Zhang et al. (1992)
Japan	1st-gen.	15–>60	2970	1.14	Watanabe et al. (1990)
Australia	RIBA-2 or -4	20–60	94 970	0.31	Archer et al. (1992)

NR, not reported
[a]RIBA-2, second-generation recombinant immunoblot assay using 5-1-1, C100-3, C33c and C22-3 antigens: a positive reaction is reactivity against any two of the four antigens; 1st-gen., first generation enzyme-linked immunosorbent assay; RIBA-2 or -4, second-generation RIBA with 5-1-1, C100-3, C33c and C22-3 antigens or only the first two: a positive reaction is reactivity against either the two antigens or the four antigens.

All three survey populations show the same pattern of infection, with rates of 1% or lower in Europe and North America when the RIBA is used, and rates of 1–3% in the Middle East and parts of Asia; only in Central Africa are higher rates seen. In all of these surveys, rates increased with age, particularly after the age of 30. The sex ratio varied from a 2:1 excess in men to an excess in women. In the study of blood donors in Australia, there was a peak prevalence in younger adults (30–34 years in each sex) (Archer et al., 1992).

Specific studies of prevalence have also been carried out in groups considered to be at increased risk. These can be divided into those in which parenteral transmission is considered a risk and those in which risk is considered to increase owing to other behaviour patterns.

1.3.1 *Parenteral exposure*

(a) *Occupation*

In Japan, all reported 'needle-stick' injuries in staff at one hospital were studied over the period 1981–89 (Kiyosawa et al., 1991). A total of 110 employees received such injuries while

Table 3. Seroprevalence of HCV antibodies in pregnant women in various regions

Country or region	Assay[a]	Age group (years)	No. of people	% with Ab	Reference
Niger	2nd-gen.	mean, 24.3	355	0	Develoux et al. (1992) (abstract)
France	RIBA-2	< 20–> 40	1089	North African, 1.9 Black African, 4.8 European, 0 Asian, 1.8	Aussel et al. (1991)
France	RIBA-2	17–45	2367	French, 0.99 African, 1.06	Roudot-Thoraval et al. (1992)
Spain	1st-gen.	Not reported	241	1.2	Esteban et al. (1989)
USA	RIBA-2	13–43	1005	1.8	van Bohman et al. (1992)
Thailand	1st-gen.	18–35	212	2.8	Boonmar et al. (1990)
Taiwan	RIBA	23–36	944	0.63	Lin et al. (1991)

RIBA-2, second-generation recombinant immunoblot assay; 1st-gen., first-generation enzyme-linked immunosorbent assay

treating HCV-seropositive individuals; four developed acute hepatitis, three seroconverted to anti-HCV, and the remainder did not seroconvert to anti-HCV. A study of 456 New York (USA) dentists in 1985–87 (Klein et al., 1991) demonstrated prevalences of anti-HCV (by ELISA confirmed with RIBA) of 1.75% in male and 1.6% in female dentists and 0.14% among blood donors with at least one year of post-graduate education. The only significant association with HCV seropositivity in this study was with oral surgery; the HCV-seropositive dentists reported having treated more AIDS patients, homosexual men, intravenous drug users and haemophiliacs than those who were seronegative. In contrast, 94 dentists in south Wales (United Kingdom) were all found to be seronegative for anti-HCV (Herbert et al., 1992). In Germany, the prevalence of antibodies to HCV (analysed by RIBA) was 0.58% among 1033 hospital employees and 0.24% among blood donor controls (Jochen, 1992). A study of 945 hospital workers in southern Italy found 4.8% to be seropositive, with a seroprevalence of 1.1% of 3575 blood donor controls (De Luca et al., 1991); 576 factory workers from the same area had a 10% seroprevalence (De Luca et al., 1992). In a haemodialysis unit in Italy, 2.5% of staff members were seropositive for antibodies to HCV (Maggi & Petrarulo, 1992).

(b) Bleeding disorders

The prevalence of HCV antibody in people with haemophilia A or B or von Willebrand's disease, who receive clotting factors, is shown in Table 4. The first-generation assays appeared to be less sensitive than the second-generation assays.

Table 4. Prevalence of antibodies to HCV in people with blood clotting disorders

Country or region	No. of people	Bleeding disorder	Assay[a]	% with Ab	Reference
Spain	97	Haemophilia	1st-gen. RIA	63.9	Esteban et al. (1989)
Australia	176	165 with haemophilia A, 5 with haemophilia B, 6 with von Willebrand's disease	1st-gen. ELISA	75.6	Fairley et al. (1990)
Germany	28	Haemophilia	ELISA	85.7	Abb (1991)
Sweden	141	112 with haemophilia A, 29 with haemophilia B	1st-gen. ELISA	86.5	Widell et al. (1991)
USA	131	117 with haemophilia A, 12 with haemophilia B, 1 asymptomatic haemophila carrier, 1 with von Willebrand's disease	1st-gen. ELISA	76.3	Brettler et al. (1990)
Scotland	78	66 with haemophilia A, 19 with haemophilia B	RIBA-2	96.2	Watson et al. (1992)
France	42	Haemophilia	EIA-2	100	Laurian et al. (1992)
Australia	392	331 with haemophilia A, 40 with haemophila B, 21 with von Willebrand's disease	1st-gen. ELISA	73.0	Leslie et al. (1992)

[a]1st-gen. RIA, first-generation radioimmunoassay; 1st-gen. ELISA, first-generation enzyme-linked immunosorbent assay; RIBA-2, second-generation recombinant immunoblot assay; EIA-2, second-generation enzyme immunoassay

(c) Renal patients

A number of studies have been carried out in patients undergoing haemodialysis for renal failure or who have received renal transplants (Table 5). These studies show a relationship between HCV seropositivity and previous blood transfusion and duration of haemodialysis. In peritoneally dialysed patients, previous haemodialysis was a significant risk factor for seropositivity; the first-generation assays had a significant rate of false-negativity.

Kidney transplant patients in France had a seroprevalence of antibodies to HCV of 23.6% (Pol et al., 1992). Of 27 patients followed prospectively, 10 (37%) were already seropositive at the time of transplantation and remained anti-HCV seropositive during follow-up, 11 (41%) patients developed antibody at an average of 95 months after renal transplantation, and six initially seropositive patients (22.2%) lost antibody at an average of 111 months after transplantation. In a similar study in Spain, 32 (48%) of 67 patients were seropositive at the time of transplantation, nine of the 32 (28%) lost antibody after transplantation and five of the remaining 35 seronegative patients (14%) became seropositive (Ponz et al., 1991).

(d) Intravenous drug users

Studies of seroprevalence for antibodies to HCV among intravenous drug users are summarized in Table 6. Rates of infection are high in all geographical areas, and, when it was

Table 5. Prevalence of antibodies to HCV in patients on renal dialysis

Country or region	Treatment	Assay[a]	No. of people	Prevalence (%)	Reference
New Zealand	Peritoneal dialysis	EIA-2	35	8.6	Blackmore et al. (1992)
	Haemodialysis		53	1.9	
	Transplantation		155	4.5	
Germany	Haemodialysis	ELISA-2	498	23.1	Schlipköter et al. (1992)
Italy	Peritoneal dialysis	RIBA	64	4.8	Brugnano et al. (1992)
	Haemodialysis		205	13.3	
Italy	Haemodialysis	ELISA C100	177	10.2	Fabrizi et al. (1992)
Italy	Haemodialysis	RIBA	146	21.9	Maggi & Petrarulo (1992)
Italy	Haemodialysis	ELISA-2	185	38.0	Mosconi et al. (1992)
Italy	Haemodialysis	RIBA	318	25.5 (mean of 3)	Vandelli et al. (1992)
Saudi Arabia	Haemodialysis	RIBA	66	45.5	Al Nasser et al. (1992)
Taiwan	Haemodialysis	EIA-2	125	47.2	Sheu et al. (1992a)
China	Peritoneal dialysis	EIA	101	29.7	Ng et al. (1991)
Japan	Haemodialysis	RIBA	393	17.8	Tamura et al. (1992)
Japan	Haemodialysis	ELISA-3	489	41.9	Fujiyama et al. (1992)
Spain	Haemodialysis	RIA	42	19.1	Esteban et al. (1989)
Australia	Dialysis (unspecified)	ELISA-2	205	5.9	Fairley et al. (1990)
	Renal transplantation		261	6.9	
Germany	Haemodyalisis	ELISA	22	9	Abb (1991)

[a]EIA-2, second-generation enzyme immunoassay; ELISA-2, second-generation enzyme-linked immunosorbent assay; RIBA, recombinant immunoblot assay; ELISA C100, ELISA with C100 antigen

examined, duration of intravenous drug use was found to be significantly associated with HCV seropositivity.

1.3.2 Non-parenteral exposure

(a) Perinatal

Inoue et al. (1991) reported on a grandmother, mother and baby in Japan, all of whom were seropositive for amplified HCV DNA fragments. The baby developed clinical hepatitis and was seropositive for HCV antibody (C100) in an ELISA; the mother and grandmother had antibodies to the nucleocapsid P22 antigen. A study of the offspring of 17 HCV antibody-seropositive women in Hong Kong (Reesink et al., 1990) revealed only one seropositive for HCV antibody, although six babies of 217 HCV-seronegative women were seropositive; the difference was not significant. A study of 13 children born to nine HCV antibody-seropositive women in Japan (Kuroki et al., 1991) showed that passively transmitted

Table 6. Prevalence of antibodies to HCV in intravenous drug users

Country	Assay[a]	No. of people	% with Ab	Reference
Spain	1st-gen. RIA	83	71.1	Esteban et al. (1989)
Australia	ELISA-2	172	86.0[b]	Bell et al. (1990)
Australia	ELISA-2	431	61.9	Fairley et al. (1990)
Italy	1st-gen. ELISA	80	67.5	Girardi et al. (1990)
Germany	1st-gen. ELISA	51	63	Abb (1991)
Sweden	1st-gen. ELISA	172	80	Widell et al. (1991)
Netherlands	1st-gen. ELISA	304	73.7	van den Hoek et al. (1990)
USA	RIBA	225	85.3	Donahue et al. (1991)
Canada	1st-gen. ELISA	76	50.0	Anand et al. (1992)

[a]1st-gen. RIA, first-generation radioimmunoassay; ELISA-2, second-generation enzyme-linked immunosorbent assay; RIBA; recombinant immunoblot assay
[b]Among people injecting drugs for more than eight years, there was 100% anti-HCV seropositivity.

antibody persisted up to six months of age; after that age, all of the babies were seronegative but 11 of the 13 children were HCV RNA seropositive. In two of these mother–child pairs, the mother had been transfused after birth and may have acquired HCV by that route. A further study of eight HCV-seropositive women (Thaler et al., 1991) confirmed that passive antibody was lost by nine months of age, but all of the children were HCV RNA seropositive. No relationship was seen with the human immunodeficiency virus (HIV) status of the mother.

A study of the infants of 43 intravenous drug users (Weintrub et al., 1991), using RIBA, showed that 17 children had passive antibody up to the age of four months. Three of 24 initially seronegative infants were persistently seropositive for antibodies to HCV up to 18 months of age.

In a study in Spain of transmission among HIV-seropositive, HCV-seropositive mothers (Perez Alvarez et al., 1992), 21 of 22 children had maternal HCV antibodies, which became undetectable by three months of age. One child had persistent antibodies and went on to develop non-A, non-B hepatitis with HIV infection. The mother of this child had advanced AIDS. In a study of eight pregnant women with HCV RNA detected by PCR (Novati et al., 1992), five of the women were seropositive for HCV (all were also seropositive for HIV). Four of eight children were seropositive for HCV RNA, three of them at birth. One child had persistent viraemia, and the other three were intermittently seropositive for HCV RNA. All three children lost antibody in the same way as the children who were not viraemic.

(b) *Familial and household transmission*

As HBV is known to be transmitted within the households of carriers, some workers have examined the prevalence of infection in households of people known to be HCV antibody seropositive. In Spain, Menéndez et al. (1991) studied 530 household contacts of 225 subjects seropositive for antibodies to HCV: 26 relatives (4.9%) were seropositive—a significantly greater proportion than among blood donors. There was no difference in prevalence between sexual and non-sexual contacts. The seroprevalence of HCV antibody in the contacts increased with age and was highly correlated with duration of contact with the index patient. A study of household contacts of seropositive haemodialysis patients in Italy (Calabrese *et al.*, 1991) showed 7% of 30 family members to be seropositive. In a second study in Italy (Mondello *et al.*, 1992), household contacts of patients with cirrhosis were examined, comprising eight husbands, eight wives, 44 children and 57 siblings of 21 patients. Two partners (12.5%), five of the children (11.3%) and 27 of the siblings (48.8%) were seropositive for antibodies to HCV (tested by RIBA-2). These prevalences were similar to those of HBV infection in the same families. In Japan, the seroprevalence of HCV antibody (by ELISA) was zero in a survey of 1442 schoolchildren (Tanaka, E. *et al.*, 1992). In Saudi Arabia (Bahakim *et al.*, 1991), however, marked geographical variation in the seroprevalence of antibody was seen in children under 10 years of age: in Riyadh, 0.9%; in Taif, 1.5%; and in Gizan, 5.7%. A report from Canada (Chaudhary *et al.*, 1992) in a home for the mentally handicapped, showed no HCV antibody (by ELISA-2) in a group of 264 children (128 with Down's syndrome), although there was a high rate of HBV infection.

(c) *Sexual transmission*

In two studies, HCV RNA was not detected by PCR in the semen of patients seropositive for HCV antibody (by ELISA) and with chronic hepatitis C (Fried *et al.*, 1992; Terada *et al.*, 1992). In contrast, in a study of 34 patients with chronic hepatitis C who were seropositive for HCV RNA, 24% of seminal fluid samples and 48% of saliva samples contained HCV RNA. Subjects who were seronegative for HCV RNA but seropositive for antibodies to HCV had no HCV RNA in body fluids (Liou *et al.*, 1992). An increased frequency of antibodies to HCV (by ELISA) was found in the semen of non-A, non-B hepatitis patients over that in controls (Kotwal *et al.*, 1992b).

Epidemiological evidence of sexual transmission has been sought by studying the prevalence of infection in sexually active people and in sexual partners of infected individuals. In Canada (Anand *et al.*, 1992), 9.3% of homosexual or bisexual men who were also HIV seropositive were found to be HCV seropositive, compared with 6.4% of a similar group who were HIV seronegative. The difference was not significant. A study of homosexual men in Italy (Gasparini *et al.*, 1991) (using first-generation ELISA) found a seroprevalence of HCV infection of 18.9%, but no association was seen with HIV or HBV seropositivity, with the type of intercourse or with sexual promiscuity. The seroprevalence of hepatitis C was 1.6% in a group of 926 homosexual or bisexual men in Baltimore, USA. Only intravenous drug use and a history of hepatitis A were associated with HCV seropositivity; there was no association with HIV-1 seropositivity or sexual behaviour variables (Donahue *et al.*, 1991). Studies of HCV antibody seroprevalence in people attending clinics for sexually transmitted diseases showed an association with such diseases, which is not as strong as that with HIV-1 or HBV (Corona *et al.*, 1991; Ranger *et al.*, 1991; Gutierrez *et al.*, 1992; Schoub *et al.*, 1992).

Studies of seroprevalence in spouses (using antibody assays) have provided little evidence of sexual transmission (Lin *et al.*, 1991; Chan, G.C.B. *et al.*, 1992). In a study of

195 spouses of Japanese patients with HCV-related chronic liver disease (Akahane *et al.*, 1992), those who had had transfusions or a history of hepatitis before marriage were excluded. The remaining 176 were tested for HCV core antibody, HCV RNA and C100 antibody (by ELISA). Of the spouses, 6% were seropositive for C100, 12% were seropositive for core antigen and seronegative for C100, and 18% were seropositive for both; 8% were HCV RNA seropositive. No controls were used in this study, but genotyping of RNA from six spouse pairs showed concordance in all of them. Studies of HCV RNA require careful interpretation.

(*d*) *Population transmission*

A number of researchers have attempted to determine the modes of transmission in populations. Alter, M.J. *et al.* (1989) carried out a case–control study in which the cases were patients with notified acute non-A, non-B hepatitis in two counties of the USA over a 12-month period. People with a known source of infection—a history within the preceding six months of blood transfusion (13%) or intravenous drug use (34%)—were excluded, leaving 74 cases. Matched controls were selected for 52 (70%) of these cases. No increased risk was found for a range of activities, including homosexual activity, health care employment, surgery, dental work or international travel; however, significant odds ratios were found for individuals with ≤ 12 years of education, more than two sexual partners and a history of hepatitis in household or sexual contacts. The last two factors were considered to be responsible for 5% and 6% of all non-A, non-B cases, respectively.

Pohjanpelto (1992) enquired about risk factors for transmission from all individuals found to be seropositive for antibodies to HCV (by enzyme immunoassay) in a laboratory in Finland. Information was obtained for 160 of 276 seropositive individuals, of whom 89% reported exposure *via* blood (64% due to intravenous drug use and 24% due to transfusion), 0.6% had a sexual partner seropositive for HCV antibody, and 8.1% had lived or travelled to countries such as Somalia, Egypt and Saudi Arabia. There were no controls in this study. In Texas, USA (van Bohman *et al.*, 1992), 23 pregnant women seropositive for HCV antibody (by ELISA; 18 with confirmation by RIBA) were compared with seronegative women, giving 1005 consecutive births. Seropositivity was significantly associated with intravenous drug use, a history of sexually transmitted disease, a history of HBV infection, sex with an intravenous drug user and more than three sexual partners during life. In a case–control study on blood donors in Sydney, Australia (Kaldor *et al.*, 1992), the cases were people who were repeatedly seropositive for antibodies to HCV (by ELISA and RIBA), and controls were those repeatedly seropositive by ELISA and seronegative by RIBA. Highly significant, independent associations with seropositivity were found for intravenous drug use, having a tattoo and the number of heterosexual contacts. Blood transfusion was not a significant risk factor in this study.

[The Working Group noted that the parenteral route is a major source of infection in some populations. They also noted that sexual and perinatal transmission can occur but that current data do not allow estimation of their relative importance in different populations.]

1.4. Clinical diseases (other than cancer)

HCV is the major cause of parenterally transmitted non-A, non-B hepatitis worldwide. Exposure to this agent often results in a clinically indolent infection, which, however, carries a risk of long-term morbidity (Mondelli & Colombo, 1991; Czaja, 1992).

1.4.1 *Acute infection*

The time-lag between exposure to HCV during transfusion and development of clinical acute hepatitis is 2–26 weeks, with a peak of onset between 6 and 12 weeks (Alter, H.J. *et al.*, 1989). Using second-generation ELISA, which detects serum antibodies against both structural and non-structural proteins of HCV, the mean time between exposure and seroconversion is 2.3 weeks (Mattsson *et al.*, 1992). In patients with transfusion-associated non-A, non-B hepatitis followed prospectively for 10–14 years, the time between exposure to HCV and onset of hepatic virus replication, detected by serum HCV RNA, is as short as one week (Farci *et al.*, 1991). The hepatitis is clinically mild during its acute phase. The range of serum alanine aminotransferase (ALT) levels is 200–600 IU/L, and 75% of cases are anicteric and relatively asymptomatic (Alter, H.J. *et al.*, 1989; Aach *et al.*, 1991). In contrast, community-acquired hepatitis C is more often symptomatic (Alter *et al.*, 1992). A likely explanation for this discrepancy is that studies of community-acquired hepatitis have as their starting point the enrolment of patients with clinically detectable disease. Thus, the occurrence of community-acquired hepatitis C is probably underestimated because of the large number of subclinical cases that escape detection.

One characteristic feature of hepatitis C is a fluctuating serum ALT pattern (Alter H.J. *et al.*, 1989; Mondelli & Colombo, 1991). Patients may have highly fluctuating ALT levels within periods of time as short as one week, and such variations may persist. A smaller number of patients have a single ALT peak and then proceed to apparent full recovery, or a plateau-like, mild elevation of ALT level. Patients with a monophasic pattern of serum ALT recovered from hepatitis more often than patients with either fluctuating or plateau-like serum ALT patterns (Tateda *et al.*, 1979). A feature of hepatitis in some patients is an apparently long-lasting normalization of serum ALT, suggesting full recovery, which is followed later by symptomless enzymatic exacerbations. Antibody against the non-structural C100-3 epitope of HCV (by first-generation ELISA) disappears from almost all patients who recover clinically and biochemically but persists in patients with chronic hepatitis (Alter, H.J. *et al.*, 1989; Alberti, 1991).

While the majority of cases of acute hepatitis C are clinically indolent, severe cases occur. Fulminant hepatic failure is seen rarely in patients who are immunosuppressed or have pre-existing liver disease. On the basis of serum HCV RNA, a marker for replicating virus, HCV may be the cause of hepatic failure in up to 18% of cases of fulminant non-A, non-B hepatitis (Theilmann *et al.*, 1992; Féray *et al.*, 1993). In some other patients with fulminant hepatitis, HCV has been implicated as a cofactor in conjunction with other hepatitis viruses (HAV, HBV or HDV) (Féray *et al.*, 1993) or with drugs.

1.4.2 *Chronic infection*

Twenty percent of all patients with chronic hepatitis C progress to cirrhosis, regardless of the route of infection (Mendenhall *et al.*, 1991; Mondelli & Colombo, 1991).

In many patients, development of chronic liver disease is heralded by persistent elevations in serum ALT activity for more than six months after the onset of acute hepatitis C, and is accompanied by persistence of serum antibodies to HCV and HCV RNA. Histological features of chronic liver disease and cirrhosis have also been detected, however, in seropositive viraemic patients with a persistently normal ALT level (Alberti *et al.*, 1992). In most patients, progression of hepatitis C to cirrhosis is a clinically indolent process, with an average length of approximately 20 years (Kiyosawa *et al.*, 1990a). Even the apparently benign disease, chronic persistent hepatitis C, entails a risk of progression to cirrhosis (Hay *et al.*, 1985). As with tranfusion-associated infection, most patients with HCV acquired by other routes had persistent infection for several years, even in the absence of active liver disease (Alter *et al.*, 1992).

Chronic HCV infection may have important clinical consequences. In a long-term multicentre follow-up study of 568 patients who developed post-transfusion hepatitis between 1967 and 1980, there was a small but significant increase in the number of deaths related to liver disease (Seeff *et al.*, 1992).

The factors that influence the severity of liver damage and the rate of progression to cirrhosis in patients with HCV infection are largely unknown. Clinical and epidemiological factors that may predict the severity of chronic hepatitis C include age at infection, duration of disease, serum ALT levels, co-occurrence of HBV infection and alcoholism. In haemophiliac patients, chronic hepatitis and cirrhosis were more often detected in those with persistently elevated serum levels of ALT (54%) than in individuals with only intermittently abnormal enzyme levels (7%) (Colombo *et al.*, 1988). In a US multicentre study of alcoholics, anti-HCV was more frequently associated with cirrhosis than with less severe hepatic lesions (Mendenhall *et al.*, 1991). Finally, studies of virus genotyping have indicated that the severity of liver disease correlates well with the predominance of the Japanese strain or with the co-occurrence of multiple strains (Takada *et al.*, 1992).

There is controversy about whether the course of HCV infection is different in immunocompromised patients. In a three-year follow-up of 97 patients with non-A, non-B hepatitis (Martin *et al.*, 1989), there was evolution to cirrhosis in 11, including the only three with HIV infection; these three patients developed symptomatic cirrhosis within three years of the onset of hepatitis. The serum titres of HCV RNA were higher in HIV-seropositive than in HIV-seronegative patients (Wright *et al.*, 1992a). Liver-graft infections recurred in almost all patients who were infected with HCV before transplantation, and accelerated hepatic histological deterioration was seen in some (Féray *et al.*, 1992; Wright *et al.*, 1992b).

1.4.3 *Extrahepatic manifestations*

Several extrahepatic manifestations of HCV infection have been described. For instance, 82% of 74 Italian patients with porphyria cutanea tarda had circulating antibodies to HCV (by RIBA) (Fargion *et al.*, 1992). A serum sickness-like syndrome has been described in patients with acute non-A, non-B hepatitis (Perrillo *et al.*, 1981). The possible link beweem HCV and such extrahepatic syndromes as polyarteritis nodosa and idiopathic pulmonary fibrosis is under debate. Antibodies to HCV were detected (by ELISA-2, confirmed by RIBA-2) in three (8%) of 38 patients with polyarteritis nodosa (Deny *et al.*, 1992). Antibodies to HCV were found in 19/66 (29%) Japanese patients with idiopathic pulmonary fibrosis by ELISA-1, whether or not there was chronic liver disease; RIBA was used to confirm the presence of antibodies in 12/19 patients (Ueda et al., 1992). HCV has been implicated in many cases of type-II cryoglobulinaemia. Agnello et al. (1992) detected HCV RNA in 16/19 such patients and antibody to HCV in eight (by RIBA). Quantitative studies in four patients showed that almost all of the HCV RNA sequences were concentrated in the cryoprecipitate. Eight patients with membranoproliferative glomerulonephritis had circulating antibodies to HCV (by RIBA), and cryoglobulin-like structures, immunoglobulin G and M and C3 antigen were demonstrated within the glomeruli (Johnson et al., 1993). In another study, 57% of 28 patients with chronic hepatitis C had histological evidence of Sjøgren's syndrome, compared with only 5% of controls with miscellaneous diseases (Haddad et al., 1992).

1.5 Therapy

No vaccine is currently available for HCV infection.

1.5.1 Acute and fulminant HCV infection

Most cases of acute HCV infection are asymptomatic and do not require medical attention. In cases of malaise and fatigue, bed rest is advised. In symptomatic acute HCV infection, therapy is aimed at relief of the signs and symptoms associated with the acute phase of the disease. It includes parenteral nutrition in cases of dehydration and inanition due to nausea and vomiting, and replacement of coagulation factors in cases of bleeding due to impaired synthetic liver function. While fulminant hepatitis C is a rare clinical entity (Wright et al., 1991; Féray et al., 1993; Liang et al., 1993), liver transplantation is a therapeutic option in advanced liver failure and hepatic coma (Maddrey & Van Thiel, 1988). Few trials of antiviral agents in acute HCV infection have been carried out with the intention of preventing the progression of acute hepatitis C to chronic liver disease. While in a study from Japan, natural β-interferon appeared to be effective (Omata et al., 1991), a study from Spain involving recombinant α-interferon showed no benefit for the long-term outcome of the disease (Viladomiu et al., 1992).

1.5.2 Chronic HCV infection

Because of the potentially severe natural course of HCV infection, several therapeutic strategies have been explored. While ribavirin therapy did not significantly affect HCV replication (Di Bisceglie et al., 1992), administration of α-interferon three times per week (Davis et al., 1989; Di Bisceglie et al., 1989; Ruiz-Moreno et al., 1992; Shindo et al., 1992a) or continuously (Carreño et al., 1992) was effective in about 50% of patients, resulting in normalization of liver function, disappearance of HCV RNA from serum and improved liver histology. Unfortunately, about 50% of patients suffer a relapse after cessation of therapy, with increased serum transaminase levels and reappearance of HCV RNA (Davis et al., 1989; Di Bisceglie et al., 1989; Carreño et al., 1992; Garson et al., 1992a; Ruiz-Moreno et al., 1992; Shindo et al., 1992a). A long-term response to α-interferon therapy therefore occurs in only about 25% of patients with chronic HCV infection. Studies are under way to explore the benefit of long-term therapy of chronic HCV infection with α-interferon.

The parameters that predict a response to α-interferon therapy are not well defined (Black & Peters, 1992). In contrast to HBV infection, co-infection with HCV and HIV does not seem to reduce the efficacy of α-interferon therapy (Boyer *et al.*, 1992), but patients immunosuppressed after organ transplantation respond poorly to α-interferon therapy (Davis, 1989; Wright *et al.*, 1992). Recent evidence suggests that response to α-interferon therapy may be related to the viral genotype and viral load in a given individual with HCV infection (Kanai *et al.*, 1992; Yoshioka *et al.*, 1992). The issue is further complicated by the fact that different genotypes have been identified within individuals (Martell *et al.*, 1992; Murakawa *et al.*, 1992; Tanaka T., *et al.*, 1992; Weiner *et al.*, 1992).

2. Studies of Cancer in Humans

2.1 Case series

Table 7 summarizes the seroprevalence of antibodies to HCV in 30 series of patients with hepatocellular carcinoma (HCC). In most, the prevalence was determined by first-generation assays. In general, the prevalence is high among Japanese cases, relatively high in European populations and relatively low in Chinese and Africans. In those series in which data were included for cases grouped by HBV surface antigen (HBsAg) status, the prevalence of antibodies to HCV was generally substantially higher among the HBsAg-seronegative cases.

2.2 Cohort studies

Kiyosawa *et al.* (1990b) studied 58 patients (41 men and 17 women) with chronic hepatitis C (by first-generation ELISA) admitted to Shinshu University Hospital, Japan, between January 1970 and April 1990. All had a history of blood transfusion, and 20 had had clinical acute hepatitis in the past. Twenty-six patients were diagnosed at the time of entry into the study with chronic active hepatitis and 28 with chronic persistent hepatitis. Serum samples were collected serially for a mean of 13.2 years. Among 54 patients who remained seropositive for HCV antibodies throughout the follow-up period, 10 (18.5%) developed HCC. Among four patients who converted from seropositivity to seronegativity, there was no case of HCC. In a further study including some of these patients, Yousuf *et al.* (1992) reported on 16 of 62 HCV-seropositive patients who developed HCC after a mean interval of 9.5 years. [Insufficient detail was provided on the selection of the cases, and no information was given on length of follow-up between the two comparison groups, precluding calculation of expected numbers.]

Seeff *et al.* (1992) studied 545 patients with post-transfusion non-A, non-B hepatitis (diagnosed by exclusion) and 930 matched controls who had received transfusions but did not develop non-A, non-B hepatitis. The subjects were drawn from among participants in five prospective studies of post-transfusion non-A, non-B hepatitis in the USA conducted between 1967 and 1980. Of the 568 cases, 76% were male. The 984 controls were similar to cases with respect to age, sex, race, treatment centre, receipt of immune globulin, history of alcoholism, number of units of blood transfused and date transfused. Cause of death was

Table 7. Prevalence of antibodies to HCV in case series of patients with hepatocellular carcinoma (HCC)

Reference	Location	Period	Assay	All HCC patients Total	%	HBsAg-positive patients Total	%	HBsAg-negative patients Total	%	Comments
Africa										
Levrero et al. (1991)	Senegal	1980–88	ELISA	93	NR	NR	27	NR	68	
Robson et al. (1991)	South Africa	NR	ELISA and confirmation by Abbott neutralization EIA; C100-3	30	7	11	37	NR		
Bukh et al. (1993)	South Africa	1987–90	HCV RNA and 2nd-gen. ELISA	128	20	71	10	57	33	
Americas										
El-Ashmawy et al. (1992)	USA	1985–88	Confirmation by RIBA	38	26	11	45	27	19	Liver transplant patients
McHutchison et al. (1992)	USA	NR	1st- and 2nd-gen. EIA and RIBA	46	52	NR		NR		
Asia										
Kiyosawa et al. (1990a)	Japan	1958–89		83	73	29	35	54	94	21 patients with a history of transfusion all seropositive before HCC developed
Ohkoshi et al. (1990)	Japan	NR	ELISA	100	58	42	19	58	86	
Nishioka et al. (1991)	Japan	NR	ELISA	180	51	75	15	105	76	
Watanabe et al. (1991)	Japan	NR	ELISA (C100) P22	125 125	55 69	23 23	4 4	102 102	67 83	

Table 7 (contd)

Reference	Location	Period	Assay	Prevalence of antibodies to HCV							Comments
				All HCV patients		HBsAg-positive patients		HBsAg-negative patients		
				Total	%	Total	%	Total	%	

Asia (contd)

Reference	Location	Period	Assay	All HCV Total	%	HBsAg+ Total	%	HBsAg− Total	%	Comments
Hagiwara et al. (1992)	Japan	NR	C100-3	NR		NR		39	74	All cases HBsAg-seronegative; 5/10 seronegatives were HCV RNA seropositive by PCR
Lee et al. (1992)	China	NR	ELISA	326	13	243	4	83	37	
Leung et al. (1992)	Hong Kong	1986–90	ELISA	424	7	341	4	83	19	
Shimizu, S. et al. (1992)	Japan	1985–89	2nd-gen. ELISA (83%) and RIBA (58%)	NR		NR		24	58	
Yuki et al. (1992)	Japan	NR	C100-3	148	70	38	32	110	83	Male to female ratio, 7:1
Chien et al. (1992)	Japan	NR	ELISA (C100-3) C25 or C100-3	NR NR		NR NR		268 268	63 83	
Sheu et al. (1992b)	China	1988–90	1st- and 2nd-gen. assays	NR		NR		31	68	
Kiyosawa & Furuta (1992)	Japan	1971–80 1981–90	NR	112 267	34 59	65 86	8 5	47 181	81 88	All cases were in alcoholics
Takeda et al. (1992)	Japan	1980–89	ELISA	100	51	27	11	73	66	
Sun et al. (1993)	China	NR	2nd-gen. ELISA	112	5	NR		NR		

Table 7 (contd)

Reference	Location	Period	Assay	All HCC patients Total	%	HBsAg-positive patients Total	%	HBsAg-negative patients Total	%	Comments
Europe										
Colombo et al. (1989)	Italy	1975–88	ELISA (C100-3)	132	65	41	54	91	70	
Simonetti et al. (1989)	Italy	1982–88	ELISA	200	76	31	58	169	79	
Amitrano et al. (1990)	Italy	1989	ELISA	29	62	NR		NR		
Sbolli et al. (1990)	Italy	1981–89	ELISA	78	61	8	13	70	64	
Vargas et al. (1990)	Spain	NR	NR	81	54	NR		NR		
Benvegnù et al. (1991)	Italy	NR	2nd-gen. RIBA	40	65	NR		NR		14 seropositives negative in 1st-gen. assay
Levrero et al. (1991)	Italy	1980–88	ELISA	74	NR	NR	30	NR	76	
Nalpas et al. (1991)	France	1982–89	ELISA	55	58	12	75	35	57	
Farinati et al. (1992)	Italy	NR	2nd-gen. ELISA and RIBA	97	64	NR	43	NR		
Garson et al. (1992b)	Switzerland	NR	2nd-gen. EIA and RIBA	40	35	7	14	33	39	
Baur et al. (1992)	Austria	NR	ELISA	54	22	22	18	32	25	Any HBV marker

NR, not reported; HBsAg, HBV surface antigen; ELISA, enzyme-linked immunosorbent assay; EIA, enzyme immunoassay; RIBA, recombinant immunoblot assay; PCR, polymerase chain reaction determined from death certificates for 545 (96.0%) of the cases and 930 (94.5%) controls as at February 1992, giving an average of 18 years of follow-up. No testing for antibodies to HCV was done. One case of HCC was found in the hepatitis group and two in the controls [estimated RR, 1.0]. [There were too few cases of HCC for the study to be informative.]

Verbaan et al. (1992) followed 566 patients (331 men and 235 women), with a mean age at entry into the study of 52.1 years, in a hospital in Malmö, Sweden, from whom liver biopsy samples were taken for assessment of chronic liver disease between 1978 and 1989. Causes of death were obtained from death certificates or autopsy records. Sera stored at the time of biopsy were tested for antibodies to HCV by first- and second-generation ELISA, and sera positive in these two tests were retested by second-generation RIBA. Of the 566 patients, 78 (13.8%) were seropositive by RIBA. Eleven cases of HCC developed over the follow-up period; two were diagnosed at the time of inclusion in the study. The proportion of deaths due to HCC in the seropositive group (5/23, 22%) was significantly different ($p = 0.01$) from that in the seronegative group (6/130, 5%).

In a cohort study from Taiwan, China, serum samples from 9691 male adults were collected and frozen during 1984–86 (Yu & Chen, 1993). A total of 35 cases of HCC were identified between 1984 and 1990 and matched individually by age, time of sample collection and residence to two HBsAg-seropositive and two HBsAg-seronegative controls from the original cohort. Samples were analysed for HBsAg status by a radioimmunoassay, for antibodies to HCV by an enzyme immunoassay and for serum testosterone level. Seven of the 35 cases and four of the 140 controls were seropositive for antibodies to HCV [crude relative risk (RR), 9] (multivariate-adjusted RR, 12; 95% confidence interval (CI), 2.4–58).

2.3 Case–control studies

For those studies in which estimated odds ratios (OR) are not provided, the Working Group calculated them using the crude data. The estimates are therefore not adjusted for other factors.

2.3.1 *First-generation assays*

Table 8 (p. 191) gives a summary of the case–control studies in which first-generation antibody tests were used (see section 1.2) and includes available information on the study period and source of control subjects.

(a) Africa

Coursaget et al. (1990) reported on 80 cases of HCC and 136 adult controls in Senegal. Sera were collected between 1982 and 1986. The seroprevalence of antibodies to HCV was 37.5% among the cases and 3% among the controls [OR = 20]. [No data were given on the age and sex distribution of subjects nor how they were selected.]

Kew et al. (1990) studied 380 southern African blacks (322 men, 58 women) with histologically confirmed HCC and compared them with 152 controls matched for race, sex, age and rural or urban status. The seroprevalence of antibodies to HCV among the cases (29%) was higher than that among the controls (1/152) [OR, 62]. Of the 196 HBsAg-seronegative cases, 32% were seropositive for HCV antibodies, compared with 26% of the 184 HBsAg-seropositive cases. [The periods of collection of data and sera were not given.]

(b) Americas

In a study conducted in the USA, Hasan *et al.* (1990) studied retrospectively a total of 87 HCC patients who had been diagnosed between January 1978 and March 1989 at the University of Miami Hospital and Clinic. Diagnosis was made either histologically, cytologically or by level of serum α-fetoprotein with at least one positive imaging study. Cases with alcoholic liver disease, haemochromatosis or α_1-antitrypsin deficiency were excluded. Controls were 200 consecutive blood donors. Forty percent of the cases and 0.5% of the controls were seropositive for antibodies to HCV (tested by the method of Kuo *et al.*, 1989, see p. 168) [OR, 134]. The seropositivity among cases varied by ethnicity, being found among the HBsAg-seronegative patients in 35% of 37 whites, 80% of 20 hispanics and the one black; the only Asian was seronegative. The seroprevalence of antibodies to HCV among the 41 cases with no evidence of past HBV infection was 49%, that among the 18 seropositive only for anti-HBc was 61%, and that among the 28 cases who were HBsAg seropositive was 14%. All cases who were HCV antibody seropositive and HBsAg seronegative had evidence of cirrhosis. [The sex and age distribution of the HBsAg-seropositive cases and of the controls were not given. It was not evident when the case blood samples were collected in relation to diagnosis or whether case and control samples were collected at different times.]

Yu *et al.* (1990) evaluated data on 51 cases (in 35 males and 16 females; mean age, 59.5 years) and 128 controls (81 males; mean age, 58.7 years) obtained in 1984–89 from Los Angeles County, California (USA) (for details, see p. 80 of the monograph on HBV). Of the cases, 29% were seropositive for antibodies to HCV, as were 4% of the controls. An OR of 11 was found for the association between HCV antibody seropositivity and HCC after adjustment for age and sex. The OR for antibodies to HCV in subjects with no HBV markers was 4.8; that for any HBV marker among the HCV seronegative subjects was 4.4. Ten cases and no control had evidence of any serological marker of HBV infection and were HCV seropositive ($p < 0.0005$). The authors noted that the serum specimens of the controls were drawn on average six years before those of the cases.

Di Bisceglie *et al.* (1991a) studied 99 cases of HCC seen at Johns Hopkins Oncology Center, Baltimore, USA, between January 1987 and May 1988 (for details, see p. 81 of the monograph on HBV). Controls consisted of 98 consecutive adult patients with other cancers seen between November 1987 and January 1988. The seroprevalence of antibodies to HCV was 13% among the cases and 2% among the controls; the OR for an association with HCC was 7.3.

(c) Asia

Saito *et al.* (1990) studied the seroprevalence of antibodies to HCV among 253 (207 men and 46 women; mean age, 61 years) patients with HCC diagnosed clinically and pathologically in several hospitals in Japan and from whom blood specimens were obtained at the time of diagnosis. For comparison, they evaluated 148 patients with other cancers (95 men, 53 women; mean age, 61.1 years). The seroprevalence of antibodies to HCV was 55% among cases and 10% among controls [OR, 11]. The prevalence among the cases varied by HBV status. The authors noted an association between history of transfusion and seropositivity for HCV antibodies in the controls [$p = 0.003$] but not in the cases, and that the control rate was higher than that seen in Japanese blood donors (about 1%). [No data were given on the period of study.]

In a case–control study in Qidong County, Jiangsu, China, 50 cases of HCC diagnosed during 1988 were compared with 50 population controls individually matched to cases by age, sex and place of residence (Xu et al., 1990). Four cases and no control were seropositive for antibodies to HCV ($p = 0.059$); one of these cases was seronegative for HBsAg, while the remaining three were seropositive.

Jeng and Tsai (1991) studied 48 HCC patients (35 men, 13 women; mean age, 62.0 years) in Taiwan, China, who were HBsAg seronegative and who had been recruited after admission to Kaohsiung Medical College Hospital between January 1988 and June 1990. Diagnosis was made histologically or cytologically. Controls were 54 HBsAg-seronegative individuals (46 men, eight women; mean age, 52.3 years) who were seen for normal physical check-ups during the same period. Seroprevalence for antibodies to HCV differed significantly between the two groups (60% versus 0 [$p = 0.0001$]). The authors also reported a significant difference between HCV antibody seroprevalence in these cases and in 81 HBsAg-seropositive HCC cases seen during the same period (23.5%; $p = 0.0001$).

Srivatanakul et al. (1991) conducted a matched case–control study on HCC in cases seen in Thailand in 1987–88 (Parkin et al., 1991; described in detail on p. 85 of the monograph of HBV). There was no association between the presence of antibodies to HCV and HCC (OR, 1.3); the prevalence among cases was 6% and that among the controls was 5%.

Yu et al. (1991) conducted a matched case–control study in Taiwan, China, of HCC cases from two major teaching general hospitals newly diagnosed between August 1986 and July 1987 on the basis of either pathological examination or serum α-fetoprotein levels, confirmed by imaging. There were 127 cases (121 men, 6 women; mean age, 50.4 years). Controls were selected from household registration lists, were matched for age, sex, ethnicity and residence and were recruited during the same period. The seroprevalence of antibodies to HCV was 11% among the cases and 2% among the controls. In a matched analysis, the univariate estimate of the OR associated with seropositivity for HCV antibody was 7.0, and the ratio remained elevated after control for HBsAg status, HBeAg status, smoking habits, habitual alcohol use and peanut consumption. The seroprevalence of antibodies to HCV was higher in the 17 HBsAg-seronegative cases (29%) than in the 110 HBsAg-seropositive cases (8%). Among the HBsAg-seronegative subjects, the OR for HCV seropositivity and HCC was 16. The OR for co-infection as compared with seropositivity for neither marker could not be estimated, with nine cases and no control observed.

HCV antibody status was measured in 1989–90 using an enzyme immunoassay in 42 cases of HCC and in 4818 blood donors enrolled from the Military Hospital in Riyadh, Saudi Arabia (Al Karawi et al., 1992). The seroprevalence of antibodies to HCV was 31% in cases and 1.5% among blood donors [crude OR, 30; 95% CI, 15–60]. The seroprevalence of antibodies to HCV was higher among HBsAg-seronegative HCC cases (42%) than among seropositive HCC cases (13%). [No information was available on the age or sex of the study subjects.]

In a study that overlapped partially with that of Yu et al. (1991), Chuang et al. (1992) studied 128 cases of HCC (in 112 men, 16 women; mean age, 54.3 years) and 384 age- and sex-matched community controls in Taiwan, China (described on p. 85 of the monograph on HBV). Twenty percent of the cases and 3% of controls were seropositive for HCV antibodies. Among the cases, the seroprevalence was 45% for the 29 who were HBsAg seronegative and 12% for the 99 who were HBsAg seropositive. The OR for HCC was 27 among the subjects seropositive for HCV antibody and HBsAg seronegative. The OR for HCC for the joint presence of HBsAg and HCV antibody seropositivity as compared with the presence of neither was 40. [The period of data collection was not given.]

(d) Europe

The first study on HCV and HCC, reported by Bruix et al. (1989), was conducted in Barcelona, Spain. The cases were 96 (67 men, 29 women; mean age, 63.4 years) consecutive patients with HCC confirmed by ultrasonography and biopsy or with elevated serum α-fetoprotein level. The control group comprised 177 hospitalized surgical controls without liver disease (119 men, 58 women; mean age, 54.3 years). The seroprevalence of antibodies to HCV was 75% among cases and 7% among controls. Among cases, the seroprevalence varied somewhat by risk category: all of four cases with porphyria and cirrhosis, 81% of 43 with cirrhosis of unknown etiology, 77% of 30 with alcoholic cirrhosis, 56% of nine HBsAg-seropositive cases, none of three with a previously normal liver and 71% of seven with previous liver status unknown. The seroprevalence of antibodies to HCV in the case group was significantly higher than that in the control group without liver disease [OR, 38]. [Data on time period of serum collection were not provided.]

Caporaso et al. (1991) reported on 332 consecutive patients with cirrhosis seen in a medical centre in Naples, Italy, between January 1988 and May 1990. HCC was diagnosed in 88 of these by ultrasonographic examination and serum α-fetoprotein levels and/or by cytology. The patients with HCC were more likely than the 244 control patients with only cirrhosis to be male (88 versus 61%) and to be older (mean age, 64.5 years versus 57.0). The seroprevalence of antibodies to HCV among the cases was 72% and that among the controls was 55% [RR, 2]. After control for age and sex, seropositivity for antibodies to HCV was a significant predictor of HCC ($p = 0.009$).

Poynard et al. (1991) studied 2015 patients admitted in 1982–89 to the hepatogastro-enterology service of the Antoine Béclère Hospital in Clamart, France, for alcoholism and alcoholic liver disease, using a uniform protocol. All patients were classified as alcoholic on the basis of a history of consumption of at least 50 g alcohol per day in the year before admission. Serum samples were available for testing for antibodies to HCV from 469 patients with documented liver cirrhosis (51 HCC cases and 418 controls). Diagnosis was made histologically or on the basis of α-fetoprotein levels, confirmed by ultrasonography and other imaging. The presence of cirrhosis was determined in all subjects either by biopsy or by use of an established algorithm. The seroprevalence of antibodies to HCV was 41% among the cases and 26% among the controls, giving an OR for an association with HCC of [2.0]; this estimate did not vary markedly with the presence of HBsAg. On multivariate analysis, age, male sex, HBsAg seropositivity and HCV antibody seropositivity were all significant risk factors for HCC; HCV antibody seropositivity was the weakest ($p = 0.04$). [Sex ratio and age range within the group were not available.]

Tzonou et al. (1991) re-evaluated subjects from an earlier case–control study (Trichopoulos et al., 1987; described on p. 88 of the monograph on HBV). As reported previously (Kaklamani et al., 1991), only strong seropositivity for antibodies to HCV (twice the recommended limit) was specifically related to HCC; weakly positive results were related to cases of metastatic liver cancer, suggesting that weakly positive results were false-positives. In the present report, subjects were categorized as strongly positive, weakly positive or negative. For 185 HCC cases and 432 hospital controls, the prevalence of strong reactivity to HCV antibodies was 39% among the cases and 7% among the controls: the OR was 6.2 after adjustment for age, sex, smoking and HBsAg status. The joint presence of sero-positivity for HCV antibodies and HBsAg gave an OR of 20; that for HCV-seropositive and HBsAg-seronegative subjects was 4.8 ($p < 0.05$). The prevalence of antibodies to HCV was lower among the 99 HBsAg-seronegative cases (28%) than among the 85 HBsAg-seropositive cases (51%).

Simonetti et al. (1992) evaluated 212 consecutive HCC patients (161 men, 51 women; mean age, 62.4 years) admitted to a hospital in Palermo, Italy, between June 1982 and December 1988. Diagnosis was based on biopsy or serum α-fetoprotein level, confirmed by ultrasonography or tomography. Controls were matched for age and sex and were drawn from among patients hospitalized for chronic non-hepatic disease during the same period (mean age, 62.2). Of the cases, 71% were seropositive for antibodies to HCV compared with 5% of the controls; the OR for an association with HCC was 69 after control for markers of HBV. Of the cases, 197 had confirmed cirrhosis (based on clinical criteria in 60 cases and by biopsy in 137 cases), and a second comparison group was assembled of 197 patients with cirrhosis matched for age and sex (mean age, 61.5), who were hospitalized during the same period. Of the cirrhotic cases of HCC, 74% were seropositive for HCV antibody, as were 62% of their controls; the OR for an association with HCC was 2.0 after control for markers of HBV and alcohol abuse.

2.3.2 *Second-generation assays*

Table 9 summarizes the case–control studies in which antibody to HCV was screened using second-generation assays.

(a) *Africa*

A case–control study was carried out in Maputo, Mozambique, on 178 HCC patients admitted to the department of gastroenterology of the central hospital of that city and 194 blood donors from the same hospital (Dazza et al., 1993). HCV antibody status was investigated using a second-generation enzyme immunoassay with confirmation by a line immunoassay. Eleven cases and four controls were seropositive for HCV antibody, yielding an age-adjusted OR of 1.1, which was substantially different from the crude OR of 3.1. The OR for seropositivity to HCV antibody was 1.4 (95% CI, 0.4–5.3) among HBsAg-seronegative individuals. The mean age of cases was 40.8 years and that of the controls, 31.3 years; the mean age of HCV antibody-seropositive cases was 53.9 and that of seronegative cases was 35.1. [The controls were substantially younger than the cases, but the age ranges were not given, and the statistical methods used to control for age were not described.]

Table 8. Summary of results of case–control studies of hepatocellular carcinoma and the prevalence of antibody to HCV as measured by first-generation assays

Reference and location	Subjects	Seroprevalence of antibodies to HCV Cases No.	Cases %	Controls No.	Controls %	OR[a]	95% CI	Study period and comments
Africa								
Coursaget et al. (1990); Senegal	NR	80	37.5	136	3	[20]	[6.9–57]	1982–86; stringent cut-off used for assay
Kew et al. (1990); South Africa	Men and women	380	29	152	0.7	[62]	[11–353]	Unmatched hospital controls
Americas								
Hasan et al. (1990); USA	NR	87	40	200	0.5	[134]	[23–787]	Cases, 1978–89; unspecified for controls; blood donor controls
Yu, et al. (1990); USA	Men and women	51	29	128	4	11	3.5–31	Cases, 1984–89; community controls, 1978–82; all estimates adjusted for age and sex
	Subjects with no evidence of HBV infection					4.8	1.3–18	
	Subjects with any HBV marker					∞	15–∞	
Di Bisceglie et al. (1991a); USA	Men and women	99	13	98	2	7.3	1.8–48	Cases, 1/1987–5/1988; controls, 11/1987–1/1988. Controls, other cancer patients
Asia								
Saito et al. (1990); Japan	Men and women	253	55	148	10	[11]	[5.9–19]	Controls, other cancer patients. Among controls, significant association of HCV seroprevalence and history of blood transfusion ($p = 0.003$)
Xu et al. (1990); China	Men and women	50	4	50	0	∞		Population controls ($p = 0.06$)

Table 8 (contd)

Reference and location	Subjects	Seroprevalence of antibodies to HCV Cases No. %	Seroprevalence of antibodies to HCV Controls No. %	OR[a]	95% CI	Study period and comments
Asia (contd)						
Jeng & Tsai (1991); Taiwan, China	Men and women	48 60	54 0	∞		[$p < 0.0001$]; 1988–90; non-hospital controls. 11 subjects were HBsAg seronegative
Srivatanakul et al. (1991); Thailand	Men and women	63 6	63 5	1.3	0.2–8.7	1987–88; hospital controls; matched analysis; subjects matched on sex, age, area of residence, hospital
Yu et al. (1991); Taiwan, China	Men and women	127 11	127 2	7.0	1.6–31	1986–87; community controls; matched analysis; subjects matched for age, sex, ethnicity and residence
				24	2.2–254	Conditional multivariate analysis with adjustment for matching factors plus HBsAg status, HBeAg status, smoking, habitual alcohol use and peanut consumption
	HCV seropositive/HBsAg seropositive versus neither			∞	14–∞	
Al Karawi et al. (1992); Saudi Arabia	NR	42 31	4818 1.5	[30]	[15–60]	1989–90; blood donor controls; no data on age or sex
Chuang et al. (1992); Taiwan, China	Men and women HBsAg seronegative HBsAg seropositive, HCV seropositive versus neither	128 20	384 3	[6.9] 27 40	3.5–14 9.8–75 13–128	Community controls
Europe						
Bruix et al. (1989); Spain	Men and women	96 75	177 7	[38]	[18–133]	Hospital controls
Caporaso et al. (1991); Italy	Men and women	88 72	244 55	[2.0]	[1.2–3.4]	1988–90; all subjects had cirrhosis

Table 8 (contd)

Reference and location	Subjects	Seroprevalence of antibodies to HCV Cases No. / %	Seroprevalence of antibodies to HCV Controls No. / %	OR[a]	95% CI	Study period and comments
Europe (contd)						
Poynard et al. (1991); France	Men and women	51 / 41	418 / 26	[2.0]	[1.1–3.7]	1982–89; all subjects were alcoholics and had cirrhosis.
Tzonou et al. (1991); Greece	Men and women	185 / 39	432 / 7	6.2	3.6–11	1976–84; hospital controls; all estimates adjusted for age, sex, residence; seropositivity for HCV based on 'strongly positive' results
	HCV seropositive/HBsAg seropositive *versus* neither			20	2.5–158	
	HBeAg seropositive or anti-HBe seropositive *versus* neither			∞	5.8–∞	
	HCC with cirrhosis			11	5.3–25	
Simonetti et al. (1992); Italy	Men and women Hospital controls	212 / 71	212 / 5	69.1	15–308	1982–88; conditional multivariate analysis with control for sex and age plus HBsAg and anti-HBc status
	Controls with cirrhosis	197 / 74	197 / 62	2.0	1.3–3.2	1982–88; conditional multivariate analysis with control for age and sex plus HBsAg and anti-HBc status and alcohol abuse

NR, not reported
[a]Cornfield limits; all estimates are unadjusted unless otherwise specified.

A series of 49 cases of HCC and 134 adult controls from the general population were re-investigated in Senegal with regard to HCV antibody status using both a first-generation ELISA test for C100 and an anti-core/anti-C33c recombinant assay (Coursaget *et al.*, 1992). Seropositivity to HCV antibody was found in six (12%) cases and two (1.5%) controls [crude OR, 9.2; 95% CI, 1.8–47]; seropositivity was confirmed by neutralization assay in two cases and one control [crude OR, 5.7]. [No details were provided on the methods or time of recruitment of cases and controls or on potential confounding variables.]

(b) Asia

Tanaka *et al.* (1991) conducted a case–control study in Fukuoka, Japan, on 91 cases of HCC (in 73 men and 18 women; median ages, 59.0 and 56.5 years, respectively) in 1985–89. A total of 410 controls (291 men, 119 women; median ages, 57.0 and 56.0, respectively) were identified during examinations at public health centres in 1986–89. Most of the cases had evidence of pre-existing liver disease (76 cirrhosis, nine chronic hepatitis). The prevalence of antibodies to HCV was measured with a first-generation enzyme immunoassay, and positive sera were re-tested using a second-generation assay (RIBA). The seropositivity rates in the initial assay were not related to duration of storage of the sera. Seropositivity to HCV antibody was 51% among cases and 3% among controls. The OR for an association with HCC was 52 after adjustment for demographic factors. The seroprevalence of antibodies to HCV was low among patients who were HBsAg seropositive (5%).

In a case–control study carried out in Hanoi, Viet Nam, described in detail in the monograph on HBV (p. 85), HCV antibody status was investigated using a confirmatory line immunoassay (Cordier *et al.*, 1993). Seropositivity to HCV antibody was seen in three of 152 male cases and two of 241 male hospital controls (OR, 2.0). All were HBsAg seronegative (OR, 38; 95% CI, 2.8–1443).

(c) Europe

Stroffolini *et al.* (1992) studied 65 cases of HCC diagnosed in four teaching hospitals in Palermo, Italy, between January and December of 1990 (described in detail on p. 89 of the monograph on HBV). All cases had cirrhosis; controls were hospitalized patients with non-hepatic chronic diseases. The seroprevalence of antibodies to HCV was determined using a second-generation enzyme immunoassay; positive samples were confirmed by RIBA. Seropositivity to HCV antibody was seen in 66% of cases and 13% of controls (OR, 27 after control for age, gender and HBV markers). Five cases and no control were seropositive for both HCV antibody and HBsAg (OR, 77); the OR for HCV antibody seropositivity alone was 21 and that for HBsAg alone, 13.

Zavitsanos *et al.* (1992) re-tested serum samples obtained during the case–control study described above in Athens, Greece (Tzonou *et al.*, 1991; see also p. 88 of the monograph on HBV). Samples from 181 HCC cases, 35 patients with metastatic liver cancer and 416 hospital controls with no malignant neoplasm or liver disease were examined. The sera had been collected between April 1976 and October 1984 at nine major hospitals in Athens. In the present study, sera were tested by second-generation enzyme immunoassay with confirmation empirically determined using a variety of supplemental enzyme immunoassays with other recombinant peptides and an inhibition assay using C100; a random sample of 32 HCC patients and 13 hospital controls was also tested by RIBA-2. The authors again assumed that the cases of metastatic liver cancer were true negatives. The final algorithm for positivity was repeated reactivity to the second-generation enzyme immunoassay at an absorbance to cut-off ratio of ≥ 3.0, with confirmation based on supplemental assays with seropositivity for antibody against another viral protein or by inhibition. On the basis of these tests, the OR for an association with HCC was 10.

2.4 Modifying effects of seropositivity for hepatitis B surface antigen

At least six case–control studies presented results according to HCV antibody status (assessed by first-generation tests) separately for HBsAg-seropositive and HBsAg-seronegative individuals, allowing analyses of the separate effects of each virus and their combined effects. A further five studies presented similar results based on second-generation tests (Table 10). With both the first- and second-generation tests, the ORs for HCC in subjects infected with HBV or HCV alone are increased. The OR associated with HCV alone is in general higher in studies based on second-generation tests [combined results: OR, 26; 95% CI, 16–43] than in other studies [combined results: OR, 14; 95% CI, 10–20]. The combined effect of the two viruses cannot be described accurately, given the small numbers of subjects.

The results summarized in Table 10 should be considered with caution, since the estimated ORs were not adjusted for confounding factors such as sex and age. Comparisons between the columns of the table may be valid if it can be assumed that the uncontrolled confounding effect of sex, age and other possible factors varies across the exposure categories.

3. Studies of Cancer in Experimental Animals

Primate

A seven-year-old male chimpanzee (*Pan troglodytes*), seronegative for HBsAg, anti-HBs and anti-HBc and seropositive for antibodies to hepatitis A virus, was inoculated with 40 ml of serum from a human patient with chronic non-A, non-B hepatitis, who was seronegative for markers of HBV and hepatitis A virus, and 10 months thereafter with 10 ml of the chimpanzee's own acute-phase serum (taken at day 34 after inoculation). Over the next six years, the chimpanzee received inoculations of several different plasma-derived products, including concentrates of coagulation factors II, VII, VIII, IX and XIII, and anti-thrombin III. Serum levels of aspartate and alanine transferase, γ glutamyl transferase and HBV markers were monitored and liver biopsies were performed. Serum transferase levels increased after the first inoculation of the human serum and the animal's acute-phase serum. Over the next six years, the levels fluctuated above normal, and serial liver biopsies showed changes ranging from histologically normal to moderate hepatitis (which included focal hepatocellular necrosis and chronic portal inflammation). The chimpanzee remained seronegative for hepatitis B markers throughout the study. Seven years after the first inoculation, liver masses were palpable, and necropsy revealed two large (16 × 8 cm and 5 × 7 cm)

Table 9. Summary of results of case–control studies of hepatocellular carcinoma and the presence of antibody to HCV as measured by second-generation assays

Reference and location	Subjects	Seroprevalence of antibodies to HCV Cases No.	Cases %	Controls No.	Controls %	OR[a]	95% CI	Study period and comments
Africa								
Dazza et al. (1993); Mozambique	NR	178	6	194	2	1.1	0.4–3.1	Blood donor controls; adjusted for age; mean age of cases, 40.8 years; controls, 31.3 years
Coursaget et al. (1992); Senegal	NR	49	4	134	1	[5.7]	[0.5–69]	General population controls
Asia								
Tanaka et al. (1991); Japan	Men and women	91	51	410	3	52	24–114	Cases, 1985–89; controls, 1986–89; general population controls; adjusted for age, sex, occupational class and education; initial screening by first-generation with confirmation by RIBA
Cordier et al. (1993); Viet Nam	Men	152	2	241	1	2.0	0.3–17	1989–92; hospital controls
Europe								
Stroffolini et al. (1992); Italy	Men and women	65	66	99	13	27	9.9–73	1990; all cases had cirrhosis and controls had non-hepatic chronic disease; adjusted for age, sex, hospital and HBV markers
	HCV antibody seropositive and HBsAg seropositive *versus* neither					77	3.8–1421	Adjusted for age, sex and hospital; 0.5 added to each entry; confirmation by RIBA
Zavitsanos et al. (1992); Greece	Men and women	181	13	446	1	10	4.2–26.0	1976–84; same subjects as Tzonou et al. (1991); unadjusted

[a]Cornfield limits

Table 10. Separate effects of HBV and HCV on risk for hepatocellular carcinoma

Reference and location	HBsAg seronegative HCV Ab seronegative Cases	HBsAg seronegative HCV Ab seronegative Controls	HBsAg seronegative HCV Ab seropositive Cases	HBsAg seronegative HCV Ab seropositive Controls	HBsAg seronegative HCV Ab seropositive OR	HBsAg seropositive HCV Ab seronegative Cases	HBsAg seropositive HCV Ab seronegative Controls	HBsAg seropositive HCV Ab seronegative OR	HBsAg seropositive HCV Ab seropositive Cases	HBsAg seropositive HCV Ab seropositive Controls	HBsAg seropositive HCV Ab seropositive OR
First-generation tests											
Yu et al. (1990); USA	24	110	5	5	4.8	12	13	4.4	10	0	∞
Kaklamani et al. (1991); Greece	71	373	29	29	[5.3]	42	29	[7.6]	43	1	[226]
Yu et al. (1991)[a]; China	12	104	5	2	16	101	21	22	9	0	∞
Chuang et al. (1992)[a]; China	16	267	13	8	27	87	104	14	12	5	40
Simonetti et al. (1992); Italy	46	197	133	11	[52]	15	4	[16]	18	0	[∞]
Di Bisceglie et al. (1991a); USA	80	56	12	2	[7.2]	6	0	[∞]	1	0	[∞]
Xu et al. (1990); China	11	46	1	0	∞	35	4	[37]	3	0	∞
Second-generation tests											
Stroffolini et al. (1992); Italy	11	80	38	13	[21]	11	6	[13]	5	0	[∞]
Cordier et al. (1993); Viet Nam	8	194	3	2	38	138	44	[76]	0	0	–
Tanaka et al. (1991); Japan	27	390	45	12	[54]	18	8	[33]	1	0	[∞]
Coursaget et al. (1992); Senegal	23	82	4	0	[∞]	20	50	[1.4]	2	2	[3.6]
Dazza et al. (1993); Mozambique	52	163	8	4	1.4	115	27	[13]	3	0	[∞]

[a]Partially overlapping

hepatic neoplasms interspersed with areas of haemorrhage, necrosis and fibrosis; a smaller tumour (4 × 4 cm) was also seen. Frozen sections of liver stained with a monoclonal antibody against non-A, non-B-infected hepatocytes revealed positive immunostaining, but no specific staining for HBV surface or core antigens was observed. Histological examination of liver tumours revealed trabecular, well-differentiated HCC. The adjacent liver tissue contained hyperplastic nodules and severely dysplastic hepatocytes, as well as chronic hepatitis, characterized by portal inflammation and bile duct proliferation (Linke et al., 1987; Muchmore et al., 1988). [HCV markers were not evaluated.]

4. Other Relevant Data

4.1 Pathology

The putative association between HCV and HCC is based primarily on large epidemiological and serological reviews and not on histological studies of the evolution of carcinoma. The course of HCV includes acute viral hepatitis (usually subclinical) with transition to chronic hepatitis and cirrhosis and to HCC.

4.1.1 Acute infection

Many of the histological features of acute viral hepatitis are common to all four hepatitis viruses (HBV, HCV and hepatitis A and D viruses), and hepatic reactions are similar, so that histological features do not distinguish a specific agent. Some patients with acute hepatitis due to HCV, however, have a milder inflammatory reaction than those with disease due to HBV or hepatitis A virus, and this reaction may resemble infectious mononucleosis. The similarity to mononucleosis is due to sinusoidal inflammatory proliferation and portal lymphoid hyperplasia, without hepatocellular cytopathic change. In follow-up biopsy samples from patients with post-transfusion hepatitis, the hepatocellular changes may be very mild, and a diagnosis of acute viral hepatitis is based on clinical and histological correlation. The histological changes of acute viral hepatitis due to HCV are often mild and include the same inflammatory and hepatocellular degenerative changes seen in acute viral hepatitis due to HBV. Most observations of histopathological changes in acute viral hepatitis were restricted to clinically apparent, icteric cases, which constitute a minority of infections in a population. The majority of cases are therefore not confirmed histologically (Alter, 1990).

4.1.2 Chronic infection

The transition of acute viral hepatitis due to HCV to a progressive form of chronic hepatitis is usually gradual and not easily recognized by clinical or histological criteria. The same histopathological terminology for chronic hepatitis used for HBV has been widely applied to chronic hepatitis due to HCV. In addition, chronic hepatitis due to HCV often has some features not common to HBV, which include: portal lymphoid hyperplasia with germinal follicles, hepatocellular fatty change, bile-duct damage and multinucleated giant cells (Lefkowitch & Apfelbaum, 1989; Lefkowitch et al., 1993). All of these features cannot be diagnosed in a single case. In a follow-up study of chronic post-transfusion non-A, non-B hepatitis, 82% of cases were related to HCV, and a spectrum of hepatic lesions was described, which included chronic active hepatitis and cirrhosis; a few patients had minimal histological changes (Di Bisceglie *et al.*, 1991b). In another series of chronic non-A, non-B hepatitis patients followed for a longer period (3–20 years; mean, 8 years), 75% were due to HCV. Multiple biopsy samples from 24 patients with chronic post-transfusion non-A, non-B hepatitis revealed a spectrum of chronic hepatitis, ranging from mild chronic persistent hepatitis (55%) to chronic active hepatitis with cirrhosis (16%); the other cases were sporadic non-A, non-B hepatitis (Hopf *et al.*, 1990). Kiyosawa *et al.* (1990a) examined 231 patients with chronic non-A, non-B hepatitis and correlated the histological features with time after transfusion. The mean time since transfusion was 10 years for 96 patients with chronic hepatitis, 21.2 years for 81 with cirrhosis and and 29 years for 54 with HCC. Histological and serological data in several of these reports showed slow sequential progression of chronic hepatitis to cirrhosis and HCC.

4.1.3 *Cirrhosis and hepatocellular carcinoma*

The pathogenesis of cirrhosis is described in detail in the monograph on HBV (pp. 114–115). In most of the surveys of chronic hepatitis C, HCC developed in cirrhotic patients and not only in those with early chronic active hepatitis. This point has not been widely studied, but the situation appears to be different from that for HBV.

The transition of regenerative nodules to HCC is also described above. Ferrell *et al.* (1992b) examined 110 sequential explant livers with cirrhosis: 19 livers had 40 distinctive nodules measuring 0.8–3.5 cm. After careful histological examination, 28 were categorized as macroregenerative nodules and 12 as small HCCs. Thirty of the 110 cirrhotic livers were from patients with antibodies to HCV, which was associated with a greater risk for distinctive nodule formation (47%) than for all causes of cirrhosis in the series. Furthermore, patients with cirrhosis who were seropositive for HCV markers had an increased risk for incidental HCC; thus, four of the eight patients with HCC were HCV seropositive.

4.2 Molecular biology

The presence of minus-strand HCV RNA (implying replication) has been demonstrated in HCC and non-tumorous tissue (Gerber *et al.*, 1992; Gerber, 1993). There is at present no experimental evidence that HCV sequences are integrated into the host cell genome or for an HCV coded *trans*-activating protein.

Comparison of the nucleotide and predicted encoded amino acid sequences of HCV isolates in chronically infected chimpanzees suggest that the HCV genome is susceptible to mutations, as has been observed frequently for other RNA viruses (Okamoto *et al.*, 1992b). Genomic mutations of HCV in the course of chronic infections might promote persistence of the virus and its pathogenicity. In chimpanzees inoculated sequentially with different HCV strains derived from five unrelated patients with transfusion-associated non-A, non-B hepatitis, infection did not elicit protective immunity against reinfection with homologous or heterologous strains (Farci *et al.*, 1992b).

4.3 Other observations relevant to possible mechanisms of action of HCV in carcinogenesis

Chimpanzees were originally the primary model for studying the biology of HCV. In eight chimpanzees infected experimentally with HCV, three patterns of hepatitis C viraemia were seen: (i) acute resolving hepatitis with transient appearance of HCV RNA, (ii) chronic hepatitis with persistent HCV RNA and (iii) chronic hepatitis with intermittent appearance of HCV RNA (Abe et al., 1992).

Analysis of serial clinical specimens obtained from chimpanzees infected experimentally with HCV revealed a relatively uniform relationship between peak expression of tissue markers of infection, appearance of HCV RNA in serum and elevated levels of serum ALT. Since the cytoplasmic antigen becomes detectable in infected chimpanzees within one week after inoculation, it was speculated that replication of HCV occurred very early in the incubation phase of hepatitis (Shimizu et al., 1990). In another study (Shindo et al., 1992b), the levels of HCV RNA in both serum and liver samples from champanzees paralleled disease activity, as measured by serum ALT levels. Serum ALT rose two days after inoculation, fell to normal levels between 10 and 14 days and rose to peak values at eight weeks. Serum HCV RNA became detectable by cDNA PCR three days after inoculation, persisted during the increase in serum ALT and was maximal at seven weeks. The first antibodies to appear, at nine weeks, were anti-C33c, directed against epitopes coded by the non-structural 3' region of the genome; anti-C100-3 appeared at 12 weeks and antibody to 5-1-1 antigen shortly thereafter. Approximately 30–75% of the infected chimpanzees developed chronic infections, detected by the presence of genomic and anti-genomic viral sequences in the liver (Abe et al., 1992; Farci et al., 1992a; Hilfenhaus et al., 1992). In the animals that developed chronic infection, both HCV RNA and anti-C100 (as detected in a first-generation test) remained persistently detectable.

5. Summary of Data Reported and Evaluation

5.1 Exposure data

Hepatitis C virus (HCV) is an RNA virus that is distantly related to flaviviruses and pestiviruses. The viral genome is a linear positive-strand RNA molecule about 9.4 kilobases long. It has a single, large open reading frame which encodes a polypeptide precursor of about 3000 amino acids. Viral isolates from different geographical regions display significant genetic diversity; in addition, different HCV genotypes can coexist in infected individuals. HCV infection has been detected only in humans, but the virus can be transmitted experimentally to chimpanzees.

HCV infection can be detected in serum by measuring antibody against HCV or directly measuring HCV RNA in blood. Seropositivity to HCV antibody correlates well with HCV infectivity; second-generation tests involving multiple antigenic epitopes show higher sensitivity and specificity than earlier methods. Measurement of HCV RNA is the most sensitive of the currently available tests and allows specific diagnosis in the early acute phase of infection. Replication of HCV in cell culture has been reported. Virus particles and identification of protective or neutralizing antibodies have not yet been demonstrated.

HCV causes most cases of non-A, non-B, post-transfusion hepatitis and a variable proportion of non-transfusion-associated, community-acquired non-A, non-B hepatitis. In most populations of the world, 0.5–2% of individuals have serological evidence of past or current infection. In most countries, prevalence increase with age in adult life and is approximately equal in men and women. A high prevalence of seropositivity is found in people with blood clotting disorders, in those on renal dialysis and in intravenous drug users. Transmission is mostly parenteral, although the route of infection in a significant proportion of cases of community-acquired infection is unknown. Both sexual and perinatal transmission occur.

The clinical course of acute HCV infection is mostly asymptomatic, but acute infection leads to chronic liver disease in about 50% of symptomatic patients and to liver cirrhosis in about 20% of those with chronic liver disease. Advanced liver disease and its complications may be the first clinical evidence of chronic HCV infection. Immunoprophylaxis for HCV infection is not available.

5.2 Human carcinogenicity data

Infection with HCV, as indicated by the presence of antibodies to HCV in serum, appeared to be associated with an increased risk for hepatocellular carcinoma in two cohorts of patients with chronic liver disease and in one cohort of the general population.

Over 20 case–control studies have evaluated the association between hepatocellular carcinoma and seropositivity for HCV antibodies, measured by either first- or second-generation tests. Odds ratio estimates ranging from 1.3 to 134 were observed in 17 studies in which first-generation tests were used and were significant in 15 of the studies. In six studies in which second-generation tests were used, the estimated odds ratios ranged from 1.1 to 52 and were significant in three of the studies.

In all 11 studies in which it could be evaluated, the risk for hepatocellular carcinoma was greater in subjects who were seropositive for antibodies to HCV and seronegative for hepatitis B surface antigen than in subjects seronegative for both. In the few studies in which the analysis took into account possible confounding of the effects of HCV by other risk factors for hepatocellular carcinoma, such as smoking and alcohol consumption, the association was not materially altered.

5.3 Animal carcinogenicity data

A single chimpanzee inoculated with serum from a human patient with non-A, non-B hepatitis developed chronic hepatitis; hepatocellular carcinoma occurred seven years after the first inoculation. Markers of hepatitis B viral infection were not found; the results of tests for HCV were not reported.

5.4 Other relevant data

HCV can replicate in hepatocellular carcinoma cells, but there is no evidence that DNA sequences are integrated into the host genome. Virtually all cases of HCV-related hepatocellular carcinoma occur in the presence of cirrhosis or significant chronic hepatitis.

5.5 Evaluation[1]

There is *sufficient evidence* in humans for the carcinogenicity of chronic infection with hepatitis C virus.

There is *inadequate evidence* in experimental animals for the carcinogenicity of hepatitis C virus.

Overall evaluation

Chronic infection with hepatitis C virus *is carcinogenic to humans (Group 1)*.

6. References

Aach, R.D., Stevens, C.E., Hollinger, F.B., Mosley, J.W., Peterson, D.A., Taylor, P.E., Johnson, R.G., Barbosa, L.H. & Nemo, G.J. (1991) Hepatitis C virus infection in post-transfusion hepatitis. An analysis with first- and second-generation assays. *New Engl. J. Med.*, 325, 1325–1329

Abb, J. (1991) Prevalence of hepatitis C virus antibodies in hospital personnel. *Zbl. Bakt.*, 274, 543–547

Abe, K., Inchauspe, G., Shikata, T. & Prince, A.M. (1992) Three different patterns of hepatitis C virus infection in chimpanzees. *Hepatology*, 15, 690–695

Aceti, A., Taliani, G., Bruni, R., Di Mauro, G. & Celestino, D. (1992) Hepatitis C virus antibody in Swaziland. *Acta trop.*, 51, 159–161

Agnello, V., Chung, R.T. & Kaplan, L.M. (1992) A role for hepatitis C virus infection in type II cryoglobulinemia. *New Engl. J. Med.*, 327, 1490–1495

Akahane, Y., Aikawa, T., Sugai, Y., Tsuda, F., Okamoto, H. & Mishiro, S. (1992) Transmission of HCV between spouses (Letter to the Editor). *Lancet*, 339, 1059–1060

Akyol, G., Dash, S., Shieh, Y.S.C., Malter, J.S. & Gerber, M.A. (1992) Detection of hepatitis C virus RNA sequences by polymerase chain reaction in fixed liver tissue. *Mod. Pathol.*, 5, 501–504

Albano, A., Pianetti, A., Biffi, M.R., Bruscolini, F., Baffone, W., Albano, V. & Salvaggio, A. (1992) Prevalence of anti-HCV in subjects of various age groups. *Eur. J. Epidemiol.*, 8, 309–311

Alberti, A. (1991) Diagnosis of hepatitis C. Facts and perspectives. *J. Hepatol.*, 12, 279–282

Alberti, A., Morsica, G., Chemello, L., Cavalletto, D., Noventa, F., Pontisso, P. & Ruol, A. (1992) Hepatitis C viraemia and liver disease in symptom-free individuals with anti-HCV. *Lancet*, 340, 697–698

Al Karawi, M.A., Shariq, S., El Shiekh Mohamed, A.R., Saeed, A.A. & Mohamed Ahmed, A.M. (1992) Hepatitis C virus infection in chronic liver disease and hepatocellular carcinoma in Saudi Arabia. *J. Gastroenterol. Hepatol.*, 7, 237–239

Al-Nakib, B., Koshy, A., Kaloui, M., Al-Ramahi, S., Al-Mafti, S., Radhakrishnan, S. & Al-Natib, W. (1992) Hepatitis C virus antibody in Kuwait (Letter to the Editor). *Vox sang.*, 63, 75–76

Al Nasser, M.N., Al Mugeiren, M.A., Assuhaimi, S.A., Obineche, E., Onwabalili, J. & Ramia, S. (1992) Seropositivity to hepatitis C virus in Saudi haemodialysis patients. *Vox sang.*, 62, 94–97

Alter, H.J. (1990) The hepatitis C virus and its relationship to the clinical spectrum of NANB hepatitis. *J. Gastroenterol. Hepatol.*, Suppl. 1, 78–94

---

[1]For definition of the italicized terms, see Preamble, pp. 30–34.

Alter, H.J., Purcell, R.H., Holland, P.V. & Popper, H. (1978) Transmissible agent in non-A, non-B hepatitis. *Lancet*, **i**, 459–463

Alter, M.J., Gerety, R.J., Smallwood, L.A., Sampliner, R.E., Tabor, E., Deinhardt, F., Frösner, G. & Matanoski, G.M. (1982) Sporadic non-A, non-B hepatitis: frequency and epidemiology in an urban US population. *J. infect. Dis.*, **145**, 886–893

Alter, H.J., Purcell, R.H., Shih, J.W., Melpolder, J.C., Houghton, M., Choo, Q.-L. & Kuo, G. (1989) Detection of antibody to hepatitis C virus in prospectively followed transfusion recipients with acute and chronic non-A, non-B hepatitis. *New Engl. J. Med.*, **321**, 1494–1500

Alter, M.J., Coleman, P.J., Alexander, W.J., Kramer, E., Miller, J.K., Mandel, E., Hadler, S.C. & Margolis, H.S. (1989) Importance of heterosexual activity in the transmission of hepatitis B and non-A, non-B hepatitis. *J. Am. med. Assoc.*, **262**, 1201–1205

Alter, M.J., Margolis, H.S., Krawczynski, K., Judson, F.N., Mares, A., Alexander, W.J., Hu, P.Y., Miller, J.K., Gerber, M.A., Sampliner, R.E., Meeks, E.L. & Beach, M.J. (1992) The natural history of community-acquired hepatitis C in the United States. *New Engl. J. Med.*, **327**, 1899–1905

Amitrano, L., Ascione, A., Canestrini, C., D'Agostino, S., Iaccarino, L., Vacca, C. & Gigliotti, T. (1990) Prevalence of antibody to hepatitis C virus (anti-HCV) in chronic liver diseases (CLD) in southern Italy. *Ital. J. Gastroenterol.*, **22**, 16–18

Anand, C.M., Fonseca, K., Walle, R.P., Powell, S. & Williams, M. (1992) Antibody to hepatitis C virus in selected groups of a Canadian urban population. *Int. J. Epidemiol.*, **21**, 142–145

Anon. (1975) Non-A, non-B? (Editorial) *Lancet*, **ii**, 64–65

Archer, G.T., Buring, M.L., Clark, B., Ismay, S.L., Kenrick, K.G., Pususothaman, K., Kaldor, J.M., Bolton, W.V. & Wylie, B.R. (1992) Prevalence of hepatitis C virus antibodies in Sydney blood donors. *Med. J. Aust.*, **157**, 225–227

Aussel, L., Denis, F., Ranger, S., Martin, P., Caillaud, M., Alain, J., Baudet, J. & Tabaste, J.L. (1991) Search for antibodies to hepatitis C virus in pregnant foreign women living in France. *Pathol. Biol.*, **39**, 991–996 (in French)

Bahakim, H.M., Bakir, T.M.F., Arif, M. & Ramia, S. (1991) Response to comment by Bernvil *et al.* (Letter to the Editor). *Vox sang.*, **61**, 280

Baur, M., Hay, U., Novacek, G., Dittrich, C. & Ferenci, P. (1992) Prevalence of antibodies to hepatitis C virus in patients with hepatocellular carcinoma in Austria. *Arch. Virol.*, **Suppl. 4**, 76–80

Beach, M.J., Meeks, E.L., Mimms, L.T., Vallari, D., DuCharme, L., Spelbring, J., Taskar, S., Schleicher, J.B., Krawczynski, K. & Bradley, D.W. (1992) Temporal relationships of hepatitis C virus RNA and antibody responses following experimental infection of chimpanzees. *J. med. Virol.*, **36**, 226–237

Bell, J., Batey, R.G., Farrell, G.C., Crewe, E.B., Cunningham, A.L. & Byth, K. (1990) Hepatitis C virus in intravenous drug users. *Med. J. Aust.*, **153**, 274–276

Belli, L.S., Alberti, A., Rondinara, G.F., De Carlis, L., Romani, F., Ideo, G. & Belli, L. (1993) Recurrent HCV hepatitis after liver transplantation (Letter to the Editor). *Lancet*, **341**, 378–379

Benvegnù, L., Cavalletto, D., Ruvoletto, M.G. & Alberti, A. (1991) Specificity and patterns of antibodies to hepatitis C virus in hepatocellular carcinoma (Letter to the Editor). *Hepatology*, **14**, 959

Bernvil, S.S., Andrews, V.J. & Kariem, A.A. (1991) Hepatitis C antibody prevalence in Saudi Arabian blood donor population. *Ann. Saudi Med.*, **11**, 563–567

Black, M. & Peters, M. (1992) Alpha-interferon treatment of chronic hepatitis C: need for accurate diagnosis in selecting patients. *Ann. intern. Med.*, **116**, 86–88

Blackmore, T.K., Maddocks, P., Stace, N.H. & Hatfield, P. (1992) Prevalence of antibodies to hepatitis C virus in patients receiving renal replacement therapy, and in the staff caring for them. *Aust. N.Z. J. Med.*, **22**, 353–357

van Bohman, R., Stettler, R.W., Little, B.B., Wendel, G.D., Sutor, L.J. & Cunningham, F.G. (1992) Seroprevalence and risk factors for hepatitis C virus antibody in pregnant women. *Obstet. Gynaecol.*, **80**, 609–613

Boonmar, S., Pojanagaroon, B., Watanabe, Y., Tanaka, Y., Saito, I. & Miyamura, T. (1990) Prevalence of hepatitis C virus antibody among healthy blood donors and non-A, non-B hepatitis patients in Thailand. *Jpn. J. med. Sci. Biol.*, **43**, 29–36

Boyer, N., Marcellin, P., Degott, C., Degos, F., Saimot, A.G., Erlinger, S., Benhamou, J.P. & the 'Comité des Anti-viraux' (1992) Recombinant interferon-alpha for chronic hepatitis C in patients positive for antibody to human immunodeficiency virus. *J. infect. Dis.*, **165**, 723–726

Bradley, D.W., Cook, E.H., Maynard, J.E., McCaustland, K.A., Ebert, J.W., Dolana, G.H., Petzel, R.A., Kantor, R.J., Heilbrunn, A., Fields, H.A. & Murphy, B.L. (1979) Experimental infection of chimpanzees with anti-hemophilic (factor VIII) materials: recovery of virus-like particles associated with with non-A, non-B hepatitis. *J. med. Virol.*, **3**, 253–269

Bradley, D.W., Krawczynski, K., Ebert, J.W., McCaustland, K.A., Choo, Q.-L., Houghton, M. & Kuo, G. (1990) Parenterally transmitted non-A, non-B hepatitis: virus-specific antibody response patterns in hepatitis C virus-infected chimpanzees. *Gastroenterology*, **99**, 1054–1060

Bresters, D., Cuypers, H.T.M., Reesink, H.W., Chamuleau, R.A.F.M., Schipper, M.E.I., Boeser-Nunnink, B.D.M., Lelie, P.N. & Jansen, P.L.M. (1992) Detection of hepatitis C viral RNA sequences in fresh and paraffin-embedded liver biopsy specimens of non-A, non-B hepatitis patients. *J. Hepatol.*, **15**, 391–395

Brettler, D.B., Alter, H.J., Dienstag, J.L., Forsberg, A.D. & Levine, P.H. (1990) Prevalence of hepatitis C virus antibody in a cohort of hemophilia patients. *Blood*, **76**, 254–256

Brugnano, R., Francisci, D., Quintaliani, G., Gaburri, M., Nori, G., Verdura, C., Giombini, L. & Buoncristiani, U. (1992) Antibodies against hepatitis C virus in hemodialysis patients in the central Italian region of Umbria: evaluation of risk factors. *Nephron*, **61**, 263–265

Bruix, J., Calvet, X., Costa, J., Ventura, M., Bruguera, M., Castillo, R., Barrera, J.M., Ercilla, G., Sanchez-Tapias, J.M., Vall, M., Bru, C. & Rodes, J. (1989) Prevalence of antibodies to hepatitis C virus in Spanish patients with hepatocellular carcinoma and hepatic cirrhosis. *Lancet*, **ii**, 1004–1006

Bukh, J., Miller, R.H., Kew, M.C. & Purcell, R.H. (1993) Hepatitis C virus RNA in southern African blacks with hepatocellular carcinoma. *Proc. natl Acad. Sci. USA*, **90**, 1848–1851

Calabrese, G., Vagelli, G., Guaschino, R. & Gonella, M. (1991) Transmission of anti-HCV within the household of haemodialysis patients (Letter to the Editor). *Lancet*, **ii**, 1466

Caporaso, N., Romano, M., Marmo, R., de Sio, I., Morisco, F., Minerva, A. & Coltorti, M. (1991) Hepatitis C virus infection is an additive risk factor for development of hepatocellular carcinoma in patients with cirrhosis. *J. Hepatol.*, **12**, 367–371

Carreño, V., Tapia, L., Ryff, J.-C., Quiroga, J.A. & Castillo, I. (1992) Treatment of chronic hepatitis C by continuous subcutaneous infusion of interferon-alpha. *J. med. Virol.*, **37**, 215–219

Caspari, G., Beyer, J., Richter, K., Gerlich, W.H. & Schmitt, H. (1991) Prevalence of antibodies to recombinant hepatitis C virus protein C100-3 and of elevated transaminase levels in blood donors from northern Germany. *Med. Microbiol. Immunol.*, **180**, 261–272

Cha, T.-A., Beall, E., Irvine, B., Kolberg, J., Chien, D., Kuo, G. & Urdea, M.S. (1992) At least five related, but distinct, hepatitis C viral genotypes exist. *Proc. natl Acad. Sci. USA*, **89**, 7144–7148

Chan, G.C.B., Lim, W. & Yeoh, E.K. (1992) Prevalence of hepatitis C infection in Hong Kong. *J. Gastroenterol. Hepatol.*, **7**, 117–120

Chan, S.-W., McOmish, F., Holmes, E.C., Dow, B., Peutherer, J.F., Follett, E., Yap, P.L. & Simmonds, P. (1992) Analysis of a new hepatitis C virus type and its phylogenetic relationship to existing variants. *J. gen. Virol.*, **73**, 1131–1141

Chaudhary, R.K., Perry, E., Hicks, F., MacLean, C. & Morbey, M. (1992) Hepatitis B and C infection in an institution of the developmentally handicapped (Letter to the Editor). *New Engl. J. Med.*, **327**, 1953

Chen, P.-J., Lin, M.-H., Tai, K.-F., Liu, P.-C., Lin, C.-J. & Chen, D.-S. (1992) The Taiwanese hepatitis C virus genome: sequence determination and mapping of the 5' termini of viral genomic and antigenomic RNA. *Virology*, **188**, 102–113

Chiba, J., Ohba, H., Matsuura, Y., Watanabe, Y., Katayama, T., Kikuchi, S., Saito, I. & Miyamura, T. (1991) Serodiagnosis of hepatitis C virus (HCV) infection with an HCV core protein molecularly expressed by a recombinant baculovirus. *Proc. natl Acad. Sci. USA*, **88**, 4641–4645

Chien, D.Y., Choo, Q.-L., Tabrizi, A., Kuo, C., McFarland, J., Berger, K., Lee, C., Shuster, J.R., Nguyen, T., Moyer, D.L., Tong, M., Furuta, S., Omata, M., Tegtmeier, G., Alter, H., Schiff, E., Jeffers, L., Houghton, M. & Kuo, G. (1992) Diagnosis of hepatitis C virus (HCV) infection using an immunodominant chimeric polyprotein to capture circulating antibodies: reevaluation of the role of HCV in liver disease. *Proc. natl Acad. Sci. USA*, **89**, 10011–10015

Choo, Q.-L., Kuo, G., Weiner, A.J., Overby, L.R., Bradley, D.W. & Houghton, M. (1989) Isolation of a cDNA clone derived from a blood-borne non-A, non-B viral hepatitis genome. *Science*, **244**, 359–362

Choo, Q.-L., Richman, K.H., Han, J.H., Berger, K., Lee, C., Dong, C., Gallegos, C., Coit, D., Medina-Selby, A., Barr, P.J., Weiner, A.J., Bradley, D.W., Kuo, G. & Houghton, M. (1991) Genetic organization and diversity of the hepatitis C virus. *Proc. natl Acad. Sci. USA*, **88**, 2451–2455

Chuang, W.-L., Chang, W.-Y., Lu, S.-N., Su, W.-P., Lin, Z.-Y., Chen, S.-C., Hsieh, M.-Y., Wang, L.-Y., You, S.-L. & Chen, C.-J. (1992) The role of hepatitis B and C viruses in hepatocellular carcinoma in a hepatitis B endemic area: a case–control study. *Cancer*, **69**, 2052–2054

Claeys, H., Volckaerts, A., De Beenhouwer, H. & Vermylen, C. (1992) Association of hepatitis C virus carrier state with the occurrence of hepatitis C virus core antibodies. *J. med. Virol.*, **36**, 259–264

Colombo, M., Rumi, M.G., Gringeri, A. & Mannucci, P.M. (1988) Etiology and outcome of chronic viral hepatitis in multitranfused hemophilic patients. In: Gentilini, P. & Dianzani, M.U., eds, *Pathophysiology of the Liver*, Amsterdam, Elsevier, pp. 73–79

Colombo, M., Kuo, G., Choo, Q.L., Donato, M.F., Del Ninno, E., Tommasini, M.A., Dioguardi, N. & Houghton, M. (1989) Prevalence of antibodies to hepatitis C virus in Italian patients with hepatocellular carcinoma. *Lancet*, **ii**, 1006–1008

Cordier, S., Thuy, Le Thi Bich, Verger, P., Bard, D., Dai, Le Cao, Larouze, B., Dazza, M.C., Quinh, Hoang Trong & Abenhaim, L. (1993) Risk factors for hepatocellular carcinoma in Vietnam. *Int. J. Epidemiol.*, **55**, 196–201

Corona, R., Prignano, G., Mele, A., Gentili, G., Caprilli, F., Franco, E., Ferrigno, L., Giglio, A., Titti, F., Bruno, C., Verani, P. & Pasquini, P. (1991) Heterosexual and homosexual transmission of hepatitis C virus: relation with hepatitis B virus and human immunodeficiency virus type 1. *Epidemiol. Infect.*, **107**, 667–672

Coursaget, P., Bourdil, C., Kastally, R., Yvonnet, B., Rampanarivo, Z., Chiron, J.-P., Bao, O., Diop-Mar, I., Perrin, J. & Ntarème, F. (1990) Prevalence of hepatitis C virus infection in Africa: anti-HCV antibodies in the general population and in patients suffering from cirrhosis or primary liver cancer. *Res. Virol.*, **141**, 449–454

Coursaget, P., Leboulleux, D., Le Cann, P., Bao, O. & Coll-Seck, A.M. (1992) Hepatitis C virus infection in cirrhosis and primary hepatocellular carcinoma in Senegal. *Trans. R. Soc. trop. Med. Hyg.*, **86**, 552–553

Czaja, A.J. (1992) Chronic hepatitis C virus infection—a disease in waiting? *New Engl. J. Med.*, **327**, 1949–1950

Dal-Ré, R., Aguilar, L. & Coronel, P. (1991) Current prevalence of hepatitis B, A and C in a healthy Spanish population. A seroepidemiological study. *Infection*, **19**, 409–413

Davis, G.L. (1989) Interferon treatment of viral hepatitis in immunocompromised patients. *Semin. Liver Dis.*, **9**, 267–272

Davis, G.L., Balart, L.A., Schiff, E.R., Lindsay, K., Bodenheimer, H.C., Jr, Perrillo, R.P., Carey, W., Jacobson, I.M., Payne, J., Dienstag, J.L., Van Thiel, D.H., Tamburro, C., Lefkowitch, J., Albrecht, J., Meschievitz, C., Ortego, T.J., Gibas, A. & the Hepatitis Interventional Therapy Group (1989) Treatment of chronic hepatitis C with recombinant interferon alfa. A multicenter randomized, controlled trial. *New Engl. J. Med.*, **321**, 1501–1506

Dazza, M.-C., Valdemar Meneses, L., Girard, P.-M., Astagneau, P., Villaroel, C., Delaporte, E. & Larouze, B. (1993) Absence of a relationship between antibodies to hepatitis C virus and hepatocellular carcinoma in Mozambique. *J. trop. Med. Hyg.*, **48**, 237–242

De Luca, M., Ascione, A., Canestrini, C., Di Costanzo, G.G., Galeota Lanza, A., Guardascione, M.A., Gallo, M.L., Perrotti, G.P., Samaritani, C.M., Utech, W., Iaccarino, L., Vacca, C., Pietroluongo, E., Schiano, S., Tarsitano, P. & Zarone, A. (1991) Prevalence of antibody to hepatitis C virus in hospital personnel. *Minerva Gastroenterol. Dietol.*, **37**, 141–149 (in Italian)

De Luca, M., Ascione, A., Vacca, C. & Zarone, A. (1992) Are health-care workers really at risk of HCV infection? (Letter to the Editor) *Lancet*, **339**, 1364–1365

Deny, P., Bonacorsi, S., Guillevin, L. & Quint, L. (1992) Association between hepatitis C virus and polyarteritis nodosa (Letter to the Editor). *Clin. exp. Rheumatol.*, **10**, 319

Develoux, M., Meynard, D. & Delaporte, E. (1992) Low rate of hepatitis C virus antibodies in blood donors and pregnant women from Niger. *Trans. R. Soc. trop. Med. Hyg*, **86**, 553

Diamantis, I.D., McGandy, C.E., Pult, I., Widmann, J.-J., Gudat, F. & Bianchi L. (1992) Detection of hepatitis C virus RNA in liver needle biopsies by polymerase chain reaction. *J. Hepatol.*, **14**, 405–406

Di Bisceglie, A.M., Martin, P., Kassianides, C., Lisker-Melman, M., Murray, L., Waggoner, J., Goodman, Z., Banks, S.M. & Hoofnagle, J.H. (1989) Recombinant interferon alfa therapy for chronic hepatitis C. A randomized, double-blind, placebo-controlled trial. *New Engl. J. Med.*, **321**, 1506–1510

Di Bisceglie, A.M., Order, S.E., Klein, J.L., Waggoner, J.G., Sjogren, M.H., Kuo, G., Houghton, M., Choo, Q.-L. & Hoofnagle, J.H. (1991a) The role of chronic viral hepatitis in hepatocellular carcinoma in the United States. *Am. J. Gastroenterol.*, **86**, 335–338

Di Bisceglie, A.M., Goodman, Z.D., Ishak, K.G., Hoofnagle, J.H., Melpolder, J.J. & Alter, H.J. (1991b) Long-term clinical and histopathological follow-up of chronic posttransfusion hepatitis. *Hepatology*, **14**, 969–974

Di Bisceglie, A.M., Shindo, M., Fong, T.-L., Fried, M.W., Swain, M.G., Bergasa, N.V., Axiotis, C.A., Waggoner, J.G., Park, Y. & Hoofnagle, J.H. (1992) A pilot study of ribavirin therapy for chronic hepatitis C. *Hepatology*, **16**, 649–654

Donahue, J.G., Nelson, K.E., Muñoz, A., Vlahov, D., Rennie, L.L., Taylor, E.L., Saal, A.J., Cohn, S., Odaka, N.J. & Farzadegan, H. (1991) Antibody to hepatitis C virus among cardiac surgery patients, homosexual men and intravenous drug users in Baltimore, Maryland. *Am. J. Epidemiol.*, **134**, 1206–1211

El-Ashmawy, L., Hassanein, T., Gavaler, J.S. & Van Thiel, D.H. (1992) Prevalence of hepatitis C virus antibody in a liver transplantation population. *Dig. Dis. Sci.*, **37**, 1110–1115

Enomoto, N., Takada, A., Nakao, T. & Date, T. (1990) There are two major types of hepatitis C virus in Japan. *Biochem. biophys. Res. Commun.*, **170**, 1021–1025

Esteban, J.I., Esteban, R., Viladomiu, L., López-Talavera, J.C., González, A., Hernández, J.M., Roget, M., Vargas, V., Genescà, J., Buti, M., Guardia, J., Houghton, M., Choo, Q.-L. & Kuo, G. (1989) Hepatitis C virus antibodies among risk groups in Spain. *Lancet*, **ii**, 294–297

Fabrizi, F., Di Filippo, S., Erba, G., Bacchini, G., Marcelli, D., Pontoriero, G., Crepaldi, M. & Locatelli, F. (1992) Hepatitis C virus infection and hepatic function in chronic hemodialysis patients (Letter to the Editor). *Nephron*, **61**, 119

Fairley, C.K., Leslie, D.E., Nicholson, S. & Gust, I.D. (1990) Epidemiology and hepatitis C virus in Victoria. *Med. J. Aust.*, **153**, 271–273

Farci, P., Alter, H.J., Wong, D., Miller, R.H., Shih, J.W., Jett, B. & Purcell, R.H. (1991) A long-term study of hepatitis C virus replication in non-A, non-B hepatitis. *New Engl. J. Med.*, **325**, 98–104

Farci, P., London, W.T., Wong, D.C., Dawson, G.J., Vallari, D.S., Engle, R. & Purcell, R.H. (1992a) The natural history of infection with hepatitis C virus (HCV) in chimpanzees: comparison of serologic responses measured with first- and second-generation assays and relationship to HCV viremia. *J. infect. Dis.*, **165**, 1006–1011

Farci, P., Alter, H.J., Govindarajan, S., Wong, D.C., Engle, R., Lesniewski, R.R., Mushahwar, I.K., Desai, S.M., Miller, R.H., Ogata, N. & Purcell, R.H. (1992b) Lack of protective immunity against reinfection with hepatitis C virus. *Science*, **258**, 135–140

Fargion, S., Piperno, A., Cappellini, M.D., Sampietro, M., Fracanzani, A.L., Romano, R., Caldarelli, R., Marcelli, R., Vecchi, L. & Fiorelli, G. (1992) Hepatitis C virus and porphyria cutanea tarda: evidence of a strong association. *Hepatology*, **16**, 1322–1326

Farinati, F., Fagiuoli, S., De Maria, N., Chiaramonte, M., Aneloni, V., Ongaro, S., Salvagnini, M. & Naccarato, R. (1992) Anti-HCV positive hepatocellular carcinoma in cirrhosis: prevalence, risk factors and clinical features. *J. Hepatol.*, **14**, 183–187

Féray, C., Samuel, D., Thiers, V., Gigou, M., Pichon, F., Bismuth, A., Reynes, M., Maisonneuve, P., Bismuth, H. & Bréchot, C. (1992) Reinfection of liver graft by hepatitis C virus after liver transplantation. *J. clin. Invest.*, **89**, 1361–1365

Féray, C., Gigou, M., Samuel, D., Reyes, G., Bernuau, J., Reynes, M., Bismuth, H. & Bréchot, C. (1993) Hepatitis C virus RNA and hepatitis B virus DNA in serum and liver of patients with fulminant hepatitis. *Gastroenterology*, **104**, 549–555

Ferrell, L.D., Wright, T.L., Roberts, J., Ascher, N. & Lake, J. (1992a) Hepatitis C viral infection in liver transplant recipients. *Hepatology*, **16**, 865–876

Ferrell, L.D., Wright, T., Lake, J., Roberts, J. & Ascher, N. (1992b) Incidence and diagnostic features of macroregenerative nodules vs. small hepatocellular carcinoma in cirrhotic livers. *Hepatology*, **16**, 1372–1381

Fong, T.-L., Shindo, M., Feinstone, S.M., Hoofnagle, J.H. & Di Bisceglie, A.M. (1991) Detection of replicative intermediates of hepatitis C viral RNA in liver and serum of patients with chronic hepatitis C. *J. clin. Invest.*, **88**, 1058–1060

Fried, M.W., Shindo, M., Fong, T.-L., Fox, P.C., Hoofnagle, J.H. & Di Bisceglie, A.M. (1992) Absence of hepatitis C viral RNA from saliva and semen of patients with chronic hepatitis C. *Gastroenterology*, **102**, 1306–1308

Fuchs, K., Motz, M., Schreier, E., Zachoval, R., Deinhardt, F. & Roggendorf, M. (1991) Characterization of nucleotide sequences from European hepatitis C virus isolates. *Gene*, **103**, 163–169

Fujiyama, S., Kawano, S., Sato, S., Tanaka, M., Goto, M., Taura, Y., Sato, T., Kawahara, T. & Mizuno, K. (1992) Prevalence of hepatitis C virus antibodies in hemodialysis patients and dialysis staff. *Hepato-gastroenterology*, **39**, 161–165

Garson, J.A., Brillanti, S., Ring, C., Perini, P., Miglioli, M. & Barbara, L. (1992a) Hepatitis C viraemia rebound after 'successful' interferon therapy in patients with chronic non-A, non-B hepatitis. *J. med. Virol.*, **37**, 210–214

Garson, J.A., Wicki, A.N., Ring, C.J.A., Joller, H., Zala, G., Schmid, M. & Buehler, H. (1992b) Detection of hepatitis C viraemia in Caucasian patients with hepatocellular carcinoma. *J. med. Virol.*, **38**, 152–156

Gasparini, V., Chiaramonte, M., Moschen, M.E., Fabris, P., Altinier, G., Majori, S., Campello, C. & Trivello, R. (1991) Hepatitis C virus infection in homosexual men: a seroepidemiological study in gay clubs in north-east Italy. *Eur. J. Epidemiol.*, **7**, 665–669

Gerber, M.A. (1993) Relation of hepatitis C virus to hepatocellular carcinoma. *J. Hepatol.*, **17** (Suppl. 3), S108–S111

Gerber, M.A., Shieh, Y.S.C., Shim, K.-S., Thung, S.N., Demetris, A.J., Schwartz, M., Akyol, G. & Dash, S. (1992) Short communication. Detection of replicative hepatitis C virus sequences in hepatocellular carcinoma. *Am. J. Pathol.*, **141**, 1271–1277

Girardi, E., Zaccarelli, M., Tossini, G., Puro, V., Narciso, P. & Visco, G. (1990) Short communication. Hepatitis C virus infection in intravenous drug users: prevalence and risk factors. *Scand. J. infect. Dis.*, **22**, 751–752

Goodrick, M.J., Anderson, N.A.B., Fraser, I.D., Rouse, A. & Pearson, V. (1992) History of previous drug misuse in HCV-positive blood donors (Letter to the Editor). *Lancet*, **339**, 502

Greenwood, B.M. & Whittle, H.C. (1981) *Immunology of Medicine in the Tropics. Current Topics in Immunology*, London, E. Arnold

Gutierrez, P., Orduña, A., Bratos, M.A., Eiros, J.M., Gonzalez, J.M., Almaraz, A., Caro-Patón, A. & Rodríguez-Torres, A. (1992) Prevalence of anti-hepatitis C virus antibodies in positive FTA-ABS non-drug abusing female prostitutes in Spain. *Sex. Transmitted Dis.*, January–February, 39–40

Haddad, J., Deny, P., Munz-Gotheil, C., Ambrosini, J.-C., Trinchet, J.-C., Pateron, D., Mal, F., Callard, P. & Beaugrand, M. (1992) Lymphocytic sialadenitis of Sjøgren's syndrome associated with chronic hepatitis C virus liver disease. *Lancet*, **339**, 321–323

Hagiwara, H., Hayashi, N., Mita, E., Hiramatsu, N., Ueda, K., Takehara, T., Yuki, N., Kasahara, A., Fusamoto, H. & Kamada, T. (1992) Detection of hepatitis C virus RNA in chronic non-A, non-B liver disease. *Gastroenterology*, **102**, 692–694

Hagiwara, H., Hayashi, N., Mita, E., Takehara, T., Kasahara, A., Fusamoto, H. & Kamada, T. (1993) Quantitative analysis of hepatitis C virus RNA in serum during interferon alfa therapy. *Gastroenterology*, **104**, 877–883

Han, J.H., Shyamala, V., Richman, K.H., Brauer, M.J., Irvine, B., Urdea, M.S., Tekamp-Olson, P., Kuo, G., Choo, Q.-L. & Houghton, M. (1991) Characterization of the terminal regions of hepatitis C viral RNA: identification of conserved sequences in the 5' untranslated region and poly(A) tails at the 3' end. *Proc. natl Acad. Sci. USA*, **88**, 1711-1715

Harada, S., Watanabe, Y., Takeuchi, K., Suzuki, T., Katayama, T., Takebe, Y., Saito, I. & Miyamura, T. (1991) Expression of processed core protein of hepatitis C virus in mammalian cells. *J. Virol.*, **65**, 3015-3021

Hasan, F., Jeffers, L.J., De Medina, M., Reddy, K.R., Parker, T., Schiff, E.R., Houghton, M., Choo, Q. & Kuo, G. (1990) Hepatitis C-associated hepatocellular carcinoma. *Hepatology*, **12**, 589-591

Hay, C.R.M., Preston, F.E., Triger, D.R. & Underwood, J.C.E. (1985) Progressive liver disease in haemophilia: an understated problem? *Lancet*, **i**, 1495-1498

Herbert, A.-M., Walker, D.M., Davies, K.J. & Bagg, J. (1992) Occupationally acquired hepatitis C virus infection (Letter to the Editor). *Lancet*, **339**, 305

Hijikata, M., Kato, N., Ootsuyama, Y., Nakagawa, M., Ohkoshi, S. & Shimotohno, K. (1991) Hypervariable regions in the putative glycoprotein of hepatitis C virus. *Biochem. biophys. Res. Commun.*, **175**, 220-228

Hilfenhaus, J., Krupka, U., Nowak, T., Cummins, L.B., Fuchs, K. & Roggendorf, M. (1992) Follow-up of hepatitis C virus infection in chimpanzees: determination of viraemia and specific humoral immune response. *J. gen. Virol.*, **73**, 1015-1019

Hiramatsu, N., Hayashi, N., Haruna, Y., Kasahara, A., Fusamoto, H., Mori, C., Fuke, I., Okayama, H. & Kamada, T. (1992) Immunohistochemical detection of hepatitis C virus-infected hepatocytes in chronic liver disease with monoclonal antibodies to core, envelope and NS3 regions of the hepatitis C virus genome. *Hepatology*, **16**, 306-311

van den Hoek, J.A.R., van Haastrecht, H.J.A., Goudsmith, J., de Wolf, F. & Coutinho, R.A. (1990) Prevalence, incidence and risk factors of hepatitis C virus infection among drug users in Amsterdam. *J. infect. Dis.*, **162**, 823-826

Hopf, U., Möller, B., Küther, D., Stemerowicz, R., Lobeck, H., Lüdtke-Handjery, A., Walter, E., Blum, H.E., Roggendorf, M. & Deinhardt, F. (1990) Long-term follow-up of posttransfusion and sporadic chronic hepatitis non-A, non-B and frequency of circulating antibodies to hepatitis C virus (HCV). *J. Hepatol.*, **10**, 69-76

Hosoda, K., Omata, M., Yokosuka, O., Kato, N. & Ohto M. (1992) Non-A, non-B chronic hepatitis is chronic hepatitis C: a sensitive assay for detection of hepatitis C virus RNA in the liver. *Hepatology*, **15**, 777-781

Houghton, M., Weiner, A., Han, J., Kuo, G. & Choo, Q.-L. (1991) Molecular biology of the hepatitis C viruses: implications for diagnosis, development and control of viral disease. *Hepatology*, **14**, 381-388

Hsieh, T.-T., Yao, D.-S., Sheen, I.-S., Liaw, Y.-F. & Pao, C.C. (1992) Hepatitis C virus in peripheral blood mononuclear cells. *Am. J. clin. Pathol.*, **98**, 392-396

Hyams, K.C., Phillips, I.A., Moran, A.Y., Tejada, A., Wignall, F.S. & Escamilla, J. (1992) Seroprevalence of hepatitis C antibody in Peru. *J. med. Virol.*, **37**, 127-131

Inchauspé, G., Zebedee, S., Lee, D.-H., Sugitani, M., Nasoff, M. & Prince, A.M. (1991) Genomic structure of the human prototype strain H of hepatitis C virus: comparison with American and Japanese isolates. *Proc. natl Acad. Sci. USA*, **88**, 10292-10296

Inoue, Y., Miyamura, T., Unayama, T., Takahashi, K. & Saito, I. (1991) Maternal transfer of HCV (Letter to the Editor). *Nature*, **353**, 609

Ito, S.-I., Ito, M., Cho, M.-J., Shimotohno, K. & Tajima, K. (1991) Massive sero-epidemiological survey of hepatitis C virus: clustering of carriers on the southwest coast of Tsushima, Japan. *Jpn. J. Cancer Res.*, **82**, 1–3

Japanese Red Cross Non-A, Non-B Hepatitis Research Group (1991) Effect of screening for hepatitis C virus antibody and hepatitis B virus core antibody on incidence of post-transfusion hepatitis. *Lancet*, **338**, 1040–1041

Jeng, J.-E. & Tsai, J.-F. (1991) Hepatitis C virus antibody in hepatocellular carcinoma in Taiwan. *J. med. Virol.*, **34**, 74–77

Jochen, A.B.B. (1992) Occupationally acquired hepatitis C virus infection (Letter to the Editor). *Lancet*, **339**, 304

Johnson, R.J., Gretch, D.R., Yamabe, H., Hart, J., Bacchi, C.E., Hartwell, P., Couser, W.G., Corey, L., Wener, M.H., Alpers, C.E. & Willson, R. (1993) Membranoproliferative glomerulonephritis associated with hepatitis C virus infection. *New Engl. J. Med.*, **328**, 465–470

Kaklamani, E., Trichopoulos, D., Tzonou, A., Zavitsanos, X., Koumantaki, Y., Hatzakis, A., Hsieh, C.C. & Hatziyannis, S. (1991) Hepatitis B and C viruses and their interaction in the origin of hepatocellular carcinoma. *J. Am. med. Assoc.*, **265**, 1974–1976

Kaldor, J.M., Archer, G.T., Buring, M.L., Ismay, S.L., Kenrick, K.G., Lien, A.S.M., Purusothaman, K., Tulloch, R., Bolton, W.V. & Wylie, B.R. (1992) Risk factors for hepatitis C virus infection in blood donors: a case–control study. *Med. J. Aust.*, **157**, 227–230

Kanai, K., Kako, M. & Okamoto, H. (1992) HCV genotypes in chronic hepatitis C and response to interferon (Letter to the Editor). *Lancet*, **339**, 1543

Kato, N., Hijikata, M., Ootsuyama, Y., Nakagawa, M., Ohkoshi, S., Sugimura, T. & Shimotohno, K. (1990) Molecular cloning of the human hepatitis C virus genome from Japanese patients with non-A, non-B hepatitis. *Proc. natl Acad. Sci. USA*, **87**, 9524–9528

Kelen, G.D., Green, G.B., Purcell, R.H., Chan, D.W., Qaqish, B.F., Sivertson, K.T. & Quinn, T.C. (1992) Hepatitis B and hepatitis C in emergency department patients. *New Engl. J. Med.*, **326**, 1399–1404

Kew, M.C., Houghton, M., Choo, Q.L. & Kuo, G. (1990) Hepatitis C virus antibodies in southern African blacks with hepatocellular carcinoma. *Lancet*, **335**, 873–874

Kiyosawa, K. & Furuta, S. (1992) Clinical aspects and epidemiology of hepatitis B and C viruses in hepatocellular carcinoma in Japan. *Cancer Chemother. Pharmacol.*, **31** (Suppl. 1), S150–S156

Kiyosawa, K., Sodeyama, T., Tanaka, E., Gibo, Y., Yoshizawa, K., Nakano, Y., Furuta, S., Akahane, Y., Nishioka, K., Purcell, R.H. & Alter, H.J. (1990a) Interrelationship of blood transfusion, non-A, non-B hepatitis and hepatocellular carcinoma: analysis by detection of antibody to hepatitis C virus. *Hepatology*, **12**, 671–675

Kiyosawa, K., Tanaka, E., Sodeyama, T., Furuta, K., Usuda, S., Yousuf, M. & Furuta, S. (1990b) Transition of antibody to hepatitis C virus from chronic hepatitis to hepatocellular carcinoma. *Jpn. J. Cancer Res.*, **81**, 1089–1091

Kiyosawa, K., Sodeyama, T., Tanaka, E., Nakano, Y., Furuta, S., Nishioka, K., Purcell, R.H. & Alter, H.J. (1991) Hepatitis C in hospital employees with needlestick injuries. *Ann. intern. Med.*, **115**, 367–369

Klein, R.S., Freeman, K., Taylor, P.E. & Stevens, C.E. (1991) Occupational risk for hepatitis C virus infection among New York City dentists. *Lancet*, **338**, 1539–1542

Koonin, E.V. (1991) The phylogeny of RNA-dependent RNA polymerases of positive-strand RNA viruses. *J. gen. Virol.*, **72**, 2197–2206

Kotwal, G.J., Baroudy, B.M., Kuramoto, I.K., McDonald, F.F., Schiff, G.M., Holland, P.V. & Zeldis, J.B. (1992a) Detection of acute hepatitis C virus infection by ELISA using a synthetic peptide comprising a structural epitope. *Proc. natl Acad. Sci. USA*, **89**, 4486–4489

Kotwal, G.J., Rustgi, V.K. & Baroudy, B.M. (1992b) Detection of hepatitis C virus-specific antigens in semen from non-A, non-B hepatitis patients. *Dig. Dis. Sci.*, **37**, 641–644

Krawczynski, K., Beach, M.J., Bradley, D.W., Kuo, G., Di Bisceglie, A.M., Houghton, M., Reyes, G.R., Kim, J.P., Choo, Q.-L. & Alter, M.J. (1992) Hepatitis C virus antigen in hepatocytes: immunomorphologic detection and identification. *Gastroenterology*, **103**, 622–629

Kremsdorf, D., Porchon, C., Kim, J.P., Reyes, G.R. & Bréchot, C. (1991) Partial nucleotide sequence analysis of a French hepatitis C virus: implications for HCV genetic variability in the E2/NS1 protein. *J. gen. Virol.*, **72**, 2557–2561

Kubo, Y., Takeuchi, K., Boonmar, S., Katayama, T., Choo, Q.-L., Kuo, G., Weiner, A.J., Bradley, D.W., Houghton, M., Saito, I. & Miyamura, T. (1989) A cDNA fragment of hepatitis C virus isolated from an implicated donor of post-transfusion non-A, non-B hepatitis in Japan. *Nucleic Acids Res.*, **17**, 10367–10372

Kumar, U., Cheng, D., Thomas, H. & Monjardino, J. (1992) Cloning and sequencing of the structural region and expression of putative core gene of hepatitis C virus from a British case of chronic sporadic hepatitis. *J. gen. Virol.*, **73**, 1521–1525

Kuo, G., Choo, Q.-L., Alter, H.J., Gitnick, G.L., Redeker, A.G., Purcell, R.H., Miyamura, T., Dienstag, J.L., Alter, M.J., Stevens, C.E., Tegtmeier, G.E., Bonino, F., Colombo, M., Lee, W.-S., Kuo, C., Berger, K., Shuster, J.R., Overby, L.R., Bradley, D.W. & Houghton, M. (1989) An assay for circulating antibodies to a major etiologic virus of human non-A, non-B hepatitis. *Science*, **244**, 362–364

Kuroki, T., Nishiguchi, S., Fukuda, K., Shiomi, S., Monna, T., Murata, R., Isshiki, G., Hayashi, N., Shikata, T. & Kobayashi, K. (1991) Mother-to-child transmission of hepatitis C virus (Letter to the Editor). *J. infect. Dis.*, **164**, 427–428

Lamas, E., Baccarini, P., Housset, C., Kremsdorf, D. & Bréchot, C. (1992) Detection of hepatitis C virus (HCV) RNA sequences in liver tissue by in situ hybridization. *J. Hepatol.*, **16**, 219–223

Laurian, Y., Blanc, A., Delaney, S.R. & Allain, J.-P. (1992) All exposed hemophiliacs have markers of HCV (Letter to the Editor). *Vox sang.*, **62**, 55–56

Lee, S.-D., Lee, F.-Y., Wu, J.-C., Hwang, S.-J., Wang, S.-S. & Lo, K.-J. (1992) The prevalence of anti-hepatitis C virus among Chinese patients with hepatocellular carcinoma. *Cancer*, **69**, 342–345

Lefkowitch, J.H. & Apfelbaum, T.F. (1989) Non-A, non-B hepatitis: characterization of liver biopsy pathology. *J. clin. Gastroenterol.*, **11**, 225–232

Lefkowitch, J.H., Schiff, E.R., Davis, G.L., Perrillo, R.P., Lindsay, K., Bodenheimer, H.C., Jr, Balart, L.A., Ortego, T.J., Payne, J., Dienstag, J.L., Gibas, A., Jacobson, I.M., Tamburro, C.H., Carey, W., O'Brien, C., Sampliner, R., Van Thiel, D.H., Feit, D., Albrecht, J., Meschievitz, C., Sanghvi, B., Vaughan, R.D. & the Hepatitis Interventional Therapy Group (1993) Pathological diagnosis of chronic hepatitis C: a multicenter comparative study with chronic hepatitis B. *Gastroenterology*, **104**, 595–603

Leslie, D.E., Rann, S., Nicholson, S., Fairley, C.K. & Gust, I.D. (1992) Prevalence of hepatitis C antibodies in patients with clotting disorders in Victoria. Relationship with other blood borne viruses and liver disease. *Med. J. Aust.*, **156**, 789–792

Leung, N.W.Y., Tam, J.S., Lai, J.Y., Leung, T.W.T., Lau, W.Y., Shiu, W. & Li, A.K.C. (1992) Does hepatitis C virus infection contribute to hepatocellular carcinoma in Hong Kong? *Cancer*, **70**, 40–44

Levrero, M., Tagger, A., Balsano, C., De Marzio, E., Avantaggiati, M.L., Natoli, G., Diop, D., Villa, E., Diodati, G. & Alberti, A. (1991) Antibodies to hepatitis C virus in patients with hepatocellular carcinoma. *J. Hepatol.*, **12**, 60–63

Li, J.-S., Tong, S.-P., Vitvitski, L., Lepot, D. & Trépo, C. (1991) Evidence of two major genotypes of hepatitis C virus in France and close relatedness of the predominant one with the prototype virus. *J. Hepatol.*, **13** (Suppl. 4), S33–S37

Liang, T.J., Jeffers, L., Reddy, R.K., Silva, M.O., Cheinquer, H., Findor, A., De Medina, M., Yarbough, P.O., Reyes, G.R. & Schiff, E.R. (1993) Fulminant or subfulminant non-A, non-B viral hepatitis: the role of hepatitis C and E viruses. *Gastroenterology*, **104**, 556–562

Lin, H.-H., Hsu, H.-Y., Chang, M.-H., Hong, K.-F., Young, Y.-C., Lee, T.-Y., Chen, P.-J. & Chen, D.-S. (1991) Low prevalence of hepatitis C virus and infrequent perinatal or spouse infections in pregnant women in Taiwan. *J. med. Virol.*, **35**, 237–240

Lin, C.K., Chu, R., Li, K.B. & Leong, S. (1992) A study of hepatitis C virus antibodies and serum alanine amino transferase in blood donors in Hong Kong Chinese. *Vox sang.*, **62**, 98–101

Linke, H.K., Miller, M.F., Peterson, D.A., Muchmore, E., Lesniewski, R.R., Carrick, R.J., Gagne, G.D. & Popper, H. (1987) Documentation of non-A, non-B hepatitis in a chimpanzee with hepatocellular carcinoma. In: Robinson, W., Koike, K. & Well, H., eds, *Hepadna Viruses*, New York, Alan R. Liss, pp. 357–370

Liou, T.-C., Chang, T.-T., Young, K.-C., Lin, X.-Z., Lin, C.-Y. & Wu, H.-L. (1992) Detection of HCV RNA in saliva, urine, seminal fluid, and ascites. *J. med. Virol.*, **37**, 197–202

Liu, K., Hu, Z., Li, H., Prince, A.M. & Inchauspé, G. (1992) Genomic typing of hepatitis C viruses in China. *Gene*, **114**, 245–250

Maddrey, W.C. & Van Thiel, D.H. (1988) Liver transplantation. An overview. *Hepatology*, **8**, 948–959

Maéno, M., Kaminaka, K., Sugimoto, H., Esumi, M., Hayashi, N., Komatsu, K., Abe, K., Sekiguchi, S., Yano, M., Mizuno, K. & Shikata, T. (1990) A cDNA clone closely associated with non-A, non-B hepatitis. *Nucleic Acids Res.*, **18**, 2685–2689

Maggi, P. & Petrarulo, F. (1992) Is transfusion the only risk factor for HCV infection among hemodialyzed patients? (Letter to the Editor). *Nephron*, **61**, 240

Martell, M., Esteban, J.I., Quer, J., Genescà, J., Weiner, A., Esteban, R., Guardia, J. & Gómez, J. (1992) Hepatitis C virus (HCV) circulates as a population of different but closely related genomes: quasispecies nature of HCV genome distribution. *J. Virol.*, **66**, 3225–3229

Martin, P., Di Bisceglie, A.M., Kassianides, C., Lisker-Melman, M. & Hoofnagle, J.H. (1989) Rapidly progressive non-A, non-B hepatitis in patients with human immunodeficiency virus infection. *Gastroenterology*, **97**, 1559–1561

Matsuura, Y., Harada, S., Suzuki, R., Watanabe, Y., Inoue, Y., Saito, I. & Miyamura, T. (1992) Expression of processed envelope protein of hepatitis C virus in mammalian and insect cells. *J. Virol.*, **66**, 1425–1431

Mattsson, L., Grillner, L. & Weiland, O. (1992) Seroconversion to hepatitis C virus antibodies in patients with acute post-transfusion non-A, non-B hepatitis in Sweden with a second-generation test. *Scand. J. infect. Dis.*, **24**, 15–20

McFarlane, I.G., Smith, H.M., Johnson, P.J., Bray, G.P., Vergani, D. & Williams, R. (1990) Hepatitis C virus antibodies in chronic active hepatitis: pathogenetic factor or false-positive result? *Lancet*, **335**, 754–757

McHutchison, J.G., Person, J.L., Govindarajan, S., Valinluck, B., Gore, T., Lee, S.R., Nelles, M., Polito, A., Chien, D., DiNello, R., Quan, S., Kuo, G. & Redeker, A.G. (1992) Improved detection of hepatitis C virus antibodies in high-risk populations. *Hepatology*, **15**, 19–25

Mencarini, P., De Luca, A., Antinori, A., Maiuro, G., Spedini, G., Bailly, C. & Tamburrini, E. (1991) Prevalence of anti-HCV antibodies in Cameroon (Short report). *Trans. R. Soc. trop. Med. Hyg.*, **85**, 654–655

Mendenhall, C.L., Seeff, L., Diehl, A.M., Ghosn, S.J., French, S.W., Gartside, P.S., Rouster, S.D., Buskell-Bales, Z., Grossman, C.J., Roselle, G.A., Weesner, R.E., Garcia-Pont, P., Goldberg, S.J., Kiernan, T.W., Tamburro, C.H., Zetterman, R., Chedid, A., Chen, T., Rabin, L. & the VA Cooperative Study Group (1991) Antibodies to hepatitis B virus and hepatitis C virus in alcoholic hepatitis and cirrhosis: their prevalence and clinical relevance. *Hepatology*, **14**, 581–589

Menéndez, S.R., Garciá, M.R., Sánchez San Román, S., Menéndez Tévar, F., Suárez Gonsález, A., Alvarez Navascués, C., Pérez Alvarez, R. & Rodrigo Sáez, L. (1991) Intrafamilial spread of hepatitis C virus. *Infection*, **19**, 431–433

Miller, R.H. & Purcell, R.H. (1990) Hepatitis C virus shares amino acid sequence similarity with pestiviruses and flaviviruses as well as members of two plant virus supergroups. *Proc. natl Acad. Sci. USA*, **87**, 2057–2061

Mishiro, S., Hoshi, Y., Takeda, K., Yoshikawa, A., Gotanda, T., Takahashi, K., Akahane, Y., Yoshizawa, H., Okamoto, H., Tsuda, F., Peterson, D.A. & Muchmore, E. (1990) Non-A, non-B hepatitis specific antibodies directed at host-derived epitope: implication for an autoimmune process. *Lancet*, **336**, 1400–1403

Mita, E., Hayashi, N., Ueda, K., Kasahara, A., Fusamoto, H., Takamizawa, A., Matsubara, K., Okayama, H. & Kamada, T. (1992) Expression of MBP-HCV NS1/E2 fusion protein in *E. coli* and detection of anti-NS1/E2 antibody in type C chronic liver disease. *Biochem. biophys. Res. Commun.*, **183**, 925–930

Mondelli, M.U. & Colombo, M. (1991) The emerging picture of hepatitis C. *Dig. Dis.*, **9**, 245-252

Mondello, P., Patti, S., Vitale, M.G., D'Accardo, A.M. & Spanó, C. (1992) Anti-HCV antibodies in household contacts of patients with cirrhosis of the liver—preliminary results. *Infection*, **20**, 51–52

Mori, S., Kato, N., Yagyu, A., Tanaka, T., Ikeda, Y., Petchclai, B., Chiewsilp, P., Kurimura, T. & Shimotohno, K. (1992) A new type of hepatitis C virus in patients in Thailand. *Biochem. biophys. Res. Commun.*, **183**, 334–342

Mosconi, G., Campieri, C., Miniero, R., Coli, L., Orsi, C., La Manna, G., De Sanctis, L.B., Stefoni, S., Sprovieri, G. & Bonomini, V. (1992) Epidemiology of hepatitis C in a population of hemodialysis patients. *Nephron*, **61**, 298–299

Muchmore, E., Popper, H., Peterson, D.A., Miller, M.F. & Lieberman, H.M. (1988) Non-A, non-B hepatitis-related hepatocellular carcinoma in a chimpanzee. *J. med. Primatol.*, **17**, 235–246

Murakawa, K., Esumi, M., Kato, T., Kambara, H. & Shikata, T. (1992) Heterogeneity within the nonstructural protein 5-encoding region of hepatitis C viruses from a single patient. *Gene*, **117**, 229–232

Nalpas, B., Driss, F., Pol, S., Hamelin, B., Housset, C., Bréchot, C. & Berthelot, P. (1991) Association between HCV and HBV infection in hepatocellular carcinoma and alcoholic liver disease. *J. Hepatol.*, **12**, 70-74

Negro, F., Pacchioni, D., Shimizu, Y., Miller, R.H., Bussolati, G., Purcell, R.H. & Bonino, F. (1992) Detection of intrahepatic replication of hepatitis C virus RNA by in situ hybridization and comparison with histopathology. *Proc. natl Acad. Sci. USA*, **89**, 2247–2251

Ng, Y.-Y., Lee, S.-D., Wu, S.-C., Yang, W.-C., Chiang, S.-S. & Huang, T.-P. (1991) Antibodies to hepatitis C virus in uremic patients on continuous ambulatory peritoneal dialysis. *J. med. Virol.*, **35**, 263–266

Nishioka, K., Watanabe, J., Furuta, S., Tanaka, E., Iino, S., Suzuki, H., Tsuji, T., Yano, M., Kuo, G., Choo, Q-L., Houghton, M. & Oda, T. (1991) A high prevalence of antibody to the hepatitis C virus in patients with hepatocellular carcinoma in Japan. *Cancer*, **67**, 429–433

Novati, R., Thiers, V., d'Arminio Monforte, A., Maisonneuve, P., Principi, N., Conti, M., Lazzarin, A. & Bréchot, C. (1992) Mother-to-child transmission of hepatitis C virus detected by nested polymerase chain reaction. *J. infect. Dis.*, **165**, 720–723

Ohkoshi, S., Kojima, H., Tawaraya, H., Miyajima, T., Kamimura, T., Asakura, H., Satoh, A., Hirose, S., Hijikata, M., Kato, N. & Shimotohno, K. (1990) Prevalence of antibody against non-A, non-B hepatitis virus in Japanese patients with hepatocellular carcinoma. *Jpn. J. Cancer Res.*, **81**, 550–553

Okamoto, H. (1992) Characterization of genomic structure of hepatitis C virus. *Igaku no Ayumi*, **161**, 298–302 (in Japanese)

Okamoto, H., Okada, S., Sugiyama, Y., Yotsumoto, S., Tanaka, T., Yoshizawa, H., Tsuda, F., Miyakawa, Y. & Mayumi, M. (1990a) The 5'-terminal sequence of the hepatitis C virus genome. *Jpn. J. exp. Med.*, **60**, 167–177

Okamoto, H., Munekata, E., Tsuda, F., Takahashi, K., Yotsumoto, S., Tanaka, T., Tachibana, K., Akahane, Y., Sugai, Y., Miyakawa, Y. & Mayumi, M. (1990b) Enzyme-linked immunosorbent assay for antibodies against the capsid protein of hepatitis C virus with a synthetic oligopeptide. *Jpn. J. exp. Med.*, **60**, 223–233

Okamoto, H., Okada, S., Sugiyama, Y., Tanaka, T., Sugai, Y., Akahane, Y., Machida, A., Mishiro, S., Yoshizawa, H., Miyakawa, Y. & Mayumi, M. (1990c) Detection of hepatitis C virus RNA by a two-stage polymerase chain reaction with two pairs of primers deduced from the 5'-noncoding region. *Jpn. J. exp. Med.*, **60**, 215–222

Okamoto, H., Okada, S., Sugiyama, Y., Kurai, K., Iizuka, H., Machida, A., Miyakawa, Y. & Mayumi, M. (1991) Nucleotide sequence of the genomic RNA of hepatitis C virus isolated from a human carrier: comparison with reported isolates for conserved and divergent regions. *J. gen. Virol.*, **72**, 2697–2704

Okamoto, H., Kurai, k., Okada, S.-I., Yamamoto, K., Iizuka, H., Tanaka, T., Fukuda, S., Tsuda, F. & Mishiro, S. (1992a) Full-length sequence of a hepatitis C virus genome having poor homology to reported isolates: comparative study of four distinct genotypes. *Virology*, **188**, 331–341

Okamoto, H., Kojima, M., Okada, S.-I., Yoshizawa, H., Iizuka, H., Tanaka, T., Muchmore, E.E., Peterson, D.A., Ito, Y. & Mishiro, S. (1992b) Genetic drift of hepatitis C virus during a 8.2-year infection in a chimpanzee: variability and stability. *Virology*, **190**, 894–899

Okamoto, H., Tsuda, F., Machida, A., Munekata, E., Akahane, Y., Sugai, Y., Mashiko, K., Mitsui, T., Tanaka, T., Miyakawa, Y. & Mayumi, M. (1992c) Antibodies against synthetic oligopeptides deduced from the putative core gene for the diagnosis of hepatitis C virus infection. *Hepatology*, **15**, 180–186

Omata, M., Yokosuka, O., Takano, S., Kato, N., Hosoda, K., Imazeki, F., Tada, M., Ito, Y. & Ohto, M. (1991) Resolution of acute hepatitis C after therapy with natural beta interferon (Short report). *Lancet*, **338**, 914–915

Parkin, D.M., Srivatanakul, P., Khlat, M., Chenvidhya, D., Chotiwan, P., Insiripong, S., L'Abbé, K.A. & Wild, C.P. (1991) Liver cancer in Thailand. I. A case–control study of cholangiocarcinoma. *Int. J. Cancer*, **48**, 323–328

Perez Alvarez, L., Gurbindo, M.D., Hernandez-Sampelayo, T., Casado, C., Leon, P., Garcia Saiz, A., De Andres, R. & Najera, R. (1992) Mother-to-infant transmission of HIV and hepatitis C infections in children born to HIV-seropositive mothers. *AIDS*, **6**, 427–440

Perrillo, R.P., Pohl, D.A., Roodman, S.T. & Tsai, C.C. (1981) Acute non-A, non-B hepatitis with serum sickness-like syndrome and aplastic anemia. *J. Am. med. Assoc.*, **245**, 494–496

van der Poel, C.L., Bresters, D., Reesink, H.W., Plaisier, A.A.D., Schaasberg, W., Leentvaar-Kuypers, A., Choo, Q.-L., Quan, S., Polito, A., Houghton, M., Kuo, G., Lelie, P.N. & Cuypers, H.T.M. (1992) Early anti-hepatitis C virus response with second-generation C200/C22 ELISA. *Vox sang.*, **62**, 208–212

Pohjanpelto, P. (1992) Risk factors connected with hepatitis C infections in Finland (Short communication). *Scand. J. infect. Dis.*, **24**, 251–252

Pol, S., Legendre, C., Saltiel, C., Carnot, F., Bréchot, C., Berthelot, P., Mattlinger, B. & Kreis, M. (1992) Hepatitis C virus in kidney recipients. Epidemiology and impact on renal transplantation. *J. Hepatol.*, **15**, 202–206

Ponz, E., Campistol, J.M., Barrera, J.M., Gil, C., Pinto, J., Andreu, J. & Bruguera, M. (1991) Hepatitis C virus antibodies in patients on hemodialysis and after kidney transplantation. *Transplant. Proc.*, **23**, 1371–1372

Poynard, T., Aubert, A., Lazizi, Y., Bedossa, P., Hamelin, B., Terris, B., Naveau, S., Dubreuil, P., Pillot, J. & Chaput, J.-C. (1991) Independent risk factors for hepatocellular carcinoma in French drinkers. *Hepatology*, **13**, 896–901

Prince, A.M., Brotman, B., Grady, G.F., Kulins, W.J., Hazzi, C., Levine, R.W. & Millian, S.J. (1974) Long-incubation post-transfusion hepatitis without serological evidence of exposure to hepatitis B virus. *Lancet*, **ii**, 241–246

Prince, A.M., Brotman, B., Huima, T., Pascual, D., Jaffery, M. & Inchauspé, G. (1992) Immunity to hepatitis C infection. *J. infect. Dis.*, **165**, 438–443

Qian, C., Camps, J., Maluenda, M.D., Civeira, M.P. & Prieto, J. (1992) Replication of hepatitis C virus in peripheral blood mononuclear cells. Effect of alpha-interferon therapy. *J. Hepatol.*, **16**, 380–383

Ranger, S., Aussel, L., Winbreck, P., Loustaud, V., Rogues, A.M., Mounier, M., Delpeyroux, C. & Denis, F. (1991) Seroprevalence of hepatitis C virus in subjects contaminated with the human immunodeficiency virus. *Pathol. biol.*, **39**, 126–130 (in French)

Rapicetta, M., Attili, A.F., Mele, A., De Santis, A., Chionne, P., Cristiano, K., Spada, E., Giuliani, E., Carli, L., Goffredo, F. & Capocaccia, L. (1992) Prevalence of hepatitis C virus antibodies and hepatitis C virus-RNA in an urban population. *J. med. Virol.*, **37**, 87–92

Read, A.E., Donegan, E., Lake, J., Ferrell, L., Galbraith, C., Kuramoto, I.K., Zeldis, J.B., Ascher, N.L., Roberts, J. & Wright, T.L. (1991) Hepatitis C in patients undergoing liver transplantation. *Ann. intern. Med.*, **114**, 282–284

Reesink, H.W., Wong, V.C.W, Ip, H.M.H., van der Poel, C.L., van Exel-Oehlers, P.J. & Lelie, P.N. (1990) Mother-to-infant transmission and hepatitis C virus (Letter to the Editor). *Lancet*, **335**, 1216–1217

Robson, S.C., Du Toit, J.M.G., Brice, E.A.W., Bird, A.R. & Brink, N.S. (1991) Hepatitis C virus antibodies in patients with liver disease. The western Cape experience. *South Afr. med. J.*, **80**, 282–284

Roudot-Thoraval, F., Deforges, L., Girollet, J.-P., Maria, B., Milliez, J., Pathier, D., Duval, J. & Dhumeaux, D. (1992) Prevalence of antibodies to hepatitis C virus in a population of pregnant women in France. *Gastroenterol. clin. Biol.*, **16**, 255–259 (in French)

Ruiz-Moreno, M., Rua, M.J., Castillo, I., García-Novo, M.D., Santos, M., Navas, S. & Carreño, V. (1992) Treatment of children with chronic hepatitis C with recombinant interferon-alpha: a pilot study. *Hepatology*, **16**, 882–885

Saito, I., Miyamura, T., Ohbayashi, A., Harada, H., Katayama, T., Kikuchi, S., Watanabe, Y., Koi, S., Onji, M., Ohta, Y., Choo, Q.-L., Houghton, M. & Kuo, G. (1990) Hepatitis C virus infection is associated with the development of hepatocellular carcinoma. *Proc. natl Acad. Sci. USA*, **87**, 6547–6549

Sbolli, G., Zanetti, A.R, Tanzi, E., Cavanna, L., Civardi, G., Fornari, F., Di Stasi, M. & Buscarini, L. (1990) Serum antibodies to hepatitis C virus in Italian patients with hepatocellular carcinoma. *J. med. Virol.*, **30**, 230–232

Schlipköter, U., Gladziwa, U., Cholmakov, K., Weise, A., Rasshofer, R., Lorbeer, B., Luz, N., Deinhardt, F. & Raggendorf, M. (1992) Prevalence of hepatitis C virus infection in dialysis patients and their contacts using a second generation enzyme-linked immunosorbent assay. *Med. Microbiol. Immunol.*, **181**, 173–180

Schoub, B.D., Johnson, S., McAnerney, J.M. & Blackburn, N.K. (1992) The role of sexual transmission in the epidemiology of hepatitis C virus in black South Africans. *Trans. R. Soc. trop. Med. Hyg.*, **86**, 431–433

Scott, D.A., Constantine, N.T., Callahan, J., Burans, J.P., Olson, J.G., Al-Fadeel, M., Al-Ozieb, H., Arunkumer, H. & Hyams, K.C. (1992) The epidemiology of hepatitis C virus antibody in Yemen. *Am. J. trop. Med. Hyg.*, **46**, 63–68

Seeff, L.B., Buskell-Bales, Z., Wright, E.C., Durako, S.J., Alter, H.J., Iber, F.L., Hollinger, F.B., Gitnick, G., Knodell, R.G., Perrillo, R.P., Stevens, C.E., Hollingsworth, C.G. & the National Heart, Lung and Blood Institute Study Group (1992) Long-term mortality after transfusion-associated non-A, non-B hepatitis. *New Engl. J. Med.*, **327**, 1906–1911

Sheu, J.-C., Lee, S.-H., Wang, J.-T., Shih, L.-N., Wang, T.-H. & Chen, D.-S. (1992a) Prevalence of anti-HCV and HCV viremia in hemodialysis patients in Taiwan. *J. med. Virol.*, **37**, 108–112

Sheu, J.-C., Huang, G.-T., Shih, L.-N., Lee, W.-C., Chou, H.-C., Wang, J.-T., Lee, P.-H., Lai, M.-Y., Wang, C.-Y., Yang, P.-M., Lee, H.-S. & Chen, D.-S. (1992b) Hepatitis C and B viruses in hepatitis B surface antigen-negative hepatocellular carcinoma. *Gastroenterology*, **103**, 1322–1327

Shieh, Y.S.C., Shim, K.-S., Lampertico, P., Balart, L.A., Jeffers, L.J., Thung, S.N., Regenstein, F., Reddy, K.R., Farr, G., Schiff, E.R. & Gerber, M.A. (1991) Detection of hepatitis C virus sequences in liver tissue by the polymerase chain reaction. *Lab. Invest.*, **65**, 408–411

Shimizu, Y.K., Weiner, A.J., Rosenblatt, J., Wong, D.C., Shapiro, M., Popkin, T., Houghton, M., Alter, H.J. & Purcell, R.H. (1990) Early events in hepatitis C virus infection in chimpanzees. *Proc. natl Acad. Sci. USA*, **87**, 6441–6444

Shimizu, S., Kiyosawa, K., Sodeyama, T., Tanaka, E. & Nakano, M. (1992) High prevalence of antibody to hepatitis C virus in heavy drinkers with chronic liver diseases in Japan. *J. Gastroenterol. Hepatol.*, **7**, 30–35

Shimizu, Y.K., Iwamoto, A., Hijikata, M., Purcell, R.H. & Yoshikura, H. (1992) Evidence for in vitro replication of hepatitis C virus genome in a human T-cell line. *Proc. natl Acad. Sci. USA*, **89**, 5477–5481

Shindo, M., Di Bisceglie, A.M. & Hoofnagle, J.H. (1992a) Long-term follow-up of patients with chronic hepatitis C treated with alpha-interferon. *Hepatology*, **15**, 1013–1016

Shindo, M., Di Bisceglie, A.M., Biswas, R., Mihalik, K. & Feinstone, S.M. (1992b) Hepatitis C virus replication during acute infection in the chimpanzee. *J. infect. Dis.*, **166**, 424–427

Simonetti, R.G., Cottone, M., Craxi, A., Pagliaro, L., Rapicetta, M., Chionne, P. & Costantino, A. (1989) Prevalence of antibodies to hepatitis C virus in hepatocellular carcinoma (Letter to the Editor). *Lancet*, **ii**, 1338

Simonetti, R.G., Cammà, C., Fiorello, F., Cottone, M., Rapicetta, M., Marino, L., Fiorentino, G., Craxì, A., Ciccaglione, A., Giuseppetti, R., Stroffolini, T. & Pagliaro, L. (1992) Hepatitis C virus infection as a risk factor for hepatocellular carcinoma in patients with cirrhosis. A case–control study. *Ann. intern. Med.*, **116**, 97–102

Spaete, R.R., Alexander, D'A., Rugroden, M.E., Choo, Q.-L., Berger, K., Crawford, K., Kuo, C., Leng, S., Lee, C., Ralston, R., Thudium, K., Tung, J.W., Kuo, G. & Houghton, M. (1992) Characterization of the hepatitis C virus E2/NS1 gene product expressed in mammalian cells. *Virology*, **188**, 819–830

Srivatanakul, P., Parkin, D.M., Khlat, M., Chenvidhya, D., Chotiwan, P., Insiripong, S., L'Abbé, K.A. & Wild, C.P. (1991) Liver cancer in Thailand. II. A case–control study of hepatocellular carcinoma. *Int. J. Cancer*, **48**, 329–332

Stroffolini, T., Chiaramonte, M., Tiribelli, C., Villa, E., Simonetti, R.G., Rapicetta, M., Stazi, M.A., Bertin, T., Croce, S.L., Trande, P., Magliocco, A. & Chionne, P. (1992) Hepatitis C virus infection, HBsAg carrier state and hepatocellular carcinoma: relative risk and population attributable risk from a case–control study in Italy. *J. Hepatol.*, **16**, 360–363

Sun, Z.T., Zhu, Y.R. & Harris, C.C. (1993) Viral chemical interaction in hepatocarcinogenesis in area of prevalence (Abstract 331/33). *Cancer Detect. Prev.*, **17**, 207

Suzuki, H. *et al.* (1991) Clinical significance of second generation anti-HCV assay kit (ELISA) and RIBA-II in liver disease. *J. Med. pharm. Sci.*, **26**, 303–312 (in Japanese)

Tabor, E., Gerety, R.J., Drucker, J.A., Seeff, L.B., Hoofnagle, J.H., Jackson, D.R., April, M., Barker, L.F. & Pineda-Tamondong, G. (1978) Transmission of non-A, non-B hepatitis from man to chimpanzee. *Lancet*, **i**, 463–466

Takada, N., Takase, S., Enomoto, N., Takada, A. & Date, T. (1992) Clinical backgrounds of the patients having different types of hepatitis C virus genomes. *J. Hepatol.*, **14**, 35–40

Takahashi, K., Okamoto, H., Kishimoto, S., Munekata, E., Tachibana, K., Akahane, Y., Yoshizawa, H. & Mishiro, S. (1992) Demonstration of a hepatitis C virus-specific antigen predicted from the putative core gene in the circulation of infected hosts. *J. gen. Virol.*, **73**, 667–672

Takamizawa, A., Mori, C., Fuke, I., Manabe, S., Murakami, S., Fujita J., Onishi, E., Andoh, T., Yoshida, I. & Okayama, H. (1991) Structure and organization of the hepatitis C virus genome isolated from human carriers. *J. Virol.*, **65**, 1105–1113

Takeda, S., Nagafuchi, Y., Tashiro, H., Abe, Y., Fukushige, H., Komori, H., Okamoto, K., Ohsato, K. & Haratake, J. (1992) Antihepatitis C virus status in hepatocellular carcinoma and the influence on clinicopathological findings and operative results. *Br. J. Surg.*, **79**, 1195–1198

Takehara, T., Hayashi, N., Mita, E., Hagiwara, H., Ueda, K., Katayama, K., Kasahara, A., Fusamoto, H. & Kamada, T. (1992) Detection of the minus strand of hepatitis C virus RNA by reverse transcription and polymerase chain reaction: implications for hepatitis C virus replication in infected tissue. *Hepatology*, **15**, 387–390

Takeuchi, K., Boonmar, S., Kubo, Y., Katayama, T., Harada, H., Ohbayashi, A., Choo, Q.-L., Kuo, G., Houghton, M., Saito, I. & Miyamura, T. (1990a) Hepatitis C viral cDNA clones isolated from a healthy carrier donor implicated to post-transfusion non-A, non-B hepatitis. *Gene*, **91**, 287–291

Takeuchi, K., Kubo, Y., Boonmar, S., Watanabe, Y., Katayama, T., Choo, Q.-L., Kuo, G., Houghton, M., Saito, I. & Miyamura, T. (1990b) Nucleotide sequence of core and envelope genes of the hepatitis C virus genome derived directly from human healthy carriers. *Nucleic Acids Res.*, **18**, 4626

Tamura, I., Koda, T., Kobayashi, Y., Ichimura, H., Kurimura, O. & Kurimura, T. (1992) Prevalence of four blood-borne viruses (HBV, HCV, HTLV-1, HIV-1) among haemodialysis patients in Japan. *J. med. Virol.*, **36**, 271–273

Tanaka, K., Hirohata, T., Koga, S., Sugimachi, K., Kanematsu, T., Ohryohji, F., Nawata, H., Ishibashi, H., Maeda, Y., Kiyokawa, H., Tokunaga, K., Irita, Y., Takeshita, S., Arase, Y. & Nishino, N. (1991) Hepatitis C and hepatitis B in the etiology of hepatocellular carcinoma in the Japanese population. *Cancer Res.*, **51**, 2842–2847

Tanaka, E., Kiyosawa, K., Sodeyama, T., Hayata, T., Ohike, V., Nakano, Y., Yoshizawa, K., Furuta, S., Watanabe, Y., Watanabe, J. & Nishioka, K. (1992) Prevalence of antibody to hepatitis C virus in Japanese schoolchildren: a comparison with adult blood donors. *Am. J. trop. Med. Hyg.*, **46**, 460–464

Tanaka, T., Kato, N., Nakagawa, M., Ootsuyama, Y., Cho, M.-J., Nakazawa, T., Hijikata, M., Ishimura, Y. & Shimotohno, K. (1992) Molecular cloning of hepatitis C virus genome from a single Japanese carrier: sequence variation within the same individual and among infected individuals. *Virus Res.*, **23**, 39–53

Tateda, A., Kikuchi, K., Numazaki, Y., Shirachi, R. & Ichida, N. (1979) Non-B hepatitis in Japanese recipients of blood transfusions: clinical and serologic studies after the introduction of laboratory screening of donor blood for hepatitis B surface antigen. *J. infect. Dis.*, **139**, 511–518

Terada, S., Kawanishi, K. & Katayama, K. (1992) Minimal hepatitis C infectivity in semen (Letter to the Editor). *Ann. intern. Med.*, **117**, 171–172

Thaler, M.M., Park, C.-K., Landers, D.V., Wara, D.W., Houghton, M., Veeremann-Wauters, G., Sweet, R.-L. & Han, J.H. (1991) Vertical transmission of hepatitis C (Short report). *Lancet*, **338**, 17–18

Theilmann, L., Solbach, C., Toex, U., Müller, H.M., Pfaff, E., Otto, G. & Goeser, T. (1992) Role of hepatitis C virus infection in German patients with fulminant and subacute hepatic failure. *Eur. J. clin. Invest.*, **22**, 569–571

Trichopoulos, D., Day, N.E., Kaklamani, E., Tzonou, A., Muñoz, N., Zavitsanos, X., Koumantaki, Y. & Trichopoulou, A. (1987) Hepatitis B virus, tobacco smoking and ethanol consumption in the etiology of hepatocellular carcinoma. *Int. J. Cancer*, **39**, 45–49

Tsukiyama-Kohara, K., Kohara, M., Yamaguchi, K., Maki, N., Toyoshima, A., Miki, K., Tanaka, S., Hattori, N. & Nomoto, A. (1991) A second group of hepatitis C viruses. *Virus Genes*, **5**, 243–254

Tzonou, A., Trichopoulos, D., Kaklamani, E., Zavitsanos, X., Koumantaki, Y. & Hsieh, C.-C. (1991) Epidemiologic assessment of interactions of hepatitis-C virus with seromarkers of hepatitis-B and -D viruses, cirrhosis and tobacco smoking in hepatocellular carcinoma. *Int. J. Cancer*, **49**, 377–380

Ueda, T., Ohta, K., Suzuki, N., Yamaguchi, M., Hirai, K., Horiuchi, T., Watanabe, J., Miyamoto, T. & Ito, K. (1992) Idiopathic pulmonary fibrosis and high prevalence of serum antibodies to hepatitis C virus. *Am. Rev. respir. Dis.*, **146**, 266–268

Vandelli, L., Medici, G., Savazzi, A.M., De Palma, M., Vecchi, C., Zanchetta, G. & Lusvarghi, E. (1992) Behavior of antibody profile against hepatitis C virus in patients on maintenance hemodialysis. *Nephron*, **61**, 260–262

Vargas, V., Castells, L. & Esteban, J.I. (1990) High frequency of antibodies to the hepatitis C virus among patients with hepatocellular carcinoma (Letter to the Editor). *Ann. intern. Med.*, **112**, 232–233

Verbaan, H., Widell, A., Lindgren, S., Lindmark, B., Nordenfelt, E. & Eriksson, S. (1992) Hepatitis C in chronic liver disease: an epidemiological study based on 566 consecutive patients undergoing liver biopsy during a 10-year period. *J. intern. Med.*, **232**, 33–42

Viladomiu, L., Genescà, J., Esteban, J.I., Allende, H., González, A., López-Talavera, J.C., Esteban, R. & Guardia, J. (1992) Interferon-alpha in acute post-transfusion hepatitis C: a randomized, controlled trial. *Hepatology*, **15**, 767–769

Wang, J.-T., Sheu, J.-C., Lin, J.-T., Wang, T.-H. & Chen, D.S. (1992) Detection of replicative form of hepatitis C virus RNA in peripheral blood mononuclear cells. *J. infect. Dis.*, **166**, 1167–1169

Wang, Y., Okamoto, H. & Mishiro, S. (1992) HCV genotypes in China (Letter to the Editor). *Lancet*, **339**, 1168

Watanabe, J., Minegishi, K., Mitsumori, T., Ishifuji, M., Oguchi, T., Ueda, M., Tokunaga, E., Tanaka, E., Kiyosawa, K., Furuta, S., Katayama, T., Kuo, G., Choo, Q.-L., Houghton, M. & Nishioka, K. (1990) Prevalence of anti-HCV antibody in blood donors in the Tokyo area. *Vox sang.*, **59**, 86–88

Watanabe, J. *et al.* (1991a) Sensitivity and specificity of assays for antibody to HCV by 2nd generation ELISA and RIBA-II in voluntary blood donors. *J. Med. pharm. Sci.*, **26**, 313–321 (in Japanese)

Watanabe, J., Matsumoto, C., Nishioka, K. & Yoshizawa, H. (1991b) Anti-GOR to screen HCV-RNA-positive blood donors (Letter to the Editor). *Lancet*, **338**, 391

Watanabe, Y., Harada, S., Saito, I. & Miyamura, T. (1991) Prevalence of antibody against the core protein of hepatitis C virus in patients with hepatocellular carcinoma. *Int. J. Cancer*, **48**, 340–343

Watanabe, J., Matsumoto, C., Fujimura, K., Shimada, T., Yoshizawa, H., Okamoto, H., Iizuka, H., Tango, T., Ikeda, H., Endo, N., Mazda, T., Nojiri, T., Aoyama, K., Kanemitsu, K., Yamano, H., Mizui, M., Yokoishi, F., Tokunaga, K. & Nishioka, K. (1993) Predictive value of screening tests for persistent hepatitis C virus infection evidenced by viraemia: Japanese experience. *Vox sang.*, **65**, 199–203

Watson, H.G., Ludlam, C.A., Rebus, S., Zhang, L.Q., Peutherer, J.F. & Simmonds, P. (1992) Use of several second generation serological assays to determine the true prevalence of hepatitis C virus infection in haemophiliacs treated with non-virus inactivated factor VIII and IX concentrates. *Br. J. Haematol.*, **80**, 514–518

Weiner, A.J., Christopherson, C., Hall, J.E., Bonino, F., Saracco, G., Brunetto, M.R., Crawford, K., Marion, C.D., Crawford, K.A., Venkatakrishna, S., Miyamura, T., McHutchinson, J., Cuypers, T. & Houghton, M. (1991) Sequence variation in hepatitis C viral isolates. *J. Hepatol.*, **13** (Suppl. 4), S6–S14

Weiner, A.J., Geysen, H.M., Christopherson, C., Hall, J.E., Mason, T.J., Saracco, G., Bonino, F., Crawford, K., Marion, C.D., Crawford, K.A., Brunetto, M., Barr, P.J., Miyamura, T., McHutchinson, J. & Houghton, M. (1992) Evidence for immune selection of hepatitis C virus (HCV) putative envelope glycoprotein variants: putative role in chronic HCV infections. *Proc. natl Acad. Sci. USA*, **89**, 3468–3472

Weintrub, P.S., Veereman-Wauters, G., Cowan, M.J. & Thaler, M.M. (1991) Hepatitis C virus infection in infants whose mothers took street drugs intravenously. *J. Pediatr.*, **119**, 869–874

Widell, A., Hansson, B.G., Berntorp, E., Moestrup, T., Johansson, H.P., Hansson, H. & Nordenfelt, E. (1991) Antibody to a hepatitis C virus related protein among patients at high risk for hepatitis B. *Scand. J. infect. Dis.*, **23**, 19–24

Wright, T.L., Hsu, H., Donegan, E., Feinstone, S., Greenberg, H., Read, A., Ascher, N.L., Roberts, J.P. & Lake, J.R. (1991) Hepatitis C virus not found in fulminant non-A, non-B hepatitis. *Ann. intern. Med.*, **115**, 111–112

Wright, H.I., Gavaler, J.S. & Van Thiel, D.H. (1992) Preliminary experience with interferon-alpha-2b therapy of viral hepatitis in liver allograft recipients. *Transplantation*, **53**, 121–124

Wright, T.L., Hollander, H., Kim, M., Wilber, J., Chan, C., Polito, A., Urdea, M., Thaler, M.M., Held, M.J. & Scharschmidt, B. (1992a) Hepatitis C viremia in human immunodeficiency virus (HIV) infected patients with and without AIDS (Abstract No. 101). *Hepatology*, **16**, 70A

Wright, T.L., Donegan, E., Hsu, H.H., Ferrell, L., Lake, J.R., Kim, M., Combs, C., Fennessy, S., Roberts, J.P., Ascher, N.L. & Greenberg, H.B. (1992b) Recurrent and acquired hepatitis C viral infection in liver transplant recipients. *Gastroenterology*, **103**, 317–322

Wyke, R.J., Tsiquaye, K.N., Thornton, A., White, Y., Portmann, B., Das, P.K., Zuckerman, A.J. & Williams, R. (1979) Transmission of non-A non-B hepatitis to chimpanzees by factor-IX concentrates after fatal complications in patients with chronic liver disease. *Lancet*, **i**, 520–524

Xu, Z., Sheng, F.-M., Xu, Z.-Y. & Wang, Q.-S. (1990) Relationship between HCV infection and primary hepatocellular carcinoma (PHC). *Tumor (Shanghai)*, **10**, 115 (in Chinese)

Yoshioka, K., Kakumu, S., Wakita, T., Ishikawa, T., Itoh, Y., Takayanagi, M., Higashi, Y., Shibata, M. & Morishima, T. (1992) Detection of hepatitis C virus by polymerase chain reaction and response to interferon-alpha therapy: relationship to genotypes of hepatitis C virus. *Hepatology*, **16**, 293–299

Yoshizawa, H., Akahane, Y., Itoh, Y., Iwakiri, S., Kitajima, K., Morita, M., Tanaka, A., Nojiri, T., Shimizu, M., Miyakawa, M. & Mayumi, M. (1980) Virus-like particles in a plasma fraction (fibrinogen) and in the circulation of apparently healthy blood donors capable of inducing non-A/non-B hepatitis in humans and chimpanzees. *Gastroenterology*, **79**, 512–520

Yousuf, M., Nakano, Y., Tanaka, E., Sodeyama, T. & Kiyosawa, K. (1992) Persistence of viremia in patients with type-C chronic hepatitis during long-term follow-up. *Scand. J. Gastroenterol.*, **27**, 812–816

Yu, M.-W. & Chen, C.-J. (1993) Elevated serum testorenone levels and risk of hepatocellular carcinoma. *Cancer Res.*, **53**, 790–794

Yu, M.C., Tong, M.J., Coursaget, P., Ross, R.K., Govindarajan, S. & Henderson, B.E. (1990) Prevalence of hepatitis B and C viral markers in black and white patients with hepatocellular carcinoma in the United States. *J. natl Cancer Inst.*, **82**, 1038–1041

Yu, M.-W., You, S.-L., Chang, A.-S., Lu, S.-N., Liaw, Y.-F. & Chen, C.-J. (1991) Association between hepatitis C virus antibodies and hepatocellular carcinoma in Taiwan. *Cancer Res.*, **51**, 5621–5625

Yuki, N., Hayashi, N., Kasahara, A., Hagiwara, H., Katayama, K., Fusamoto, H. & Kamada, T. (1992) Hepatitis B virus markers and antibodies to hepatitis C virus in Japanese patients with hepatocellular carcinoma. *Dig. Dis. Sci.*, **37**, 65–72

Zaaijer, H.L., Cuypers, H.T.M., Reesink, H.W., Winkel, I.N., Gerken, G. & Lelie, P.N. (1993) Reliability of polymerase chain reaction for detection of hepatitis C virus (Short report). *Lancet*, **341**, 722–724

Zavitsanos, X., Hatzakis, A., Kaklamani, E., Tzonou, A., Toupadaki, N., Broeksma, C., Chrispeels, J., Troonen, H., Hadziyannis, S., Hsieh, C.-C., Alter, H. & Trichopoulos, D. (1992) Association between hepatitis C virus and hepatocellular carcinoma using assays based on structural and nonstructural hepatitis C virus peptides. *Cancer Res.*, **52**, 5364–5367

Zhang, Y.-Y., Hansson, B.G., Widell, A. & Nordenfelt, E. (1992) Hepatitis C virus antibodies and hepatitis C virus RNA in Chinese blood donors determined by ELISA, recombinant immunoblot assay and polymerase chain reaction. *Acta pathol. microbiol. immunol. scand.*, **100**, 851–855

Zignego, A.L., Macchia, D., Monti, M., Thiers, V., Mazzetti, M., Foschi, M., Maggi, E., Romagnani, S., Gentilini, P. & Bréchot, C. (1992) Infection of peripheral mononuclear blood cells by hepatitis C virus. *J. Hepatol.*, **15**, 382–386

HEPATITIS D VIRUS

1. Exposure Data

1.1 Structure and biology of hepatitis D virus (HDV)

1.1.1 *Structure of the virus*

Hepatitis delta antigen (HDAg) was first described by Rizzetto *et al.* (1977). Hepatitis D virus (HDV), also known as the 'delta agent', is a satellite agent of hepatitis B virus (HBV). HDV does not synthezise its own coat; it is enveloped by hepatitis B surface antigen (HBsAg), which occurs as large (L), middle (M) and small or major (S) surface proteins, differing in the length of the amino-terminal extension (Ueda *et al.*, 1991). In infectious hepatitis B virions, the ratio of the three HBsAgs L:M:S in the envelope is 1:1:4 (Bruss & Ganem, 1991). In comparison, the ratio L:M:S in HDV particles is 1:5:95 (Taylor, 1992). In this respect, HDV envelopes are very similar to empty spherical HBsAg particles, suggesting that HDV uses the excess production of empty HBsAg particles. It has been shown *in vitro* that the smallest HBsAg (S) is sufficient to package the HDV genome (Wang *et al.*, 1991). Interestingly, HDAg could also be packaged by woodchuck hepatitis virus (WHV) surface antigen, even in the absence of HDV RNA (Ryu *et al.*, 1992).

Naturally occurring HDV particles have a diameter of about 36 nm (Wang *et al.*, 1986) but are somewhat heterogeneous in size. Inside the HBsAg particle is the HDAg and the viral RNA genome. HDV RNA and HDAg exist as a ribonucleoprotein complex (Taylor, 1992).

1.1.2 *Structure of HDV genome and gene products*

The viral genome was first identified in 1986 in sera and liver tissue from HBV–HDV infected chimpanzees and was found to be a single-stranded (Taylor, 1990), circular RNA molecule of about 1700 base pairs (Chen *et al.*, 1986; Denniston *et al.*, 1986; Kos *et al.*, 1986; Wang *et al.*, 1986). Subsequently, HDV RNA was isolated from human sera (Makino *et al.*, 1987; Imazeki *et al.*, 1990; Saldanha *et al.*, 1990; Dény *et al.*, 1991; Imazeki *et al.*, 1991) and from liver tissue of experimentally infected woodchucks (Kuo *et al.*, 1988a; Dény *et al.*, 1991). The complete HDV RNA sequence is known for isolates from humans (Makino *et al.*, 1987; Saldanha *et al.*, 1990; Dény *et al.*, 1991; Imazeki *et al.*, 1991), chimpanzees (Wang *et al.*, 1986) and woodchucks (Kuo *et al.*, 1988a; Dény *et al.*, 1991). The domains of the HDV genome have been divided into primarily *cis*-acting sequences involved in genome replication and a region that encodes HDAg (Branch *et al.*, 1989; Chao *et al.*, 1990; Taylor, 1992). Through extensive base pairing (about 70%; Taylor, 1990), the circular HDV RNA genome forms an unbranched, rod-like structure (Kos *et al.*, 1986; Wang *et al.*, 1986; Makino *et al*, 1987; Kuo *et al.*, 1988a).

HDV is the only known animal virus with a circular RNA genome (Taylor, 1990): circular RNAs have so far been found only in higher plants, where they exist as subviral pathogens, called viroids, or as viroid-like satellite RNAs. Viroids are non-encapsidated, short, circular RNA molecules with a rod-like secondary structure, which replicate autonomously in susceptible cells and do not code for any protein. Viroid-like satellite RNAs are found within the capsid of specific helper viruses required for their replication. Phylogenetic analyses revealed that HDV RNA carries a viroid-like domain which is closely related to the viroid-like satellite RNAs of plants (Elena et al., 1991).

HDV particles contain a single species of RNA, called genomic RNA. In infected liver cells, significant amounts of two other RNA species are detected: an RNA species representing the full-length complement of the genome, known as antigenomic RNA; and complementary RNAs of less than full length which encode the HDAg (Chen et al., 1986, 1989; Hsieh et al., 1990). Self-processing properties were first described for pre-rRNA of tetrahymena (a ciliated protozoan) (Cech & Bass, 1986); both genomic and antigenomic HDV RNAs have been shown to contain well-defined, self-cleaving, self-ligating sequences (Kuo et al., 1988b; Sharmeen et al., 1988, 1989; Wu & Lai, 1989; Wu et al., 1989). The structural and biochemical requirements for self-cleavage and self-ligation have been defined (Wu et al., 1989; Wu & Lai, 1990; Perrotta & Been, 1991; Kumar et al., 1992; Suh et al., 1992). Self-cleavage of HDV RNA is believed to be a central feature for the processing of viral RNA during replication (Taylor, 1990).

HDAg is the only known protein encoded by HDV RNA (Taylor et al., 1992). HDAg is found not only inside the HDV particles but also within the nuclei of infected cells. Human HDAg has been shown to be a highly basic nuclear phosphoprotein with RNA binding activity, specific for HDV RNA (Chang et al., 1988). The RNA binding activity depends, at least in part, on the rod-like structure of HDV RNA (Chao et al., 1991). There are two related forms of HDAg (Bergmann & Gerin, 1986; Wang et al., 1986; Weiner et al., 1988): the small form (S), 195 amino acids long, which is essential for delta replication (Kuo et al., 1988a, 1989); and the large form (L), 214 amino acids long (Makino et al., 1987), which represents a 19-amino acid carboxy-terminal extension of the small form. During HDV replication, initiated by the S genome, a population of modified HDV genomes appears that encodes the L protein. The mutation responsible for the switch from S to L protein synthesis is an A to G mutation in the termination codon of the S form. The substrate for the sequence change is the viral genomic RNA rather than the antigenomic RNA (Luo et al., 1990; Casey et al., 1992; Zheng et al., 1992).

The small form of HDAg (S) is required for HDV RNA replication, however, it is not sufficient for HDV virion production. While both antigenic isoforms of HDAg (S and L) have an HDV genome binding domain and are packaged into HBsAg envelopes, presence of the L form of HDAg is required for virion synthesis; this protein itself can be packaged into HBsAg particles in the complete absence of HDV RNA (Chen et al., 1992). The L protein not only fails to support HDV replication but acts as a *trans*-dominant inhibitor of viral replication (Glenn & White, 1991). Experimental evidence suggests that the two main functions of the L form of HDAg, i.e. in packaging and *trans*-dominant inhibition of HDV replication, are located in different domains of the large HDAg (Chen et al., 1992).

Thus, the small form of HBsAg is sufficient for HDV particle assembly; the large form of HDAg is required for HDV virion production; the small form of HDAg is necessary for HDV replication; and the large form of HDAg inhibits HDV replication.

1.1.3 *Replication of HDV*

Since the HDV genome does not carry a polymerase gene and purified preparations of HDV are not associated with polymerase activity (Wang *et al.*, 1986), the exact mode of replication of HDV and consequently the extent of the helper function of the hepadnaviruses is not known. In-situ hybridization analyses suggest that replication of HDV RNA is closely associated with HDAg expression and is located primarily in nuclei of infected cells (Gowans *et al.*, 1988).

HDV replication does not require hepatocytes and also occurs in mouse fibroblasts (Taylor, 1992) and COS7 monkey kidney cells (Kuo *et al.*, 1989). The only known HDV protein required for viral replication is the small form of HDAg (Taylor, 1992).

Studies of HDV-related nucleic acids from livers of infected hosts show clearly that HDV replicates without a DNA intermediate. Instead, HDV replicates *via* RNA-directed RNA synthesis (Taylor, 1990). The replication of HDV is in many ways similar to that of the plant viroids, virusoids and satellite RNAs (Branch *et al.*, 1990; Elena *et al.*, 1991): replication occurs in the cell nucleus (Gowans *et al.*, 1988); the enzyme is probably a redirected RNA polymerase II (MacNaughton *et al.*, 1991); and both self-cleavage and self-ligation of RNA are involved (Kuo *et al.*, 1988b; Sharmeen *et al.*, 1988, 1989; Wu & Lai, 1989; Wu *et al.*, 1989; Wu & Lai, 1990; Perrotta & Been, 1991; Kumar *et al.*, 1992; Suh *et al.*, 1992). Models have been proposed for the regulation of RNA processing and for HDV replication (Taylor, 1990; Hsieh & Taylor, 1991; Taylor *et al.*, 1992).

A number of in-vitro systems allow analysis of HDV replication. A system for the continuous replication and gene expression of the HDV genome has been established (Chen *et al.*, 1990).

1.1.4 *HDV-related animal models*

HDV has been successfully transmitted to chimpanzees (Rizzetto *et al.*, 1980a,b, 1981a; Purcell *et al.*, 1987). Serial passage of HDV in chronically HBV-seropositive chimpanzees resulted in increasingly severe liver disease without increasing markers of HDV replication or gene expression (Ponzetto *et al.*, 1988a). In addition, HDV has been propagated in WHV-infected woodchucks (Ponzetto *et al.*, 1984a, 1987a; Negro *et al.*, 1989; Dourakis *et al.*, 1991) and has been reported in ducks infected with duck hepatitis B virus (Ponzetto *et al.*, 1987b). The available evidence indicates that HDV infection does not occur naturally in these animal models, and humans are the only known natural host.

1.1.5 *HDV mutants*

Heterogeneity of HDV genomes exists between isolates from different geographic regions as well as in given isolates. A comparison of published HDV sequences from different geographic regions revealed a homology of 85–90%, regardless of their geographic origin (Lai *et al.*, 1991). The extremes are the high degree of homology (about 95%) between an HDV isolate from southern California (Makino *et al.*, 1987) and one from England (Saldanha *et al.*, 1990) and the low degree of homology (about 80%) between two isolates from Japan (Imazeki *et al.*, 1990). Sequence divergence has also been noted within the same geographic area (Lai *et al.*, 1991). It is highest in the genome region between nucleotides 0 and 650 (Saldanha *et al.*, 1990) where no biologically important function has been localized.

HDV sequence variations are also seen in individual patients. In a study from Japan (Imazeki *et al.*, 1990), the mutation rate of HDV was calculated to be about 0.6 per kilobase and year; and in one from southern California (USA) (Lai *et al.*, 1991), the rate was 7–20 mutations per kilobase and year. This mutation frequency, inherently high for RNA viruses owing to lack of a proof-reading function of RNA polymerases, results in the coexistence of different genotypes, called quasispecies, in HDV-infected individuals. The significance of HDV mutations and HDV mutants is unknown.

1.1.6 *HDV–HBV interaction*

HDV replication can proceed in the absence of a hepadnavirus both *in vitro* (Taylor *et al.*, 1987) and *in vivo* (Ottobrelli *et al.*, 1991). For propagation and expression of its pathogenetic potential, HDV requires the presence of genetic information that encodes the major HBsAg (Wang *et al.*, 1991) from a hepadnavirus. Therefore, concurrent infection with a hepadnavirus is a prerequisite for the natural life cycle of HDV. Although HBV expression is a prerequisite for HDV propagation, it is significantly reduced by HDV both *in vivo* (Arico *et al.*, 1985; Hadziyannis *et al.*, 1985; Krogsgaard *et al.*, 1987; Chen *et al.*, 1988; Chu & Liaw, 1988; Wu *et al.*, 1990a) and *in vitro* (Wu *et al.*, 1991).

Clinically, the highest levels of HDV replication are found in patients with the highest level of HBV replication, usually in the serological setting of HBsAg and HBeAg positivity; these patients also had the most serious course of liver disease (Smedile *et al.*, 1991a).

In patients who had undergone liver tranplantation for end-stage HDV-associated chronic liver disease, HDV reinfection was detected early with no evidence of HBV infection or liver pathology. Reappearance of liver disease was preceded by reactivation of HBV replication and by intrahepatic propagation of HDV (Ottobrelli *et al.*, 1991). These findings suggest that HDV–HBV cooperation is necessary for HDV-associated liver disease. Therefore, a third mechanism in addition to HDV coinfection with HBV and HDV superinfection of HBV carriers may be HBV superinfection of HDV carriers. Whether HDV infection exists in HBV-seronegative individuals who are potentially at risk of becoming superinfected with HBV is unclear.

1.1.7 *Host range and target cells of HDV infection*

The host range of HDV is very narrow and follows that of HBV. Current evidence indicates that natural HDV infection occurs only in humans. This host range is believed to reflect the specificity of the liver-cell receptor for the HBV envelope protein, which binds to an epitope in the pre-S1 region 21–47 (Neurath *et al.*, 1986) and which is also found on cells of extrahepatic origin (Neurath *et al.*, 1990). It is not clear whether the ligand on HDV used for virus adsorption is identical to HBV.

In infected individuals, HDAg and nucleic acids are found primarily in liver cells. HDV RNA copy numbers are estimated to be about 300 000 per infected cell (Taylor, 1990). In infected chimpanzees, as many as 10^{11} virions can be detected per millilitre of blood (Ponzetto et al., 1988a). In contrast to HBV (Blum et al., 1983; Halpern et al., 1983; Tagawa et al., 1985; Yoffe et al., 1990), HDAg and HDV RNA have not been detected conclusively in tissues other than liver.

1.2 Methods of detection

1.2.1 In serum and plasma

Infection is detected on the basis of assays for viral antibodies or viral RNA in serum or HDAg in liver tissue. Typical serological markers of acute and chronic hepatitis D are shown in Figure 1.

Fig. 1. Typical serological markers of acute and chronic hepatitis D

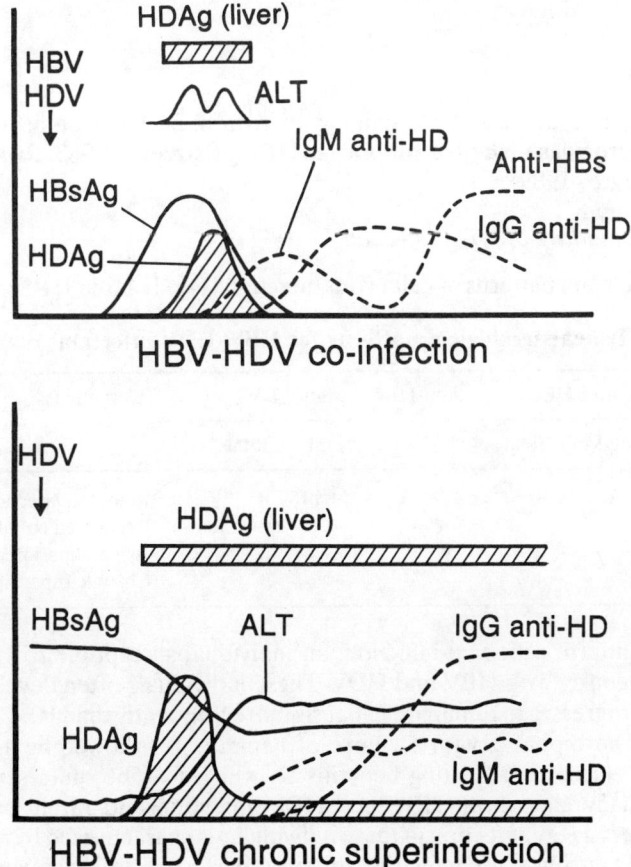

HBV, hepatitis B virus; HDV, hepatitis D virus; HDAg, hepatitis D antigen; HBsAg, hepatitis B surface antigen; Ig, immunoglobulin; anti-HD, hepatitis D antibody; anti-HBs, hepatitis B surface antibody; ALT, alanine aminotransferase

(a) Hepatitis D antigen

Several commercial assay systems are available for the detection of HDAg but are not used clinically (Rizzetto et al., 1991). HDAg can be detected by alternative western blot assay (Rizzetto et al., 1991) or by blocking radioimmunoassay (Smedile et al., 1981).

(b) Hepatitis D antibody

Hepatitis D antibody (anti-HD) immunoglobulin (Ig) M class or total anti-HD is detected by enzyme immunoassay and radioimmunoassay (Rizzetto et al., 1981b).

(c) HDV RNA

HDV RNA can be detected by dot (northern) blot hybridization (Smedile et al., 1986) or reverse transcriptase with the polymerase chain reaction (PCR). PCR is much more sensitive than conventional hybridization techniques or immunological analysis. PCR also allows cloning and sequencing of HDV in order to determine genomic structure (Denniston et al., 1986; Zignego et al., 1992).

1.2.2 In liver tissues

Liver HDAg can be tested by staining in frozen or fixed paraffin sections using fluorescence or peroxidase-labelled antibody to HDAg (Rizzetto, 1983; Rizzetto et al., 1983; Di Biceglie & Negro, 1989).

1.2.3 Serological markers of HDV infection

There are two main patterns of delta virus infection (Fig. 1; Table 1; Rizzetto et al., 1991).

Table 1. Typical serological patterns for HBV–HDV infection

HBsAg	Anti-HBc		Anti-HBs	Anti-HDV		Comments
	IgM	Total		IgM	Total	
+	+	+	−	+	+	Acute co-infection
−	−	+	+	−	(+ then −)	Recovered co-infection
+	−	+	−	+	+	Acute superinfection
+	−	+	−	−	+	Chronic superinfection

In the first pattern, called co-infection, an individual susceptible to HBV infection is infected simultaneously with HBV and HDV. These individuals often develop severe acute hepatitis, which progresses to fulminant hepatitis more frequently than HBV infection alone. The disease may be biphasic, with a course of hepatitis B followed by a brief period of recovery, and a relapse representing hepatitis D, which may be quite severe. If patients recover, they usually clear both HBV and HDV infection and rarely become HBV or HBV–HDV carriers. HDV infection in these individuals is characterized by seropositivity for IgM class anti-HD during acute infection, followed by a weak IgG class anti-HD response (measured as total anti-HDV), which persists for one to five years. For this reason, serological surveys of anti-HD prevalence do not reflect adequately past history of HDV coinfection.

In the second pattern, called superinfection, an HBV carrier is infected with HDV. At this point, the patient may develop clinical, biochemical and histological signs and symptoms of acute viral hepatitis; however, most patients are unable to clear the virus and become chronic carriers of both HBV and HDV, with a clinical course of chronic active hepatitis progressing to cirrhosis, which may be much more aggressive than HBV infection alone. Total anti-HDV antibodies persist at high titres for prolonged periods, often for life, in these patients. HDV infection may suppress HBV replication, and some patients become HBsAg seronegative, leading to potential diagnostic confusion unless testing for anti-HBc and anti-HDV is done concurrently. HDV RNA may be used to follow these patients; HDAg is not routinely measured in serum (Salassa *et al.*, 1991).

1.3 Epidemiology of infection

1.3.1 *Prevalence*

The interpretation of epidemiological studies of infection should take into account the fact that it requires the presence of HBV. In many studies, only those individuals seropositive for HBV are tested for HDV. Since HDV infection suppresses the expression of HBsAg, the prevalence of infection may be underestimated. Secondly, in people who resolve their HDV infection, there is no long-lasting serological marker of past infection. Thus, prevalence studies reflect only recent and chronic infection. Superinfection is associated with significantly increased morbidity and mortality from chronic liver disease, and this effect on survival also influences the interpretation of prevalence data. For these reasons, the studies of geographic variation described below indicate the characteristics of the groups being tested.

Since HDV infection is so dependent on HBV infection, the descriptive data have been classified by level of infection with HBV. Table 2 shows the prevalence of infection with HDV in countries with a low endemicity of hepatitis B. There was no significant difference in infection rates between men and women in these studies. The reports from Norway and Sweden both showed no HDV infection in populations of intravenous drug users in the early 1970s but a rise in the prevalence of infection from the mid-70s onwards. HDV was introduced in Scandinavia in 1970–75 (Hansson *et al.*, 1982; Siebke *et al.*, 1986). The study of blood donors in the USA showed no association between seroprevalence for HDV and age, sex or blood group, but there was a significantly higher prevalence of anti-HD in HBV-carrier donors from California (12.1%) than from other areas of the USA (1.4–6.7%) (Nath *et al.*, 1985).

Table 3 shows the prevalence of infection with HDV in various populations in countries with intermediate levels of hepatitis B endemicity. There is a consistently higher prevalence among people with chronic hepatitis than among asymptomatic carriers. There is also marked geographical variability. HDV was introduced in Greece in 1965; a decrease in HDV infection has been observed subsequently (Hadziyannis *et al.*, 1991).

The prevalences of HDV in countries with a high endemicity for hepatitis B are shown in Table 4. There is again geographical variability between countries and also marked varia-

Table 2. Prevalence of HDV antibody (HDAg) in various hepatitis B surface antigen (HBsAg)-seropositive populations of countries and regions with low endemicity of hepatitis B

Country or region	Period	Group studied	No. of HBsAg carriers	Prevalence (%) of HDAg sero-positivity among HBsAg sero-positives	Reference
France	1984–88	Pregnant women	52	13.5	Ranger et al. (1990)
Germany	1982–84	Blood donors	301	0.3	Roggendorf et al. (1986)
		Haemodialysis patients	298	0.7	
		Chronic liver disease patients	220	2.7	
		Intravenous drug users	13	38.5	
		Haemophiliacs	16	50.0	
Northern Ireland	1970–89	Haemophiliacs	28	7.1	Curran et al. (1991)
		Foreign-born adults/contacts	153	2.6	
Sweden	1970–81	Chronic carriers			Hansson et al. (1982)
		Intravenous drug users	80	51.3	
		Non-intravenous drug users	101	3.0	
		Acute carriers			
		Intravenous drug users	291	17.2	
		Non-intravenous drug users	308	1.6	
Norway	1972–82	Chronic carriers	108	0	Siebke et al. (1986)
		Intravenous drug users	64	32.8	
Poland	NR	Asymptomatic carriers	123	1.6	Boron et al. (1987)
		Acute hepatitis B patients	35	2.8	
		Chronic hepatitis B or cirrhosis patients	15	6.6	
Canada	1983–85	Chronic carriers	121	0	Ratnam et al. (1986)
		Acute hepatitis B patients	22	0	
USA	1979	Blood donors	1915	3.8	Nath et al. (1985)

NR, not reported

bility within countries both geographically and between ethnic groups. Thus, Greenfield et al. (1986) in 1982–84 found virtually no HDV infection in 123 HBsAg-seropositive patients from the southern part of Kenya but a prevalence of 31% among healthy individuals in the north. Among these northern tribes, there was marked variation in the prevalence of HDV infection: 22% in the Turkana, 65% in the Rendille and 72% in the Samburn. A study in Djibouti in 1987 (Abbatte et al., 1989) found marked differences by ethnic group, with a prevalence of HDV of 7.7% in male Afars and 0.7% in the remainder of the population. In China (Roggendorf et al., 1987), prevalences of HDV infection in the general population vary by province, from 0 to 9%, in HBsAg-seropositive individuals. The reasons for these local variations are not understood. HDV infection, and particularly superinfection of HBV carriers, appears to be an ominous occurrence that may develop in populations among whom

HBV infection is endemic, e.g. in Venezuela. The age at infection in these populations is dependent on the usual age at infection with HBV (Hadler et al., 1984). In the study of Bensabath et al. (1987) in the Amazon Basin, Brazil, children were infected under the age of 10 years, clearly indicating that a horizontal, non-sexual route is involved.

Table 3. Prevalence of HDV antibody (HDAg) in various hepatitis B surface antigen (HBsAg)-seropositive populations of countries or regions with intermediate endemicity of hepatitis B

Country or region	Period	Group studied	No. of HBsAg carriers	Prevalence (%) of HDAg seropositivity among HBsAg seropositives	Reference
Former USSR	NR	Asymptomatic carriers			Ketiladze et al. (1987)
		European	274	3.3	
		Asian	257	14.4	
		Chronic hepatitis B patients			
		European	36	13.9	
		Asian	63	41.3	
Greece	1983	General population	260	27.3	Hadziyannis et al. (1987)
Spain	1974–86	Acute hepatitis B patients			Buti et al. (1988)
		Intravenous drug users	155	65	
		Non-intravenous drug users	102	8.8[a]	
		Chronic hepatitis B patients			
		Intravenous drug users	105	67	
		Non-intravenous drug users	319	5.6	
		Asymptomatic carriers	68	0	
Italy	1975–85	Asymptomatic carriers	210	6.0	Smedile et al. (1987)
		Acute hepatitis B patients	238	5.4	
		Chronic hepatitis B patients	171	16.3	
Argentina	NR	Blood donors	1168	1.4	Fay et al. (1987)
		Acute hepatitis B patients	130	0.77	
		Chronic hepatitis B patients	135	2.2	
		Cirrhosis patients	52	5.8	
Jordan	1978–85	Asymptomatic carriers	136	1.5	Toukan et al. (1987)
		Acute hepatitis B patients	108	15.7	
		Chronic hepatitis B patients	79	22.8	
Egypt	1986	Chronic hepatitis B patients	44	47.7	El Zayadi et al. (1988)
		Asymptomatic carriers	48	8.3	
Yemen	1988	General population	112	1.8	Scott et al. (1990)
Saudi Arabia	NR	Pregnant women	185	9.7	Ramia & Bahakim (1988)
India	NR	Commercial donors	135	5.9	Arankalle et al. (1992)
		Voluntary donors	243	2.1	

NR, not reported
[a]HDAg or anti-HD

Table 4. Prevalence of HDV antibody (HDAg) in various hepatitis B surface antigen (HBsAg)-seropositive populations of countries or regions with high endemicity of hepatitis B

Country or region	Period	Group studied	No. of HBsAg carriers	Prevalence (%) of HDAg seropositivity among HBsAg seropositives	Reference
China	1983–85	Asymptomatic carriers	246	0.4	Wang et al. (1987)
		Acute hepatitis B patients	65	3.1	
		Chronic hepatitis B patients	104	0.9	
Indonesia	1986	Pregnant women	26	0	Vranckx et al. (1988)
Pacific Islands	1985–86	General population	646	33	Brindle et al. (1988)
Somalia	NR	General population	220	16.8	Aceti et al. (1989)
Kenya	1986–87	General population	132	42.4	Okoth et al. (1991)
Central African Republic	1984–88	Hospital patients	34	41.2	Crovari et al. (1991)
Brazil (Amazon)	NR	General population	232	45.2	da Fonseca et al. (1987)
Brazil (Amazon)	NR	Asymptomatic carriers	99	24	Bensabath et al. (1987)
		Acute hepatitis B patients	25	28	
		Chronic hepatitis B patients	21	100	
		Fulminant hepatitis B patients	27	74	

1.3.2 Transmission

In all populations studied, intravenous drug users have some of the highest prevalences of infection with HDV. In the USA, some 42% of HBsAg-seropositive intravenous drug users were found to be infected with HDV in the early 1970s (Ponzetto et al., 1984b), 35% of imprisoned intravenous drug users who were HBV carriers in Greece were positive for HDV (Roumeliotou-Karayannis et al., 1987) and 65% of a similar group in Scotland. As in Scandinavia, the virus appears to have first affected intravenous drug users in Scotland around 1975 (McCruden & Follett, 1989). In Poland, serial prevalence studies of intravenous drug users suggest that introduction was later, in the mid-1980s (Laskus et al., 1992). The introduction of HDV into the intravenous drug user population has been shown to have led to outbreaks of infection among the non-user population (Mijch et al., 1987) through both non-sexual and sexual routes (Lettau et al., 1987).

Sexual transmission of HDV infection appears to be relatively inefficient. A study of 1368 US female prostitutes, ≥ 18 years old, showed that only 6% of the 18 non-drug users who were HBV carriers were seropositive for HDV; seropositivity rose to 21% of the 21 HBV carriers among intravenous drug users (Rosenblum et al., 1992). A study of acute hepatitis due to HDV in Taiwanese men showed a significant association with sexual contact with prostitutes (odds ratio, 5.5); the prevalence of HDV infection amongst HBV-carrier prostitutes was 59% (Wu *et al.*, 1990b). In a similar study in Taiwan, which included women with acute HDV hepatitis, one of the four women seropositive for HDV was a prostitute and another was the wife of a patient with active HDV infection (Liaw *et al.*, 1990). These studies suggest that the major risk for HDV infection of the general population in some parts of the world is heterosexual transmission.

The prevalence of HDV among male homosexual HBV carriers in Italy was 40% (4/10) and that in male heterosexual HBV carriers was 17% (6/36) (Mele *et al.*, 1988). Studies of four cohorts of homosexual men in the USA showed that rates of HDV infection among HBsAg-seropositive men varied significantly by geographic location, from 15.1% in Los Angeles to 0 in Chicago. HDV infection was associated with intravenous drug use, number of sexual partners and rectal trauma (Solomon *et al.*, 1988). Incident studies of homosexual male participants in HBV vaccine trials and in the 'Sentinel Counties Study' of acute hepatitis in the USA revealed three men with HDV infections among 290 with newly diagnosed HBV in the trials and none among 63 men with acute HBV infections in the Sentinel Counties Study, suggesting that HDV is an infrequent cause of acute hepatitis in homosexual men in the USA (Weisfuse *et al.*, 1989).

Blood transfusion and in particular administration of pooled blood products carried a high risk of HDV infection, as attested by the prevalence of 17–100% HDV infection in HBsAg-seropositive haemophiliacs (Lemon *et al.*, 1991; see also Table 2). The risk for transfusion-associated HDV infection has been estimated at one in 3000 transfusions, on the basis of sensitive tests for HBV markers (Rosina *et al.*, 1985).

Familial transmission of HDV was studied in Italy. Female sex of the index case in a household (odds ratio, 5.5) and HDV infection in that index HBV carrier (odds ratio, 71) were both independently associated with HDV superinfection of household members (Craxì *et al.*, 1991).

A study of 1556 HBV carriers who first presented to 35 liver units in Italy showed that the prevalence of HDV was independently related to young age (peak, 30–40 years), residence in the south of the country, intravenous drug use, large families and household contact with a HDV carrier. No association was found with blood transfusion or male homosexuality (Sagnelli *et al.*, 1992).

1.4 Clinical diseases (other than cancer)

HDV can either co-infect with HBV or superinfect HBV carriers (Rizzetto, 1983). In early studies, a link between HDV and severe liver disease was consistently demonstrated, leading to the widely accepted concept that this virus was invariably a highly pathogenic agent (Rizzetto *et al.*, 1983). Contrary to that hypothesis was a recent observation that patients in Greece (Hadziyannis *et al.*, 1991) and several liver transplant recipients in Italy and Belgium (Ottobrelli *et al.*, 1991) had clinically latent HDV infections which were associated with minor liver damage and even normal histology (Rizzetto *et al.*, 1992).

1.4.1 *Acute infection*

Acute hepatitis D results either from coinfection or superinfection and is of differing degrees of clinical severity. Many patients with acute HDV–HBV co-infection have a delayed immune response to HDV (anti-HD), requiring that serial blood samples be tested over months after the onset of hepatitis in order to establish the correct diagnosis (Salassa et al., 1991). In these patients, the hepatitis had a biphasic course, characterized by two peaks in serum alanine aminotransferase levels a few weeks apart (Caredda et al., 1987). Co-occurrence of IgM anti-HBc and IgM anti-HD is a typical serological feature of acute co-infection (Di Bisceglie & Negro, 1989) (see also Table 1). HDV superinfection of HBsAg carriers often results in a monophasic hepatitis with seroconversion to IgM anti-HD. Severe hepatitis is common in both co-infected and superinfected patients (Craig et al., 1986; Caredda et al., 1987).

Fulminant hepatitis is more frequent in HDV-infected patients than in patients with hepatitis B alone (Smedile et al., 1982). During the years 1979–82, 55 cases of fulminant hepatitis were seen in a unit in Milan, Italy: 28 were serologically related to HDV, and four of these were cases of superinfection of chronic HBsAg carriers (Rizzetto et al., 1992). During the period 1986–88, HDV infection was found to account for 13 of 25 cases (52%) of fulminant hepatitis B in adults seen at the Western Attica General Hospital in Athens, Greece; five of the 13 were intravenous drug users (Tassopoulos et al., 1990). Of the 71 patients admitted to the University of Southern California Liver Service (USA) in 1969–83 with fulminant hepatitis B, HDV infection was demonstrated in 33.8%, and 79% of these cases were due to HBV–HDV co-infection (Govindarajan et al., 1984a).

1.4.2 Chronic infection

In Milan, hepatitis progressed to chronicity in 1.2% of patients with acute hepatitis B alone, in 2.4% of HBV–HDV co-infected patients and in as many as 91% of those super-infected with HDV (Caredda et al., 1987). While progression to chronicity was frequent in the superinfected patients, the risk in the co-infected patients was the same as for patients with HBV infection alone.

Several lines of evidence support the existence of carriers of HBsAg and anti-HD with persistently normal serum alanine aminotransferase and essentially normal livers (Hadziyannis et al., 1991; Rizzetto et al., 1992). Follow-up of 27 HDV-seropositive liver transplant recipients showed that HDV recurred in 22 (81%); in nine patients, the virus recurred without recrudescence of liver disease (Ottobrelli et al., 1991).

Anti-HD was commoner in patients with chronic active hepatitis or cirrhosis than in other patient groups (Sagnelli et al., 1992). In highly endemic areas, chronic liver failure was largely caused by HDV superinfection and exposure to HDV early in life (Bensabath et al., 1987). Chronic hepatitis D presents a wide range of symptoms, none of which is sufficiently specific to provide a diagnosis. Characteristic features of these patients are the prevalence of anti-HBe in serum and a frequent history of acute hepatitis. In contrast, a clinical episode of hepatitis was reported in fewer than 5% of the HDV-seronegative carriers with anti-HBe in Mediterranean countries (Rizzetto et al., 1983). Additional features noted in southern European patients were the presence of splenomegaly and, in advanced cases, the presence of cholestasis out of proportion to other indices of liver failure (Rizzetto et al., 1992).

A long-term study of 176 Italian patients with chronic hepatitis D showed that the course of the disease is bimodal (Bonino et al., 1987). In about 15% of the patients, the disease progressed to liver failure within two years; in about 70%, the disease evolved slowly over

10–20 years; and the remainder had spontaneous remission of the disease. Using an HDV RNA riboprobe to detect the serum virological pattern and PCR for amplification of serum HBV DNA, chronic hepatitis D patients were divided into three groups: those with simultaneously replicating HDV and HBV, those with replicating HDV alone and those with neither HDV nor HBV replication (Smedile et al., 1991b). Histological examination showed active disease in all patients of the first group, with a tendency for rapid evolution to cirrhosis and liver failure. More cases of inactive cirrhosis were observed in the second and third groups. It is possible that the virological states of the three subgroups represent different phases of the same disease course.

These data clearly indicate that active infection with HBV and HDV results in more severe liver damage than with either virus alone. Studies of liver transplant patients demonstrated that HDV infection in the transplanted liver is not in itself pathogenic and the virus becomes hepatotoxic only when HBV is reactivated (Ottobrelli et al., 1991). Serial analyses in patients demonstrate rapid development of genotypic heterogeneity of HDV. The rates of evolution of the HDV isolates may correlate with the changes in the clinical pictures of hepatitis: the more drastic the change in the symptom of hepatitis, the more nucleotide changes were detected (Lee et al., 1992).

1.5 Therapy and immunoprophylaxis

1.5.1 *Therapy*

(a) Acute fulminant HDV infection

In symptomatic acute fulminant HDV infection, therapy is aimed at relieving the signs and symptoms associated with the acute phase of the disease. Therapy includes parenteral nutrition in cases of dehydration and inanition due to nausea and vomiting, replacement of coagulation factors in cases of bleeding due to impaired synthetic liver functions and liver transplantation in cases of advanced liver failure and hepatic coma (Maddrey & Van Thiel, 1988). Except for an anecdotal report on the use of adenosine arabinoside monophosphate (Garcia et al., 1990), no trial of antiviral agents in acute HDV infection has been published.

(b) Chronic HDV infection

Because of the severe natural course of HDV infection, several therapeutic modalities have been explored: prednisone, azathioprine, levamisole (Arrigoni et al., 1983; Rizzetto et al., 1983) and adenine arabinoside (Rosina et al., 1991) were shown to be ineffective. Interferon-α has been explored in several trials (Hoofnagle et al., 1986, 1987; Rosina et al., 1987; Thomas et al., 1987; Rosina & Rizzetto, 1989; Rosina et al., 1991). While interferon-α was of some value for the treatment of chronic hepatitis D, long-term follow-up of HDV carriers revealed a high relapse rate after cessation of therapy.

1.5.2 *Immunoprophylaxis*

There is no specific vaccine against HDV. Vaccines against hepatitis B provide protection to individuals susceptible to both HBV and HDV but provide protection to HBV carriers against HDV. The degree of protection afforded by HBV vaccine is presumed to be similar to that against HBV carriage, but the protective efficacy against HDV has never been evaluated. HBV immunoglobulin does not prevent superinfection with HDV.

2. Studies of Cancer in Humans

2.1 Case series

Studies of hepatocellular carcinoma (HCC) and seropositivity for anti-HD in case series are summarized in Table 5. The prevalence of anti-HD seropositivity varied from 0 to 88%, but the findings are difficult to interpret because of the highly variable prevalence of HDV infection in the source populations.

2.2 Case–control studies

Kew *et al.* (1984) detected neither anti-HD nor HDAg in sera from 107 HBsAg-seropositive black South Africans with HCC (101 men, six women); testing was by radioimmunoassay. Moreover, tissue HDAg was not found in neoplastic and non-neoplastic liver samples from an additional 80 cases of HCC by the direct immunoperoxidase technique. Serum anti-HD and HDAg were not present in the HBsAg-positive chronic carriers or in the renal transplant recipients tested.

Cronberg *et al.* (1984) conducted a study of 130 clinically diagnosed cases of HCC, 83 patients with other liver disorders and 50 controls in Senegal. Most of the subjects were seen at Le Dantec Hospital; the controls were primarily healthy relatives of patients. The 88 cases who were considered 'highly probable' to have HCC on the basis of an α-fetoprotein level ≥ 100 μg/L were compared with 31 controls with a level ≤ 15 μg/L. Anti-HD was found by solid-phase radioimmunoassay in 13 (20%) of the 65 HBsAg-seropositive 'highly probable' HCC cases. The investigators compared this prevalence with that of those HBsAg-seropositive people without HCC, combining the eight controls and 26 other subjects with liver disorders who had an α-fetoprotein level ≤ 15 μg/L in order to obtain a figure of 21%. The anti-HD prevalence was 0 in the eight HBsAg-seropositive controls and 27% in the 26 other patients. [No further details were given as to subject selection or study timing.]

Liaw *et al.* (1987) reported a 4% prevalence of HDV seropositivity among 124 HBV-carrier cases of HCC in Taiwan, China; none had a history of drug abuse or multiple blood transfusions. Two percent of asymptomatic HBsAg carriers and 14% of HBsAg-seropositive liver cirrhosis patients were also seropositive for anti-HD. Anti-HD antibody in serum was analysed by radioimmunoassay and HDAg in liver by direct immunofluorescence.

Trichopoulos *et al.* (1987a), in a study described in the monograph on HBV (p. 88; Trichopoulos *et al.*, 1987b), tested for the presence of HDAg and anti-HD in the sera of 87 HBsAg-seropositive HCC cases and 29 HBsAg-seropositive hospital controls, using ELISA for HDAg and radioimmunoassay for anti-HD. No HDAg was detected; 10% of cases and no control were reactive to anti-HD (exact p = 0.067). Adjustment for age and sex had no effect on the comparison. Among HCC cases, no association was found for the presence of cirrhosis and anti-HD seropositivity. A later re-analysis of these subjects for a possible interaction between HDV and HCV found no association with respect to HCC (Tzonou

Table 5. Hepatocellular carcinoma (HCC) and HDV infection in case series

Reference and location	Period	No of HCC cases	No. HBsAg seropositive	No. anti-HD seropositive	No. HDAg seropositive	% HBsAg seropositivity among HDAg seropositives	Assay for HDAg[a]
Africa							
Kew et al. (1984); South Africa	NR	107	107	0	0	0	RIA (serum), IP (liver)
Cenac et al. (1987); Niger	1982–85	29	21	14	NT	67	RIA (serum)
Americas							
Govindarajan et al. (1984b); USA	1971–82	39	39	1	1	3	Solid-phase blocking RIA (serum)
Asia							
Chen et al. (1984); Taiwan, China	NR	11	11	0	0	0	Solid-phase blocking RIA (serum), IF (liver)
Yong-Yuan et al. (1990); China	NR	20	16	NT	0	0	IF and IP (liver) (anti-HD IgG)
Ashraf et al. (1986); Saudi Arabia	1984–85	30	30	5	NT	17	RIA (serum)
Shobokshi & Serebour (1987); Saudi Arabia	NR	116 (serum) 200 (liver)	NR NR	5 NT	NT 12	NR NR	ELISA for total antibody (serum), IF (liver)
Toukan et al. (1987); Jordan	1978–85	15	15	10	NT	67	RIA (serum)
Rezvan et al. (1990); Iran (Islamic Republic of)	1986–88	8	8	5	NT	63	EIA

Table 5 (contd)

Reference and location	Period	No. of HCC cases	No. HBsAg seropositive	No. anti-HD seropositive	No. HDAg seropositive	% HBsAg seropositivity among HDAg seropositives	Assay for HDAg[a]
Europe							
Craxi et al. (1983); Raimondo et al. (1984); Italy	1977–83	79	79	8	0/18	10.1	RIA (serum), IF (liver)
Tapalaga et al. (1987); Romania	NR	8	8	7	NT	87.5	NR (serum)
Oliveri et al. (1991); Italy	1986–89	91	35	10	NT	29	IP (liver)
Verme et al. (1991); Italy	1986–88	62	25	9	NT	36	
Tassopoulos et al. (1989); Greece	1978–85	47	20	0	0	0	RIA (serum)
Hadziyannis et al. (1991); Greece	1970–89	303	303	59	0	19.5	RIA, ELISA (serum)

HBsAg, hepatitis B surface antigen; anti-HD, antibody to HDV; HDAg, hepatitis D antigen; NR, not reported; NT, not tested
[a]RIA, radioimmunoassay; IP, immunoperoxidase; IF, immunofluorescence; ELISA, enzyme-linked immunosorbent assay; EIA, enzyme immunoassay

et al., 1991). Of the 75 anti-HD-seronegative HCC cases tested, 52% were seropositive for anti-HC; in contrast, of the nine anti-HD-seropositive HCC cases, 33% were positive for anti-HC.

In another study, also summarized in the monograph on HBV (p. 81; Di Bisceglie *et al.*, 1991), radioimmunoassay of 99 HCC cases and 98 controls detected none with anti-HD, regardless of seropositivity for HBsAg.

These studies are summarized in Table 6.

Table 6. Case–control studies of HDV in relation to hepatocellular carcinoma among hepatitis B virus carriers[a]

Reference	Location	Cases No.	Cases %	Controls No.	Controls %	RR	95% CI
Trichopoulos *et al.* (1987a)	Greece	87	10	29	0	∞	[0.9–∞]
Cronberg *et al.* (1984)	Senegal	65	20	8	0	∞	[0.4–∞]
Liaw *et al.* (1987)	Taiwan, China	124	4.0	137	2.2	[1.9]	[0.4–12]

[a]In the studies of Kew *et al.* (1984) and Di Bisceglia *et al.* (1991), none of the cases or controls were anti-HD seropositive.

3. Studies of Cancer in Experimental Animals

The only available study (Ponzetto *et al.*, 1988b) was reported as an abstract and could not be used to evaluate the carcinogenicity of HDV.

4. Other Relevant Data

4.1 Pathology

HCC evolves through chronic HDV infection, which usually begins as acute viral hepatitis and may not be apparent clinically. Many patients with chronic HDV are identified through screening programmes, and the acute event is not documented. The transition of chronic hepatitis to cirrhosis may also be inapparent clinically.

4.1.1 *Acute infection*

The hepatocellular degenerative change and inflammatory reaction of HDV superimposed on chronic HBV (usually chronic persistent hepatitis) appear as acute viral hepatitis, and the underlying carrier state is masked and not apparent by histological review. Prior biopsy samples may be available to demonstrate chronic active hepatitis or cirrhosis in some cases, but the acute HDV infection stimulates marked degenerative and inflammatory reactions (Govindarajan *et al.*, 1986a). Some patients with acute HDV have a fulminant course (Govindarajan *et al.*, 1984a). Some have combined acute viral infection with HBV and HDV, but the histological features are similar. Serological data and the clinical course are needed to identify patients with combined HBV and HDV infection, as the histopathology is not diagnostic.

4.1.2 *Chronic infection*

Prolonged inflammation and necrosis are common in patients with chronic hepatitis B and subsequent superinfection with HDV. During this prolonged inflammatory reaction, mild chronic liver disease often proceeds to cirrhosis. In a group of 106 consecutive chronic HBV carriers, 20 had HDV, were younger than the group without HDV and had more severe chronic liver lesions than those without HDV infection. Cirrhosis occurred in 55% and chronic active hepatitis in 45% of the patients with combined infection, whereas cirrhosis was documented in only 19% of the group with chronic HBV (Lok *et al.*, 1985; Govindarajan *et al.*, 1986a). In another group of 57 patients with chronic hepatitis B, 18 also had chronic HDV infection. In this group, the portal inflammation, lobular inflammation and necrosis were more severe in the presence of HDV. HDV staining in hepatocytes indicated current HDV replication, but the intensity of staining did not correlate with the inflammation and necrosis (Kanel *et al.*, 1984).

4.1.3 *Cirrhosis*

The continual necrotizing effect of chronic active hepatitis leads to cirrhosis within a few years in many patients with HBV–HDV co-infection. These patients may succumb to severe inflammatory and necrotizing reactions rather than have silent chronic liver disease, as is common with pure chronic HBV infection (Govindarajan *et al.*, 1986a).

4.2 Other observations relevant to possible mechanisms of action of HDV in carcinogenesis

HDV infection was transmitted experimentally to chimpanzees (Rizzetto *et al.*, 1980a) and eastern woodchucks (Ponzetto *et al.*, 1984a). Following experimental infection, the chimpanzees usually developed acute hepatitis of varying degree (Ponzetto *et al.*, 1987c; Negro *et al.*, 1988). The severity of the damage was not dependent on the infecting dose but rather on changes in the genotypes, favoured by serial passages in the host (Ponzetto *et al.*, 1988a). Characteristically, with increasing passage number there was a decrease in the incubation period for hepatitis, together with an increase in pathogenicity. During the peak levels of HDV, 90% of viral genomes were either defective or non-infectious particles. The acute phase of liver damage was characterized by fluctuations in serum alanine aminotransferase levels, which lasted for up to seven months (Ponzetto *et al.*, 1991). Long-term follow-up of infected chimpanzees revealed that 54% of the animals were still infectious and circulating low levels of serum HDV RNA in the absence of significant histological liver damage (Negro *et al.*, 1988). Those animals that apparently had cleared HDV were still susceptible to reinfection with HDV, indicating lack of vigorous immune protection (Govindarajan et al., 1986b).

Woodchucks persistently infected with WHV showed biological and pathological features similar to those seen in humans, with some differences. As in humans, superinfection of chronic WHV carriers resulted in persistent HDV infection of all animals. Viraemia developed after incubation periods of one to seven weeks, depending on the infecting dose, followed by cyclic fluctuations coincident with HDV RNA expression within the liver-cell nuclei. In the course of serial transmission, an increase in the degree of the infectious potential for HDV was observed (Ponzetto et al., 1991). Animals immunized with purified cloned HDAg were not protected against infectious HDV inoculates (Karayiannis et al., 1992).

5. Summary of Data Reported and Evaluation

5.1 Exposure data

Hepatitis D virus (HDV) exists as a satellite agent of hepatitis B virus (HBV). The viral genome is a circular RNA molecule about 1700 bases long, and HDV antigen is the only known protein that it encodes. The antigen is required for viral replication in hepatocytes. Because hepatitis B surface antigen forms the envelope of HDV, HBV infection is a prerequisite for formation of HDV particles. HDV infection has been detected only in humans, although the agent can be transmitted to HBV-infected chimpanzees and to woodchucks infected with woodchuck hepatitis virus.

HDV infection can be identified in serum by detecting antibody to HDV (anti-HD) and/or HDV RNA; HDV antigen can also be detected immunohistochemically in hepatocytes. In co-infection, HDV RNA and immunoglobulin M class anti-HD appear, followed by the transient appearance of immunoglobulin G class anti-HD. Superinfection usually results in chronic infection, viraemia and persistence of anti-HD.

In countries where endemicity for HBV is low, the prevalence of HDV infection is low, except among intravenous drug users and recipients of blood products. In areas of intermediate and high endemicity for HBV, the prevalence of HDV infection is highly variable: In general, it is rare in Asia, but up to one-half of individuals with chronic HBV infection in parts of southern Europe, the Middle East, Africa, the Pacific Basin and the Amazon region may be infected with HDV. Marked variations in the prevalence of HDV infection are found within countries and sometimes between ethnic groups.

The predominant route of transmission in countries of high endemicity is unknown, that in countries of low endemicity appears to be parenteral. Sexual transmission also occurs.

HDV co- or superinfection generally results in a more severe clinical course than HBV infection alone. HDV superinfection is associated more frequently with progressive liver disease and cirrhosis than HBV infection alone.

Immunoprophylaxis with HBV vaccine is presumed to protect the individual against co-infection but cannot protect HBV carriers against superinfection with HDV. Immune globulin does not protect against HDV superinfection, and no specific HDV vaccine is available.

5.2 Human carcinogenicity data

Several case series showed no evidence of HDV infection among cases of hepatocellular carcinoma, while others reported high levels of infection.

In two case-control studies of hepatocellular carcinoma and HDV infection among subjects seropositive for hepatitis B surface antigen, there were no anti-HD-seropositive individuals among cases or controls. Three further case-control studies suggested a positive association but had limited statistical power.

5.3 Animal carcinogenicity data

No adequate data were available to the Working Group.

5.4 Other relevant data

Case series suggest that chronic hepatitis and cirrhosis develop more rapidly in patients infected with both HBV and HDV than in those infected with HBV alone.

5.5 Evaluation[1]

There is *inadequate evidence* in humans for the carcinogenicity of infection with hepatitis D virus.

There is *inadequate evidence* in experimental animals for the carcinogenicity of infection with hepatitis D virus.

Overall evaluation

Infection with hepatitis D virus *is not classifiable as to its carcinogenicity to humans (Group 3)*.

6. References

Abbatte, E.A., Fox, E., Said, S., Constantine, N.T. & Wassef, H.H. (1989) Ethnic differences in the prevalence of hepatitis delta agent in Djibouti. *Trans. R. Soc. trop. Med. Hyg.*, **83**, 107–108

Aceti, A., Paparo, B.S., Celestino, D., Pennica, A., Caferro, M., Grilli, A., Sebastiani, A., Mohamud, O.M., Abdirahman, M. & Bile, K. (1989) Sero-epidemiology of hepatitis delta virus infection in Somalia. *Trans. R. Soc. trop. Med. Hyg.*, **83**, 399–400

Arankalle, V.A., Ramamoorthy, C.L. & Banerjee, K. (1992) Seroepidemiology of hepatitis delta virus infection in Pune, India. *Trans. R. Soc. trop. Med. Hyg.*, **86**, 89

Arico, S., Aragona, M., Rizzetto, M., Caredda, F., Zanetti, A., Marinucci, G., Diana, S., Farci, P., Arnone, M., Caporaso, N., Ascione, A., Dentico, P., Pastore, G., Raimondo, G. & Craxì, A. (1985) Clinical significance of antibody to the hepatitis delta virus in symptomless HBsAg carriers. *Lancet*, **ii**, 356–358

---

[1]For definition of the italicized terms, see Preamble, pp. 30–34.

Arrigoni, A., Ponzetto, A., Actis, G. & Bonino, F. (1983) Levamisole and chronic delta hepatitis (Letter to the Editor). *Ann. intern. Med.*, **98**, 1024

Ashraf, S.J., Arya, S.C., Parande, C.M., Sahay, R. & Ageel, A.R. (1986) Anti-delta antibody in primary hepatocellular carcinoma patients in the Gizan area of Saudi Arabia. *Infection*, **14**, 250–251

Bensabath, G., Hadler, S.C., Soares, P., Fields, H., Dias, L.B., Popper, H. & Maynard, J.E. (1987) Hepatitis delta virus infection and Labrea hepatitis. Prevalence and role in fulminant hepatitis in the Amazon basin. *J. Am. med. Assoc.*, **258**, 479–483

Bergmann, K.F. & Gerin, J.L. (1986) Antigens of hepatitis delta virus in the liver and serum of humans and animals. *J. infect. Dis.*, **154**, 702–706

Blum, H.E., Stowring, L., Figus, A., Montgomery, C.K., Haase, A.T. & Vyas, G.N. (1983) Detection of hepatitis B virus DNA in hepatocytes, bile duct epithelium, and vascular elements by in situ hybridization. *Proc. natl Acad. Sci. USA*, **80**, 6685–6688

Bonino, F., Negro, F., Baldi, M., Brunetto, M.R., Chiaberge, E., Capalbo, M., Maran, E., Lavarini, C., Rocca, N. & Rocca, G. (1987) The natural history of chronic delta hepatitis. *Prog. clin. biol. Res.*, **234**, 145–152

Boroń, P., Boroń-Kaczmarska, A., Bobrowska, E., Kamińska, H. & Łapiński, W. (1987) Prevalence of anti-delta antibodies in selected populations of HBsAg carriers in the Bialystok region, Poland. *Prog. clin. biol. Res.*, **234**, 427

Branch, A.D., Benenfeld, B.J., Baroudy, B.M., Wells, F.V., Gerin, J.L. & Robertson, H.D. (1989) An ultraviolet-sensitive RNA structural element in a viroid-like domain of the hepatitis delta virus. *Science*, **243**, 649–652

Branch, A.D., Levine, B.J. & Robertson, H.D. (1990) The brotherhood of circular RNA pathogens: viroids, circular satellites, and the delta agent. *Semin. Virol.*, **1**, 143–152

Brindle, R.J., Eglin, R.P., Parsons, A.J., Hill, A.V.S. & Selkon, J.B. (1988) HTLV-1, HIV-1, hepatitis B and hepatitis delta in the Pacific and South-east Asia: a serological survey. *Epidemiol. Inf.*, **100**, 153–156

Bruss, V. & Ganem, D. (1991) The role of envelope proteins in hepatitis B virus assembly. *Proc. natl Acad. Sci. USA*, **88**, 1059–1063

Buti, M., Esteban, R., Jardi, R., Allende, H., Baselgam J.M. & Guardia, J. (1988) Epidemiology of delta infection in Spain. *J. med. Virol.*, **26**, 327–332

Caredda, F., Antinori, S., Re, T., Pastecchia, C. & Moroni, M. (1987) Course and prognosis of acute HDV hepatitis. *Prog. clin. biol. Res.*, **234**, 267–276

Casey, J.L., Bergmann, K.F., Brown, T.L. & Gerin, J.L. (1992) Structural requirements for RNA editing in hepatitis delta virus: evidence for a uridine-to-cytidine editing mechanism. *Proc. natl Acad. Sci. USA*, **89**, 7149–7153

Cech, T.R. & Bass, B.L. (1986) Biological catalysis by RNA. *Ann. Rev. Biochem.*, **55**, 599–629

Cenac, A., Develoux, M., Lamothe, F., Soubiran, G., Vetter, J.M., Soumana, I. & Trépo, C. (1987) Delta superinfection in patients with chronic hepatitis liver cirrhosis and hepatocellular carcinoma in a Sahelian area. Study of 112 cases versus 46 controls. *Trans. R. Soc. trop. Med. Hyg.*, **81**, 994–997

Chang, M.-F., Baker, S.C., Soe, L.H., Kamahora, T., Keck, J.G., Makino, S., Govindarajan, S. & Lai, M.M.C. (1988) Human hepatitis delta antigen is a nuclear phosphoprotein with RNA-binding activity. *J. Virol.*, **62**, 2403–2410

Chao, Y.-C., Chang, M.-F., Gust, I. & Lai, M.M.C. (1990) Sequence conservation and divergence of hepatitis δ virus RNA. *Virology*, **178**, 384–392

Chao, M., Hsieh, S.-Y. & Taylor, J. (1991) The antigen of hepatitis delta virus: examination of in vitro RNA-binding specificity. *J. Virol.*, **65**, 4057–4062

Chen, D.-S., Lai, M.-Y. & Sung, J.-L. (1984) Delta agent infection in patients with chronic liver diseases and hepatocellular carcinoma—an infrequent finding in Taiwan. *Hepatology*, **4**, 502–503

Chen, P.-J., Kalpana, G., Goldberg, J., Mason, W., Werner, B., Gerin, J. & Taylor, J. (1986) Structure and replication of the genome of the hepatitis delta virus. *Proc. natl Acad. Sci. USA*, **83**, 8774–8778

Chen, P.-J., Chen, D.-S., Chen, C.-R., Chen, Y.-Y., Chen, H.-M. H., Lai, M.-Y. & Sung, J.-L. (1988) Delta infection in asymptomatic carriers of hepatitis B surface antigen: low prevalence of delta activity and effective suppression of hepatitis B virus replication. *Hepatology*, **8**, 1121–1124

Chen, P.-J., Yang, P.-M., Chen, C.-R. & Chen, D.-S. (1989) Characterization of the transcripts of hepatitis D and B viruses in infected human livers. *J. infect. Dis.*, **160**, 944–947

Chen, P.-J., Kuo, M.Y.-P., Chen, M.-L., Tu, S.-J., Chiu, M.-N., Wu, H.-L., Hsu, H.-C. & Chen, D.-S. (1990) Continuous expression and replication of the hepatitis delta virus genome in Hep G2 hepatoblastoma cells transfected with cloned viral DNA. *Proc. natl Acad. Sci. USA*, **87**, 5253–5257

Chen, P.-J., Chang, F.-L., Wang, C.-J., Lin, C.-J., Sung, S.-Y. & Chen, D.-S. (1992) Functional study of hepatitis delta virus large antigen in packaging and replication inhibition: role of the amino-terminal leucine zipper. *J. Virol.*, **66**, 2853–2859

Chu, C.-M. & Liaw, Y.-F. (1988) Acute delta superinfection in a previously unrecognised HBsAg carrier with transient loss of HBsAg simulating acute non-A, non-B hepatitis. *Gut*, **29**, 1013–1015

Craig, J.R., Govindarajan, S. & DeCock, K.M. (1986) Delta viral hepatitis. Histopathology and course. *Pathol. Ann.*, **21**, 1–21

Craxì, A., Raimondo, G., Giannuoli, G., Longo, G., Caltagirone, M., Aragona, M., Squadrito, G. & Pagliaro, L. (1983) Delta agent and hepatocellular carcinoma. *Prog. clin. biol. Res.*, **143**, 231–234

Craxì, A., Tinè, F., Vinci, M., Almasio, P., Cammà, C., Garofalo, G. & Pagliaro, L. (1991) Transmission of hepatitis B and hepatitis delta viruses in the households of chronic hepatitis B surface antigen carriers: a regression analysis of indicators of risk. *Am. J. Epidemiol.*, **134**, 641–650

Cronberg, S., Hansson, B.-G., Thermos, M., Moestrup, T. & Sow, A.M. (1984) Hepatitis D (delta agent) in primary hepatocellular carcinoma and liver disease in Senegal. *Liver*, **4**, 275–279

Crovari, P., Santolini, M., Bandettini, R., Bonanni, P., Branca, P. & Coppola, R.C. (1991) Epidemiology of HBV and HDV infections in a rural area of Central African Republic. *Prog. clin. biol. Res.*, **364**, 69–73

Curran, R.A., O'Neill, H.J. & Connolly, J.H. (1991) Hepatitis delta virus infection in Northern Ireland 1970–1989. *Ulster med. J.*, **60**, 159–163

Denniston, K.J., Hoyer, B.H., Smedile, A., Wells, F.V., Nelson, J. & Gerin, J.L. (1986) Cloned fragment of the hepatitis delta virus RNA genome: sequence and diagnostic application. *Science*, **232**, 873–875

Dény, P., Zignego, A.L., Rascalou, N., Ponzetto, A., Tiollais, P. & Bréchot, C. (1991) Nucleotide sequence analysis of three different hepatitis delta viruses isolated from a woodchuck and humans. *J. gen. Virol.*, **72**, 735–739

Di Bisceglie, A.M. & Negro, F. (1989) Diagnosis of hepatitis delta virus infection. *Hepatology*, **10**, 1014–1016

Di Bisceglie, A.M., Order, S.E., Klein, J.L., Waggoner, J.G., Sjogren, M.H., Kuo, G., Houghton, M., Choo, Q.-L. & Hoofnagle, J.H. (1991) The role of chronic viral hepatitis in hepatocellular carcinoma in the United States. *Am. J. Gastroenterol.*, **86**, 335–338

Dourakis, S., Karayiannis, P., Goldin, R., Taylor, M., Monjardino, J. & Thomas, H.C. (1991) An in situ hybridization, molecular biological and immunohistochemical study of hepatitis delta virus in woodchucks. *Hepatology*, **14**, 534–539

Elena, S.F., Dopazo, J., Flores, R., Diener, T.O. & Moya, A. (1991) Phylogeny of viroids, viroidlike satellite RNAs, and the viroidlike domain of hepatitis delta virus RNA. *Proc. natl Acad. Sci. USA*, **88**, 5631–5634

El Zayadi, A., Ponzetto, A., Selim, O., Forzani, B., Lavarini, C. & Rizzetto, M. (1988) Prevalence of delta antibodies among urban HBsAg-positive chronic liver disease patients in Egypt. *Hepato-gastroenterology*, **35**, 313–315

Fay, O., Tanno, H., Palazzi, J. & Gatti, H. (1987) Anti-delta antibody in various HBsAg positive Argentine populations. *Prog. clin. biol. Res.*, **234**, 517–518

da Fonseca, J.C.F. & Simonetti, J.P. (1987) Epidemiology of the hepatitis delta virus (HDV) in Brazil. *Prog. clin. Biol. Res.*, **234**, 507–514

Garcia, G., Smedile, A., Bergmann, K.F., Gerin, J.L., Gregory, P.B., Merigan, T.C. & Robinson, W.S. (1990) Acute delta hepatitis during treatment with adenosine arabinoside monophosphate with resolution of the HBsAg carrier state. *West. J. Med.*, **153**, 80–82

Glenn, J.S. & White, J.M. (1991) *trans*-Dominant inhibition of human hepatitis delta virus genome replication. *J. Virol.*, **65**, 2357–2361

Govindarajan, S., Chin, K.P., Redeker, A.G. & Peters, R.L. (1984a) Fulminant B viral hepatitis: role of delta agent. *Gastroenterology*, **86**, 1417–1420

Govindarajan, S., Hevia, F.J. & Peters, R.L. (1984b) Prevalence of delta antigen/antibody in B-viral-associated hepatocellular carcinoma. *Cancer*, **53**, 1692–1694

Govindarajan, S., deCock, K.M. & Redeker, A.G. (1986a) Natural course of delta superinfection in chronic hepatitis B virus-infected patients: histopathologic study with multiple liver biopsies. *Hepatology*, **6**, 640–644

Govindarajan, S., Fields, H.A., Humphrey, C.D. & Margolis, H.S. (1986b) Pathologic and ultrastructural changes of acute and chronic delta hepatitis in an experimentally infected chimpanzee. *Am. J. Pathol.*, **122**, 315–322

Gowans, E.J., Baroudy, B.M., Negro, F., Ponzetto, A., Purcell, R.H. & Gerin, J.L. (1988) Evidence for replication of hepatitis delta virus RNA in hepatocyte nuclei after in vivo infection. *Virology*, **167**, 274–278

Greenfield, C., Farci, P., Osidiana, V., MacPherson, C.N.L., Romig, T., Zeyhle, E., French, M., Johnson, B., Tukei, P., Wankya, B.M. & Thomas, H.C. (1986) Hepatitis delta virus infection in Kenya. Its geographic and tribal distribution. *Am. J. Epidemiol.*, **123**, 416–23

Hadler, S.C., De Monzon, M., Ponzetto, A., Anzola, E., Rivero, D., Mondolfi, A., Bracho, A., Francis, D.P., Gerber, M.A., Thung, S., Gerin, J., Maynard, J.E., Popper, H. & Purcell, R.H. (1984) Delta virus infection and severe hepatitis. An epidemic in the Yupca Indians of Venezuela. *Ann. intern. Med.*, **100**, 339–344

Hadziyannis, S.J., Sherman, M., Lieberman, H.M. & Shafritz, D.A. (1985) Liver disease activity and hepatitis B virus replication in chronic delta antigen-positive hepatitis B virus carriers. *Hepatology*, **5**, 544–547

Hadziyannis, S.J., Hatzakis, A., Papaioannou, C., Anastassakos, C. & Vassiliadis, E. (1987) Endemic hepatitis delta virus in a Greek community. *Prog. clin. biol. Res.*, **234**, 181–202

Hadziyannis, S.J., Papaioannou, C. & Alexopoulou, A. (1991) The role of the hepatitis delta virus in acute hepatitis and in chronic liver disease in Greece. *Prog. clin. biol. Res.*, **364**, 51–62

Halpern, M.S., England, J.M., Deery, D.T., Petcu, D.J., Mason, W.S. & Molnar-Kimber, K.L. (1983) Viral nucleic acid synthesis and antigen accumulation in pancreas and kidney of Pekin ducks infected with duck hepatitis B virus. *Proc. natl Acad. Sci. USA*, **80**, 4865–4869

Hansson, B.G., Moestrup, T., Widell, A. & Nordenfelt, E. (1982) Infection with delta agent in Sweden: introduction of a new hepatitis agent. *J. infect. Dis.*, **146**, 472–478

Hoofnagle, J.H., Mullen, K.D., Peters, M., Avigan, M.I., Park, Y., Waggoner, J.G., Gerin, J.L., Smedile, A. & Hoyer, B. (1986) Treatment of chronic delta hepatitis with recombinant alpha interferon. In: Stewart, W.E. & Schellekens, H., eds, *The Biology of the Interferon System*, New York, Elsevier, pp. 493–495

Hoofnagle, J.H., Mullen, K., Peters, K., Avigan, M., Park, Y., Waggoner, J., Gerin, J.L., Hoyer, B. & Smedile, A. (1987) Treatment of chronic delta hepatitis with recombinant human alpha interferon. *Prog. clin. biol. Res.*, **234**, 291–298

Hsieh, S.-Y. & Taylor, J.M. (1991) Regulation of polyadenylation of hepatitis delta virus antigenomic RNA. *J. Virol.*, **65**, 6438–6446

Hsieh, S.-Y., Chao, M., Coates, L. & Taylor, J. (1990) Hepatitis delta virus genome replication: a polyadenylated mRNA for delta antigen. *J. Virol.*, **64**, 3192–3198

Imazeki, F., Omata, M. & Ohto, M. (1990) Heterogeneity and evolution rates of delta virus RNA sequences. *J. Virol.*, **64**, 5594–5599

Imazeki, F., Omata, M. & Ohto, M. (1991) Complete nucleotide sequence of hepatitis delta virus RNA in Japan (Short communication). *Nucleic Acids Res.*, **19**, 5439

Kanel, G.C., Govindarajan, S. & Peters, R.L. (1984) Chronic delta infection and liver biopsy changes in chronic active hepatitis B. *Ann. intern. Med.*, **101**, 51–54

Karayiannis, P., Goldin, R., Luther, S., Carman, W.F., Monjardino, J. & Thomas, H.C. (1992) Effect of cyclosporin-A in woodchucks with chronic hepatitis delta virus infection. *J. med. Virol.*, **36**, 316–321

Ketiladze, E.S., Vyazov, S.O., Chernovetsky, M.A., Mikhailov, M.I., Bugayeva, N.P. & Kozlova, T.P. (1987) Delta infection in patients and HBsAg carriers. *Prog. clin. biol. Res.*, **234**, 461–466

Kew, M.C., Dusheiko, G.M., Hadziyannis, S.J. & Patterson, A. (1984) Does delta infection play a part in the pathogenesis of hepatitis B virus related hepatocellular carcinoma? *Br. med. J.*, **288**, 1727

Kos, A., Dijkema, R., Arnberg, A.C., van der Meide, P.H. & Schellekens, H. (1986) The hepatitis delta (δ) virus possesses a circular RNA. *Nature*, **323**, 558–560

Krogsgaard, K., Kryger, P., Aldershvile, J., Andersson, P., Sørensen, T.I.A., Nielsen, J.O. & the Copenhagen Hepatitis Acuta Programme (1987) Delta-infection and suppression of hepatitis B virus replication in chronic HBsAg carriers. *Hepatology*, **7**, 42–45

Kumar, P.K.R., Suh, Y.-A., Miyashiro, H., Nishikawa, F., Kawakami, J., Taira, K. & Nishikawa, S. (1992) Random mutations to evaluate the role of bases at two important single-stranded regions of genomic HDV ribozyme. *Nucleic Acids Res.*, **20**, 3919–3924

Kuo, M.Y.-P., Goldberg, J., Coates, L., Mason, W., Gerin, J. & Taylor, J. (1988a) Molecular cloning of hepatitis delta virus RNA from an infected woodchuck liver: sequence, structure, and applications. *J. Virol.*, **62**, 1855–1861

Kuo, M.Y.-P., Sharmeen, L., Dinter-Gottlieb, G. & Taylor, J. (1988b) Characterization of self-cleaving RNA sequences on the genome and antigenome of human hepatitis delta virus. *J. Virol.*, **62**, 4439–4444

Kuo, M.Y.-P., Chao, M. & Taylor, J. (1989) Initiation of replication of the human hepatitis delta virus genome from cloned DNA: role of delta antigen. *J. Virol.*, **63**, 1945–1950

Lai, M.M.C., Lee, C.-M., Bih, F.-Y. & Govindarajan, S. (1991) The molecular basis of heterogeneity of hepatitis delta virus. *J. Hepatol.*, **13** (Suppl. 4), S121–S124

Laskus, T., Radkowski, M., Lupa, E., Cianciara, J., Slusarczyk, J., Halama, G. & Horban, A. (1992) Introduction of hepatitis delta virus into Polish drug community. *Infection*, **20**, 43–44

Lee, C.-M., Bih, F.-Y., Chao, Y.-C., Govindarajan, S. & Lai, M.M.C. (1992) Evolution of hepatitis delta virus RNA during chronic infection. *Virology*, **188**, 265–273

Lemon, S.M., Becherer, P.R., Wang, J.-C., White, G.C., Lesesne, H., Janco, R.L., Hanna, W.T., Davis, C., Johnson, C.A., Poon, M.C. & Andes, A. (1991) Hepatitis delta infection among multiply-transfused hemophiliacs. *Prog. clin. biol. Res.*, **364**, 351–360

Lettau, L.A., McCarthy, J.G., Smith, M.H., Hadler, S.C., Morse, L.J., Ukena, T., Bessette, R., Gurwitz, A., Irvine, W.G., Fields, H.A., Grady, G.F. & Maynard, J.E. (1987) Outbreak of severe hepatitis due to delta and hepatitis B viruses in parenteral drug abusers and their contacts. *New Engl. J. Med.*, **317**, 1256–1262

Liaw, Y.-F., Lin, H.-H., Chu, C.-M., Sheen, I.-S. & Huang, M.-J. (1987) Hepatitis delta virus infection in Taiwan. *Prog. clin. biol. Res.*, **234**, 479–483

Liaw, Y.-F., Chiu, K.-W., Chu, C.-M., Sheen, I.-S. & Huang, M.-J. (1990) Heterosexual transmission of hepatitis delta virus in the general population of an area endemic for hepatitis B virus infection: a prospective study. *J. infect. Dis.*, **162**, 1170–1172

Lok, A., Lindsay, I., Scheuer, P.J. & Thomas, H.C. (1985) Clinical and histological features of delta infection in chronic hepatitis B virus carriers. *J. clin. Pathol.*, **38**, 530–533

Luo, G., Chao, M., Hsieh, S.-Y., Sureau, C., Nishikura, K. & Taylor, J. (1990) A specific base transition occurs on replicating hepatitis delta virus RNA. *J. Virol.*, **64**, 1021–1027

MacNaughton, T.B., Gowans, E.J., McNamara, S.P. & Burrell, C.J. (1991) Hepatitis δ antigen is necessary for access of hepatitis δ virus RNA to the cell transcriptional machinery but is not part of the transcriptional complex. *Virology*, **184**, 387–390

Maddrey, W.C. & Van Thiel, D.H. (1988) Liver transplantation: an overview. *Hepatology*, **8**, 948–959

Makino, S., Chang, M.-F., Shieh, C.-K., Kamahora, T., Vannier, D.M., Govindarajan, S. & Lai, M.M.C. (1987) Molecular cloning and sequencing of a human hepatitis delta (δ) virus RNA. *Nature*, **329**, 343–346

McCruden, E.A.B. & Follett, E.A.C. (1989) Hepatitis delta virus infections in intravenous drug abusers with hepatitis B in the west of Scotland. *J. med. Virol.*, **29**, 59–62

Mele, A., Franco, E., Caprilli, F., Gentili, G., Stazi, M.A., Zaratti, L., Capitanio, B., Crescimbeni, E., Corona, R., Pana, A. & Pasquini, P. (1988) Hepatitis B and delta virus infection among heterosexuals, homosexuals and bisexual men. *Eur. J. Epidemiol.*, **4**, 488–491

Mijch, A.M., Barnes, R., Crowe, S.M., Dimitrakakis, M. & Lucas, C.R. (1987) An outbreak of hepatitis B and D in butchers. *Scand. J. infect. Dis.*, **19**, 179–184

Nath, N., Mushahwar, I.K., Fang, C.T., Barberian, H. & Dodd, R.Y. (1985) Antibodies to delta antigen in asymptomatic hepatitis B surface antigen-reactive blood donors in the United States and their association with other markers of hepatitis B virus. *Am. J. Epidemiol.*, **122**, 218–225

Negro, F., Bergmann, K.F., Baroudy, B.M., Satterfield, W.C., Popper, H., Purcell, R.H. & Gerin, J.L. (1988) Chronic hepatitis D virus (HDV) infection in hepatitis B virus carrier chimpanzees experimentally superinfected with HDV. *J. infect. Dis.*, **158**, 151–159

Negro, F., Korba, B.E., Forzani, B., Baroudy, B.M., Brown, T.L., Gerin, J.L. & Ponzetto, A. (1989) Hepatitis delta virus (HDV) and woodchuck hepatitis virus (WHV) nucleic acids in tissues of HDV-infected chronic WHV carrier woodchucks. *J. Virol.*, **63**, 1612–1618

Neurath, A.R., Kent, S.B.H., Strick, N. & Parker, K. (1986) Identification and chemical synthesis of a host cell receptor binding site on hepatitis B virus. *Cell*, **46**, 429–436

Neurath, A.R., Strick, N., Sproul, P., Ralph, H.E. & Valinsky, J. (1990) Detection of receptors for hepatitis B virus on cells of extrahepatic origin. *Virology*, **176**, 448–457

Okoth, F.A., Kobayashi, M., Kaptich, D.C., Kaiguri, P.M., Tukei, P.M., Takayanagi, T. & Yamanaka, T. (1991) Seroepidemiological study for HBV markers and anti-delta in Kenya. *East Afr. med. J.*, **68**, 515–525

Oliveri, F., Brunetto, M.R., Baldi, M., Piantino, P., Ponzetto, A., Forzani, B., Smedile, A., Verme, G. & Bonino, F. (1991) Hepatitis delta virus (HDV) infection and hepatocellular carcinoma (HCC). *Prog. clin. biol. Res.*, **364**, 217–222

Ottobrelli, A., Marzano, A., Smedile, A., Recchia, S., Salizzoni, M., Cornu, C., Lamy, M.E., Otte, J.B., de Hemptinne, B., Geubel, A., Grendele, M., Colledan, M., Galmarini, D., Marinucci, G., di Giacomo, C., Agnes, S., Bonino, F. & Rizzetto, M. (1991) Patterns of hepatitis delta virus reinfection and disease in liver transplantation. *Gastroenterology*, **101**, 1649–1655

Perrotta, A.T. & Been, M.D. (1991) A pseudoknot-like structure required for efficient self-cleavage of hepatitis delta virus RNA. *Nature*, **350**, 434–436

Ponzetto, A., Cote, P.J., Popper, H., Hoyer, B.H., London, W.T., Ford, E.C., Bonino, F., Purcell, R.H. & Gerin, J.L. (1984a) Transmission of the hepatitis B virus-associated delta agent to the eastern woodchuck. *Proc. natl Acad. Sci. USA*, **81**, 2208–2212

Ponzetto, A., Seeff, L.B., Buskell-Bales, Z., Ishak, K.G., Hoofnagle, J.H., Zimmerman, H.J., Purcell, R.H., Gerin, J.L. & the Veterans Administration Hepatitis Cooperative Study Group (1984b) Hepatitis B markers in United States drug addicts with special emphasis on the delta hepatitis virus. *Hepatology*, **4**, 1111–1115

Ponzetto, A., Forzani, B., Smedile, A., Hele, C., Avanzini, L., Novara, R. & Canese, M.G. (1987a) Acute and chronic delta infection in the woodchuck. *Prog. clin. biol. Res.*, **234**, 37–46

Ponzetto, A., Rapicetta, M., Forzani, B., Smedile, A., Hele, C., Morace, G., di Rienzo, A.M., Palladino, P., Avanzini, L., Gerin, J.L. & Verme, G. (1987b) Hepatitis delta virus infection in Pekin ducks chronically infected by the duck hepatitis B virus. *Prog. clin. biol. Res.*, **234**, 47–49

Ponzetto, A., Hoyer, B.H., Popper, H., Engle, R., Purcell, R.H. & Gerin, J.L. (1987c) Titration of the infectivity of hepatitis D virus in chimpanzees. *J. infect. Dis.*, **155**, 72–78

Ponzetto, A., Negro, F., Popper, H., Bonino, F., Engle, R., Rizzetto, M., Purcell, R.H. & Gerin, J.L. (1988a) Serial passage of hepatitis delta virus in chronic hepatitis B virus carrier chimpanzees. *Hepatology*, **8**, 1655–1661

Ponzetto, A., Forzani, B., Hele, C., Negro, F., Avanzini, L., Callea, F., Bonetti, M.G., Rapicetta, M., Gerin, J.L. & Verme, G. (1988b) Hepatocellular carcinoma and hepatitis delta virus in the woodchuck animal model (Abstract). *Gastroenterology*, **94**, A583

Ponzetto, A., Negro, F., Gerin, J.L. & Purcell, R.H. (1991) Experimental hepatitis delta virus infection in the animal model. *Prog. clin. biol. Res.*, **364**, 147–157

Purcell, R.H., Satterfield, W.C., Bergmann, K.F., Smedile, A., Ponzetto, A. & Gerin, J.L. (1987) Experimental hepatitis delta virus infection in the chimpanzee. *Prog. clin. biol. Res.*, **234**, 27–36

Raimondo, G., Craxì, A., Longo, G., Giannuoli, G., Caltagirone, M., Aragona, M., Pecoraro, G., Squadrito, G. & Pagliaro, L. (1984) Delta infection in hepatocellular carcinoma positive for hepatitis B surface antigen (Brief report). *Ann. intern. Med.*, **101**, 343–344

Ramia, S. & Bahakim, H. (1988) Perinatal transmission of hepatitis B virus-associated hepatitis D virus. *Ann. Inst. Pasteur/Virol.*, **139**, 285–290

Ranger, S., Mounier, M., Denis, F., Alain, J., Baudet, J., Tabaste, J.L., Delpeyroux, C. & Roussanne, M.C. (1990) Prevalence of markers for hepatitis B (HBsAg, HBeAg, DNA) and delta viruses in about 10 000 pregnant women in Limoges (France). *Pathol. biol.*, **38**, 694–699 (in French)

Ratnam, S., Head, C.B. & Butler, R.W. (1986) Lack of evidence of hepatitis D (delta) infection in Newfoundland and Labrador. *Can. med. Assoc. J.*, **134**, 905–907

Rezvan, H., Forouzandeh, B., Taroyan, S., Fadaiee, S. & Azordegan, F. (1990) A study on delta virus infection and its clinical impact in Iran. *Infection*, **18**, 34–36

Rizzetto, M. (1983) The delta agent. *Hepatology*, **3**, 729–737

Rizzetto, M., Canese, M.G., Aricò, S., Crivelli, O., Trepo, C., Bonino, F. & Verme, G. (1977) Immunofluorescence detection of new antigen-antibody system (δ/anti-δ) associated to hepatitis B virus in liver and in serum of HBsAg carriers. *Gut*, **18**, 997–1003

Rizzetto, M., Canese, M.G., Gerin, J.L., London, W.T., Sly, D.L. & Purcell, R.H. (1980a) Transmission of the hepatitis B virus-associated delta antigen to chimpanzees. *J. infect. Dis.*, **141**, 590–602

Rizzetto, M., Hoyer, B., Canese, M.G., Shih, J.W.-K., Purcell, R.H. & Gerin, J.L. (1980b) Delta agent: association of delta antigen with hepatitis B surface antigen and RNA in serum of delta-infected chimpanzees. *Proc. natl Acad. Sci. USA*, **77**, 6124–6128

Rizzetto, M., Canese, M.G., Purcell, R.H., London, W.T., Sly, L.D. & Gerin, J.L. (1981a) Experimental HBV and delta infections of chimpanzees: occurrence and significance of intrahepatic immune complexes of HBcAg and delta antigen. *Hepatology*, **1**, 567–574

Rizzetto, M., Morello, C., Mannucci, P.M., Gocke, D.J., Spero, J.A., Lewis, J.H., Van Thiel, D.H., Scaroni, C. & Peyretti, F. (1981b) Delta infection and liver disease in hemophilic carriers of hepatitis B surface antigen. *J. infect. Dis.*, **145**, 18–22

Rizzetto, M., Verme, G., Recchia, S., Bonino, F., Farci, P., Aricò, S., Calzia, R., Picciotto, A., Colombo, M. & Popper, H. (1983) Chronic hepatitis in carriers of hepatitis B surface antigen, with intrahepatic expression of the delta antigen. An active and progressive disease unresponsive to immunosuppressive treatment. *Ann. intern. Med.*, **98**, 437–441

Rizzetto, M., Ponzetto, A. & Forzani, I. (1991) Epidemiology of hepatitis delta virus: overview. *Prog. clin. biol. Res.*, **364**, 1–20

Rizzetto, M., Hadziyannis, S., Hansson, B.G., Toukan, A. & Gust, I. (1992) Hepatitis delta virus infection in the world: epidemiological patterns and clinical expression. *Gastroenterol. int.*, **5**, 18–32

Roggendorf, M., Gmelin, K., Zoulek, G., Wolf, P., Schlipköter, U., Jilg, W., Theilmann, L. & Deinhardt, F. (1986) Epidemiological studies on the prevalence of hepatitis delta virus infections in the Federal Republic of Germany. *J. Hepatol.*, **2**, 230–236

Roggendorf, M., Mai, K., Thian, G., Hu, M., Zhuang, C., Gmelin, K., Bernhardt, R. & Deinhardt, F. (1987) Prevalence of hepatitis delta virus infection in different provinces of China. *Prog. clin. biol. Res.*, **234**, 487–491

Rosenblum, L., Darrow, W., Witte, J., Cohen, J., French, J., Gill, P.S., Potterat, J., Sikes, K., Reich, R. & Hadler, S. (1992) Sexual practices in the transmission of hepatitis B virus and prevalence of hepatitis delta virus infection in female prostitutes in the United States. *J. Am. med. Assoc.*, **267**, 2477–2481

Rosina, F. & Rizzetto, M. (1989) Treatment of chronic type D (delta) hepatitis with alpha interferon. *Semin. Liver Dis.*, **9**, 264–266

Rosina, F., Saracco, G. & Rizzetto, M. (1985) Risk of post-transfusion infection with the hepatitis delta virus: a multi-centre study. *New Engl. J. Med.*, **312**, 1488–1491

Rosina, F., Saracco, G., Lattore, V., Quartarone, V., Rizzetto, M., Verme, G., Trinchero, P., San Salvadore, F. & Smedile, A. (1987) Alpha-2 recombinant interferon in the treatment of chronic delta virus (HDV) hepatitis. *Prog. clin. biol. Res.*, **234**, 299-303

Rosina, F., Pintus, C., Meschievitz, C. & Rizzetto, M. (1991) A randomized controlled trial of a 12-month course of recombinant human interferon-alfa in chronic delta (type D) hepatitis: a multicenter Italian study. *Hepatology*, **13**, 1052-1056

Roumeliotou-Karayannis, A., Tassopoulos, N., Karpodini, E., Trichopoulou, E., Kotsianopoulou, M. & Papaevangelou, G. (1987) Prevalence of HBV, HDV and HIV infections among intravenous drug addicts in Greece. *Eur. J. Epidemiol.*, **3**, 143-146

Ryu, W.-S., Mayer, M. & Taylor, J. (1992) Assembly of hepatitis delta virus particles. *J. Virol.*, **66**, 2310-2315

Sagnelli, E., Stroffolini, T., Ascione, A., Bonino, F., Chiaramonte, M., Colombo, M., Craxì, A., Giusti, G., Manghisi, O.G., Pastore, G., Piccinino, F., Rizzetto, M., Stazi, M.A., Loti, M. & Verme, G. (1992) The epidemiology of hepatitis delta infection in Italy. *J. Hepatol.*, **15**, 211-215

Salassa, B., Daziano, E., Bonino, F., Lavarini, C., Smedile, A., Chiaberge, E., Rosina, F., Brunetto, M.R., Pessione, E., Spezia, C., Bramato, C. & Soranzo, M.L. (1991) Serological diagnosis of hepatitis B and delta virus (HBV/HDV) coinfection. *J. Hepatol.*, **12**, 10-13

Saldanha, J.A., Thomas, H.C. & Monjardino, J.P. (1990) Cloning and sequencing of RNA of hepatitis delta virus isolated from human serum. *J. gen. Virol.*, **71**, 1603-1606

Scott, D.A., Burans, J.P., Al-Ouzeib, H.D., Arunkumar, B.K., Al-Fadeel, M., Nigad, Y.R., Al-Hadad, A., Elyazeed, R.R.A., Hyams, K.C. & Woody, J.N. (1990) A seroepidemiological survey of viral hepatitis in the Yemen Arab Republic. *Trans. R. Soc. trop. Med. Hyg.*, **84**, 288-291

Sharmeen, L., Kuo, M. Y.-P., Dinter-Gottlieb, G. & Taylor, J. (1988) Antigenomic RNA of human hepatitis delta virus can undergo self-cleavage. *J. Virol.*, **62**, 2674-2679

Sharmeen, L., Kuo, M.Y.-P. & Taylor, J. (1989) Self-ligating RNA sequences on the antigenome of human hepatitis delta virus. *J. Virol.*, **63**, 1428-1430

Shobokshi, O.A. & Serebour, F.E. (1987) Prevalence of delta antigen/antibody in various HBsAg positive patients in Saudi Arabia. *Prog. clin. biol. Res.*, **234**, 471-475

Siebke, J.C., von der Lippe, B., Hansson, B.-G., Nordenfelt, E. & Degré, M. (1986) Prevalence and clinical effects of delta agent. Infections in Norwegian population subgroups. *Scand. J. infect. Dis.*, **18**, 33-36

Smedile, A., Dentico, P., Zanetti, A., Sagnelli, E., Nordenfeldt, E., Actis, G.C. & Rizzetto, M. (1981) Infection with the delta agent (δ) in chronic HBsAg carriers. *Gastroenterology*, **81**, 992-997

Smedile, A., Farci, P., Verme, G., Caredda, F., Cargnel, A., Caporaso, N., Dentico, P., Trepo, C., Opolon, P., Gimson, A., Vergani, D., Williams, R. & Rizzetto, M. (1982) Influence of delta infection on severity of hepatitis B. *Lancet*, **ii**, 945-947

Smedile, A., Rizzetto, M., Denniston, K., Bonino, F., Wells, F., Verme, G., Consolo, F., Hoyer, B., Purcell, R.H. & Gerin, J.L. (1986) Type D hepatitis: the clinical significance of hepatitis D virus RNA in serum as detected by a hybridization-based assay. *Hepatology*, **6**, 1297-1302

Smedile, A., Freni, M.A., Caruso, L., Ajello, A., Trischitta, C., Resta, M.L., Bertino, G., Berlinghieri, G., Rapisarda, S., Di Geronimo, L., Spadaro, A. & Ferrau, O. (1987) Delta infection in eastern Sicily. *Eur. J. Epidemiol.*, **3**, 386-389

Smedile, A., Rosina, F., Saracco, G., Chiaberge, E., Lattore, V., Fabiano, A., Brunetto, M.R., Verme, G., Rizzetto, M. & Bonino, F. (1991a) Hepatitis B virus replication modulates pathogenesis of hepatitis D virus in chronic hepatitis D. *Hepatology*, **13**, 413-416

Smedile, A., Rosina, F., Chiaberge, E., Lattore, V., Saracco, G., Brunetto, M.R., Bonino, F., Verme, G. & Rizzetto, M. (1991b) Presence and significance of hepatitis B virus replication in chronic type D hepatitis. *Prog. clin. biol. Res.*, **364**, 185–195

Solomon, R.E., Kaslow, R.A., Phair, J.P., Lyter, D., Visscher, B., Lyman, D., Vanraden, M.T. & Gerin, J. (1988) Human immunodeficiency virus and hepatitis delta virus in homosexual men. *Ann. intern. Med.*, **108**, 51–54

Suh, Y.-A., Kumar, P.K.R., Nishikawa, F., Kayano, E., Nakai, S., Odai, O., Uesugi, S., Taira, K. & Nishikawa, S. (1992) Deletion of internal sequence on the HDV-ribozyme: elucidation of functionally important single-stranded loop regions. *Nucleic Acids Res.*, **20**, 747–753

Tagawa, M., Omata, M., Yokosuka, D., Uchiumi, K., Imazeki, F. & Okuda, K. (1985) Early events in duck hepatitis B virus infection. Sequential appearance of viral deoxyribonucleic acid in liver, pancreas, kidney and spleen. *Gastroenterology*, **89**, 1224–1229

Tapalaga, D., Forzani, B., Hele, C., Paravacini, P., Ponzetto, A. & Theilmann, L. (1987) HDV infection in Romania. *Prog. clin. biol. Res.*, **234**, 425

Tassopoulos, N.C., Theodoropoulos, G., Sjogren, M.H., Engle, R. & Purcell, R.H. (1989) Serological markers of hepatitis B virus and hepatitis D virus infections in Greek adults with primary hepatocellular carcinoma. *Infection*, **17**, 17–19

Tassopoulos, N.C., Koutelou, M.G., Macagno, S., Zorbas, P. & Rizzetto, M. (1990) Diagnostic significance of IgM antibodies to hepatitis delta virus in fulminant hepatitis B. *J. med. Virol.*, **30**, 174–177

Taylor, J.M. (1990) Hepatitis delta virus: *cis* and *trans* functions required for replication. *Cell*, **61**, 371–373

Taylor, J.M. (1992) The structure and replication of hepatitis delta virus. *Ann. Rev. Microbiol.*, **46**, 253–276

Taylor, J., Mason, W., Summers, J., Goldberg, J., Aldrich, C., Coates, L., Gerin, J.L. & Gowans, E. (1987) Replication of human hepatitis delta virus in primary cultures of woodchuck hepatocytes. *J. Virol.*, **61**, 2891–2895

Taylor, J., Negro, F. & Rizzetto, M. (1992) Hepatitis delta virus: from structure to disease expression. *Rev. med. Virol.*, **2**, 161–167

Thomas, H.C, Farci, P., Shein, R., Karayiannis, P., Smedile, A., Caruso, L. & Gerin, J.L. (1987) Inhibition of hepatitis delta virus (HDV) replication by lymphoblastoid human alpha interferon. *Prog. clin. biol. Res.*, **234**, 277–290

Toukan, A.U., Abu-El-Rub, O.A., Abu-Laban, S.A., Tarawneh, M.S., Kamal, M.F., Hadler, S.C., Krawczynski, K., Margolis, H.S. & Maynard, J.E. (1987) The epidemiology and clinical outcome of hepatitis D virus (delta) infection in Jordan. *Hepatology*, **7**, 1340–1345

Trichopoulos, D., Day, N.E., Tzonou, A., Hadziyannis, S., Kaklamani, E., Sparos, L., Muñoz, N. & Hatzakis, A. (1987a) Delta agent and the etiology of hepatocellular carcinoma. *Int. J. Cancer*, **39**, 283–286

Trichopoulos, D., Day, N.E., Kaklamani, E., Tzonou, A., Muñoz, N., Zavitsanos, X., Koumantaki, Y. & Trichopoulou, A. (1987b) Hepatitis B virus, tobacco smoking and ethanol consumption in the etiology of hepatocellular carcinoma. *Int. J. Cancer*, **39**, 45–49

Tzonou, A., Trichopoulos, D., Kaklamani, E., Zavitsanos, X., Koumantaki, Y. & Hsieh, C.-C. (1991) Epidemiologic assessment of interactions of hepatitis-C virus with seromarkers of hepatitis-B and -D viruses, cirrhosis and tobacco smoking in hepatocellular carcinoma. *Int. J. Cancer*, **49**, 377–380

Ueda, K., Tsurimoto, T. & Matsubara, K. (1991) Three envelope proteins of hepatitis B virus: large S, middle S, and major S proteins needed for the formation of Dane particles. *J. Virol.*, **65**, 3521–3529

Verme, G., Brunetto, M.R., Oliveri, F., Baldi, M., Forzani, B., Piantino, P., Ponzetto, A. & Bonino, F. (1991) Role of hepatitis delta virus infection in hepatocellular carcinoma. *Dig. Dis. Sci.*, **36**, 1134–1136

Vranckx, R., Reniers, J., Alisjahbana, A., Ngantung, W., Sugita, E. & Meheus, A. (1988) Prevalence of anti-delta antibodies in pregnant women in Bandung, Indonesia. *Trop. geogr. Med.*, **40**, 17–19

Wang, K.-S., Choo, Q.-L., Weiner, A.J., Ou, J.-H., Najarian, R.C., Thayer, R.M., Mullenbach, G.T., Denniston, K.J., Gerin, J.L. & Houghton, M. (1986) Structure, sequence and expression of the hepatitis delta viral genome. *Nature*, **323**, 508–514

Wang, D.-Q., Cheng, H.-H., Minuk, G.Y., Liu, L.-H., Anand, C.M., Stowe, T.C., Wang, H.-X., Ying, D.-C., Tu, Y.-R. & Buchan, K.A. (1987) Delta hepatitis virus infection in China. *Int. J. Epidemiol.*, **16**, 79–83

Wang, C.-J., Chen, P.-J., Wu, J.-C., Patel, D. & Chen, D.-S. (1991) Small-form hepatitis B surface antigen is sufficient to help in the assembly of hepatitis delta virus-like particles. *J. Virol.*, **65**, 6630–6636

Weiner, A.J., Choo, Q.-L., Wang, K.-S., Govindarajan, S., Redeker, A.G., Gerin, J.L. & Houghton, M. (1988) A single antigenomic open reading frame of the hepatitis delta virus encodes the epitope(s) of both hepatitis delta antigen polypeptides p24$^\delta$ and p27$^\delta$. *J. Virol.*, **62**, 594–599

Weisfuse, I.B., Hadler, S.C., Fields, H.A., Alter, M.J., O'Malley, P.M., Judson, F.N., Ostrow, D.G. & Altman, N.L. (1989) Delta hepatitis in homosexual men in the United States. *Hepatology*, **9**, 872–874

Wu, H.-N. & Lai, M.M.C. (1989) Reversible cleavage and ligation of hepatitis delta virus RNA. *Science*, **243**, 652–654

Wu, H.-N. & Lai, M.M.C. (1990) RNA conformational requirements of self-cleavage of hepatitis delta virus RNA. *Mol. cell. Biol.*, **10**, 5575–5579

Wu, H.-N., Lin, Y.-J., Lin, F.-P., Makino, S., Chang, M.-F. & Lai, M.M.C. (1989) Human hepatitis delta virus RNA subfragments contain an autocleavage activity. *Proc. natl Acad. Sci. USA*, **86**, 1831–1835

Wu, J.-C., Lee, S.-D., Govindarajan, S., Kung, T.-W., Tsai, Y.-T., Lo, K.-J. & Ting, L.-P. (1990a) Correlation of serum delta RNA with clinical course of acute hepatitis delta virus superinfection in Taiwan: a longitudinal study. *J. infect. Dis.*, **161**, 1116–1120

Wu, J.-C., Lee, S.-D., Govindarajan, S., Lin, H.-C., Chou, P., Wang, Y.-J., Lee, S.-Y., Tsai, Y.-T., Lo, K.-J. & Ting, L.-P. (1990b) Sexual transmission of hepatitis D virus infection in Taiwan. *Hepatology*, **11**, 1057–1061

Wu, J.-C., Chen, P.-J., Kuo, M.Y.-P., Lee, S.-D., Chen, D.-S. & Ting, L.-P. (1991) Production of hepatitis delta virus and suppression of helper hepatitis B virus in a human hepatoma cell line. *J. Virol.*, **65**, 1099–1104

Yoffe, B., Burns, D.K., Bhatt, H.S. & Combes, B. (1990) Extrahepatic hepatitis B virus DNA sequences in patients with acute hepatitis B infection. *Hepatology*, **12**, 187–192

Yong-Yuan, Z., Rizzetto, M., Bonino, F., Verme, G. & Lien-Jie, H. (1990) Immunohistochemical research of HDV infection in Chinese patients with chronic liver disease. *Hepato-gastroenterology*, **37**, 411–412

Zheng, H., Fu, T.-B., Lazinski, D. & Taylor, J. (1992) Editing on the genomic RNA of human hepatitis delta virus. *J. Virol.*, **66**, 4693–4697

Zignego, A.L., Deny, P., Gentilini, P. & Bréchot, C. (1992) Polymerase chain reaction for hepatitis delta virus RNA identification and characterization In: Becker, Y. & Darai, G., eds, *Frontiers of Virology*, Berlin, Springer Verlag, pp. 101–116

SUMMARY OF FINAL EVALUATIONS

Agent	Degree of evidence of carcinogenicity		Overall evaluation of carcinogenicity to humans
	Human	Animal	
Hepatitis B virus (chronic infection with)	S		1
Hepatitis B virus		I	
Hepatitis C virus (chronic infection with)	S		1
Hepatitis C virus		I	
Hepatitis D virus (infection with)	I	I	3

S, sufficient evidence; I, inadequate evidence; for definitions, see preamble, pp. 30–34

SUPPLEMENTARY CORRIGENDA TO VOLUMES 1–58

Corrigenda to Volumes 1–41 are listed in Volume 42, pp. 251–264; additional corrigenda are given in Volume 43, p. 261, in Volume 45, p. 283, in Volume 46, p. 419, in Volume 47, p. 505, in Volume 50, p. 385, in Volume 51, p. 483, in Volume 52, p. 513 and in Volume 57, p. 399.

Volume 50 p. 271 4.2 *Replace the three last lines by*: ...polypoid hyperplasia of the colon were observed. In rats, dantron increased the combined incidence of adenomas and adenocarcinomas of the colon and caecum.

CUMULATIVE CROSS INDEX TO *IARC MONOGRAPHS ON THE EVALUATION OF CARCINOGENIC RISKS TO HUMANS*

The volume, page and year are given. References to corrigenda are given in parentheses.

A

A-α-C	*40*, 245 (1986); *Suppl. 7*, 56 (1987)
Acetaldehyde	*36*, 101 (1985) (*corr. 42*, 263); *Suppl. 7*, 77 (1987)
Acetaldehyde formylmethylhydrazone (*see* Gyromitrin)	
Acetamide	*7*, 197 (1974); *Suppl. 7*, 389 (1987)
Acetaminophen (*see* Paracetamol)	
Acridine orange	*16*, 145 (1978); *Suppl. 7*, 56 (1987)
Acriflavinium chloride	*13*, 31 (1977); *Suppl. 7*, 56 (1987)
Acrolein	*19*, 479 (1979); *36*, 133 (1985); *Suppl. 7*, 78 (1987)
Acrylamide	*39*, 41 (1986); *Suppl. 7*, 56 (1987)
Acrylic acid	*19*, 47 (1979); *Suppl. 7*, 56 (1987)
Acrylic fibres	*19*, 86 (1979); *Suppl. 7*, 56 (1987)
Acrylonitrile	*19*, 73 (1979); *Suppl. 7*, 79 (1987)
Acrylonitrile-butadiene-styrene copolymers	*19*, 91 (1979); *Suppl. 7*, 56 (1987)
Actinolite (*see* Asbestos)	
Actinomycins	*10*, 29 (1976) (*corr. 42*, 255); *Suppl. 7*, 80 (1987)
Adriamycin	*10*, 43 (1976); *Suppl. 7*, 82 (1987)
AF-2	*31*, 47 (1983); *Suppl. 7*, 56 (1987)
Aflatoxins	*1*, 145 (1972) (*corr. 42*, 251); *10*, 51 (1976); *Suppl. 7*, 83 (1987); *56*, 245 (1993)
Aflatoxin B$_1$ (*see* Aflatoxins)	
Aflatoxin B$_2$ (*see* Aflatoxins)	
Aflatoxin G$_1$ (*see* Aflatoxins)	
Aflatoxin G$_2$ (*see* Aflatoxins)	
Aflatoxin M$_1$ (*see* Aflatoxins)	
Agaritine	*31*, 63 (1983); *Suppl. 7*, 56 (1987)
Alcohol drinking	*44* (1988)
Aldicarb	*53*, 93 (1991)
Aldrin	*5*, 25 (1974); *Suppl. 7*, 88 (1987)
Allyl chloride	*36*, 39 (1985); *Suppl. 7*, 56 (1987)
Allyl isothiocyanate	*36*, 55 (1985); *Suppl. 7*, 56 (1987)
Allyl isovalerate	*36*, 69 (1985); *Suppl. 7*, 56 (1987)
Aluminium production	*34*, 37 (1984); *Suppl. 7*, 89 (1987)
Amaranth	*8*, 41 (1975); *Suppl. 7*, 56 (1987)

5-Aminoacenaphthene   *16*, 243 (1978); *Suppl. 7*, 56 (1987)
2-Aminoanthraquinone   *27*, 191 (1982); *Suppl. 7*, 56 (1987)
para-Aminoazobenzene   *8*, 53 (1975); *Suppl. 7*, 390 (1987)
ortho-Aminoazotoluene   *8*, 61 (1975) (*corr. 42*, 254);
                                                    Suppl. 7, 56 (1987)
para-Aminobenzoic acid   *16*, 249 (1978); *Suppl. 7*, 56 (1987)
4-Aminobiphenyl   *1*, 74 (1972) (*corr. 42*, 251);
                                                    Suppl. 7, 91 (1987)
2-Amino-3,4-dimethylimidazo[4,5-*f*]quinoline (*see* MeIQ)
2-Amino-3,8-dimethylimidazo[4,5-*f*]quinoxaline (*see* MeIQx)
3-Amino-1,4-dimethyl-5*H*-pyrido[4,3-*b*]indole (*see* Trp-P-1)
2-Aminodipyrido[1,2-*a*:3′,2′-*d*]imidazole (*see* Glu-P-2)
1-Amino-2-methylanthraquinone   *27*, 199 (1982); *Suppl. 7*, 57 (1987)
2-Amino-3-methylimidazo[4,5-*f*]quinoline (*see* IQ)
2-Amino-6-methyldipyrido[1,2-*a*:3′,2′-*d*]imidazole (*see* Glu-P-1)
2-Amino-1-methyl-6-phenylimidazo[4,5-*b*]pyridine (*see* PhIP)
2-Amino-3-methyl-9*H*-pyrido[2,3-*b*]indole (*see* MeA-α-C)
3-Amino-1-methyl-5*H*-pyrido[4,3-*b*]indole (*see* Trp-P-2)
2-Amino-5-(5-nitro-2-furyl)-1,3,4-thiadiazole   *7*, 143 (1974); *Suppl. 7*, 57 (1987)
4-Amino-2-nitrophenol   *16*, 43 (1978); *Suppl. 7*, 57 (1987)
2-Amino-4-nitrophenol   *57*, 167 (1993)
2-Amino-5-nitrophenol   *57*, 177 (1993)
2-Amino-5-nitrothiazole   *31*, 71 (1983); *Suppl. 7*, 57 (1987)
2-Amino-9*H*-pyrido[2,3-*b*]indole (*see* A-α-C)
11-Aminoundecanoic acid   *39*, 239 (1986); *Suppl. 7*, 57 (1987)
Amitrole   *7*, 31 (1974); *41*, 293 (1986) (*corr.*
                                                    52, 513; *Suppl. 7*, 92 (1987)
Ammonium potassium selenide (*see* Selenium and selenium compounds)
Amorphous silica (*see also* Silica)   *42*, 39 (1987); *Suppl. 7*, 341 (1987)
Amosite (*see* Asbestos)
Ampicillin   *50*, 153 (1990)
Anabolic steroids (*see* Androgenic (anabolic) steroids)
Anaesthetics, volatile   *11*, 285 (1976); *Suppl. 7*, 93 (1987)
Analgesic mixtures containing phenacetin (*see also* Phenacetin)   *Suppl. 7*, 310 (1987)
Androgenic (anabolic) steroids   *Suppl. 7*, 96 (1987)
Angelicin and some synthetic derivatives (*see also* Angelicins)   *40*, 291 (1986)
Angelicin plus ultraviolet radiation (*see also* Angelicin and some   *Suppl. 7*, 57 (1987)
    synthetic derivatives)
Angelicins   *Suppl. 7*, 57 (1987)
Aniline   *4*, 27 (1974) (*corr. 42*, 252);
                                                    27, 39 (1982); *Suppl. 7*, 99 (1987)
ortho-Anisidine   *27*, 63 (1982); *Suppl. 7*, 57 (1987)
para-Anisidine   *27*, 65 (1982); *Suppl. 7*, 57 (1987)
Anthanthrene   *32*, 95 (1983); *Suppl. 7*, 57 (1987)
Anthophyllite (*see* Asbestos)
Anthracene   *32*, 105 (1983); *Suppl. 7*, 57 (1987)
Anthranilic acid   *16*, 265 (1978); *Suppl. 7*, 57 (1987)
Antimony trioxide   *47*, 291 (1989)
Antimony trisulfide   *47*, 291 (1989)
ANTU (*see* 1-Naphthylthiourea)
Apholate   *9*, 31 (1975); *Suppl. 7*, 57 (1987)
Aramite®   *5*, 39 (1974); *Suppl. 7*, 57 (1987)

Areca nut (*see* Betel quid)
Arsanilic acid (*see* Arsenic and arsenic compounds)
Arsenic and arsenic compounds   *1*, 41 (1972); *2*, 48 (1973);
                                                                  23, 39 (1980); *Suppl. 7*, 100 (1987)

Arsenic pentoxide (*see* Arsenic and arsenic compounds)
Arsenic sulfide (*see* Arsenic and arsenic compounds)
Arsenic trioxide (*see* Arsenic and arsenic compounds)
Arsine (*see* Arsenic and arsenic compounds)
Asbestos   *2*, 17 (1973) (*corr. 42*, 252);
                                                                  14 (1977) (*corr. 42*, 256); Suppl. 7,
                                                                  106 (1987) (*corr. 45*, 283)
Atrazine   *53*, 441 (1991)
Attapulgite   *42*, 159 (1987); *Suppl. 7*, 117 (1987)
Auramine (technical-grade)   *1*, 69 (1972) (*corr. 42*, 251); *Suppl. 7*,
                                                                  118 (1987)
Auramine, manufacture of (*see also* Auramine, technical-grade)   *Suppl. 7*, 118 (1987)
Aurothioglucose   *13*, 39 (1977); *Suppl. 7*, 57 (1987)
Azacitidine   *26*, 37 (1981); *Suppl. 7*, 57 (1987);
                                                                  50, 47 (1990)
5-Azacytidine (*see* Azacitidine)
Azaserine   *10*, 73 (1976) (*corr. 42*, 255);
                                                                  Suppl. 7, 57 (1987)
Azathioprine   *26*, 47 (1981); *Suppl. 7*, 119 (1987)
Aziridine   *9*, 37 (1975); *Suppl. 7*, 58 (1987)
2-(1-Aziridinyl)ethanol   *9*, 47 (1975); *Suppl. 7*, 58 (1987)
Aziridyl benzoquinone   *9*, 51 (1975); *Suppl. 7*, 58 (1987)
Azobenzene   *8*, 75 (1975); *Suppl. 7*, 58 (1987)

B

Barium chromate (*see* Chromium and chromium compounds)
Basic chromic sulfate (*see* Chromium and chromium compounds)
BCNU (*see* Bischloroethyl nitrosourea)
Benz[*a*]acridine   *32*, 123 (1983); *Suppl. 7*, 58 (1987)
Benz[*c*]acridine   *3*, 241 (1973); *32*, 129 (1983);
                                                                  Suppl. 7, 58 (1987)
Benzal chloride (*see also* α-Chlorinated toluenes)   *29*, 65 (1982); *Suppl. 7*, 148 (1987)
Benz[*a*]anthracene   *3*, 45 (1973); *32*, 135 (1983);
                                                                  Suppl. 7, 58 (1987)
Benzene   *7*, 203 (1974) (*corr. 42*, 254); *29*, 93,
                                                                  391 (1982); *Suppl. 7*, 120 (1987)
Benzidine   *1*, 80 (1972); *29*, 149, 391 (1982);
                                                                  Suppl. 7, 123 (1987)
Benzidine-based dyes   *Suppl. 7*, 125 (1987)
Benzo[*b*]fluoranthene   *3*, 69 (1973); *32*, 147 (1983);
                                                                  Suppl. 7, 58 (1987)
Benzo[*j*]fluoranthene   *3*, 82 (1973); *32*, 155 (1983); *Suppl. 7*,
                                                                  58 (1987)
Benzo[*k*]fluoranthene   *32*, 163 (1983); *Suppl. 7*, 58 (1987)
Benzo[*ghi*]fluoranthene   *32*, 171 (1983); *Suppl. 7*, 58 (1987)
Benzo[*a*]fluorene   *32*, 177 (1983); *Suppl. 7*, 58 (1987)
Benzo[*b*]fluorene   *32*, 183 (1983); *Suppl. 7*, 58 (1987)

Benzo[c]fluorene	32, 189 (1983); Suppl. 7, 58 (1987)
Benzo[ghi]perylene	32, 195 (1983); Suppl. 7, 58 (1987)
Benzo[c]phenanthrene	32, 205 (1983); Suppl. 7, 58 (1987)
Benzo[a]pyrene	3, 91 (1973); 32, 211 (1983); Suppl. 7, 58 (1987)
Benzo[e]pyrene	3, 137 (1973); 32, 225 (1983); Suppl. 7, 58 (1987)
para-Benzoquinone dioxime	29, 185 (1982); Suppl. 7, 58 (1987)
Benzotrichloride (see also α-Chlorinated toluenes)	29, 73 (1982); Suppl. 7, 148 (1987)
Benzoyl chloride	29, 83 (1982) (corr. 42, 261); Suppl. 7, 126 (1987)
Benzoyl peroxide	36, 267 (1985); Suppl. 7, 58 (1987)
Benzyl acetate	40, 109 (1986); Suppl. 7, 58 (1987)
Benzyl chloride (see also α-Chlorinated toluenes)	11, 217 (1976) (corr. 42, 256); 29, 49 (1982); Suppl. 7, 148 (1987)
Benzyl violet 4B	16, 153 (1978); Suppl. 7, 58 (1987)
Bertrandite (see Beryllium and beryllium compounds)	
Beryllium and beryllium compounds	1, 17 (1972); 23, 143 (1980) (corr. 42, 260); Suppl. 7, 127 (1987); 58, 41 (1993)
Beryllium acetate (see Beryllium and beryllium compounds)	
Beryllium acetate, basic (see Beryllium and beryllium compounds)	
Beryllium–aluminium alloy (see Beryllium and beryllium compounds)	
Beryllium carbonate (see Beryllium and beryllium compounds)	
Beryllium chloride (see Beryllium and beryllium compounds)	
Beryllium–copper alloy (see Beryllium and beryllium compounds)	
Beryllium–copper–cobalt alloy (see Beryllium and beryllium compounds)	
Beryllium fluoride (see Beryllium and beryllium compounds)	
Beryllium hydroxide (see Beryllium and beryllium compounds)	
Beryllium–nickel alloy (see Beryllium and beryllium compounds)	
Beryllium oxide (see Beryllium and beryllium compounds)	
Beryllium phosphate (see Beryllium and beryllium compounds)	
Beryllium silicate (see Beryllium and beryllium compounds)	
Beryllium sulfate (see Beryllium and beryllium compounds)	
Beryl ore (see Beryllium and beryllium compounds)	
Betel quid	37, 141 (1985); Suppl. 7, 128 (1987)
Betel-quid chewing (see Betel quid)	
BHA (see Butylated hydroxyanisole)	
BHT (see Butylated hydroxytoluene)	
Bis(1-aziridinyl)morpholinophosphine sulfide	9, 55 (1975); Suppl. 7, 58 (1987)
Bis(2-chloroethyl)ether	9, 117 (1975); Suppl. 7, 58 (1987)
N,N-Bis(2-chloroethyl)-2-naphthylamine	4, 119 (1974) (corr. 42, 253); Suppl. 7, 130 (1987)
Bischloroethyl nitrosourea (see also Chloroethyl nitrosoureas)	26, 79 (1981); Suppl. 7, 150 (1987)
1,2-Bis(chloromethoxy)ethane	15, 31 (1977); Suppl. 7, 58 (1987)
1,4-Bis(chloromethoxymethyl)benzene	15, 37 (1977); Suppl. 7, 58 (1987)
Bis(chloromethyl)ether	4, 231 (1974) (corr. 42, 253); Suppl. 7, 131 (1987)
Bis(2-chloro-1-methylethyl)ether	41, 149 (1986); Suppl. 7, 59 (1987)
Bis(2,3-epoxycyclopentyl)ether	47, 231 (1989)
Bisphenol A diglycidyl ether (see Glycidyl ethers)	
Bisulfites (see Sulfur dioxide and some sulfites, bisulfites and metabisulfites)	

Bitumens	35, 39 (1985); *Suppl. 7*, 133 (1987)
Bleomycins	26, 97 (1981); *Suppl. 7*, 134 (1987)
Blue VRS	16, 163 (1978); *Suppl. 7*, 59 (1987)
Boot and shoe manufacture and repair	25, 249 (1981); *Suppl. 7*, 232 (1987)
Bracken fern	40, 47 (1986); *Suppl. 7*, 135 (1987)
Brilliant Blue FCF, disodium salt	16, 171 (1978) (*corr. 42*, 257); *Suppl. 7*, 59 (1987)
Bromochloroacetonitrile (*see* Halogenated acetonitriles)	
Bromodichloromethane	52, 179 (1991)
Bromoethane	52, 299 (1991)
Bromoform	52, 213 (1991)
1,3-Butadiene	39, 155 (1986) (*corr. 42*, 264); *Suppl. 7*, 136 (1987); 54, 237 (1992)
1,4-Butanediol dimethanesulfonate	4, 247 (1974); *Suppl. 7*, 137 (1987)
n-Butyl acrylate	39, 67 (1986); *Suppl. 7*, 59 (1987)
Butylated hydroxyanisole	40, 123 (1986); *Suppl. 7*, 59 (1987)
Butylated hydroxytoluene	40, 161 (1986); *Suppl. 7*, 59 (1987)
Butyl benzyl phthalate	29, 193 (1982) (*corr. 42*, 261); *Suppl. 7*, 59 (1987)
β-Butyrolactone	11, 225 (1976); *Suppl. 7*, 59 (1987)
γ-Butyrolactone	11, 231 (1976); *Suppl. 7*, 59 (1987)

C

Cabinet-making (*see* Furniture and cabinet-making)	
Cadmium acetate (*see* Cadmium and cadmium compounds)	
Cadmium and cadmium compounds	2, 74 (1973); 11, 39 (1976) (*corr. 42*, 255); *Suppl. 7*, 139 (1987); 58, 119 (1993)
Cadmium chloride (*see* Cadmium and cadmium compounds)	
Cadmium oxide (*see* Cadmium and cadmium compounds)	
Cadmium sulfate (*see* Cadmium and cadmium compounds)	
Cadmium sulfide (*see* Cadmium and cadmium compounds)	
Caffeic acid	56, 115 (1993)
Caffeine	51, 291 (1991)
Calcium arsenate (*see* Arsenic and arsenic compounds)	
Calcium chromate (*see* Chromium and chromium compounds)	
Calcium cyclamate (*see* Cyclamates)	
Calcium saccharin (*see* Saccharin)	
Cantharidin	10, 79 (1976); *Suppl. 7*, 59 (1987)
Caprolactam	19, 115 (1979) (*corr. 42*, 258); 39, 247 (1986) (*corr. 42*, 264); *Suppl. 7*, 390 (1987)
Captafol	53, 353 (1991)
Captan	30, 295 (1983); *Suppl. 7*, 59 (1987)
Carbaryl	12, 37 (1976); *Suppl. 7*, 59 (1987)
Carbazole	32, 239 (1983); *Suppl. 7*, 59 (1987)
3-Carbethoxypsoralen	40, 317 (1986); *Suppl. 7*, 59 (1987)
Carbon blacks	3, 22 (1973); 33, 35 (1984); *Suppl. 7*, 142 (1987)
Carbon tetrachloride	1, 53 (1972); 20, 371 (1979); *Suppl. 7*, 143 (1987)

Carmoisine	8, 83 (1975); Suppl. 7, 59 (1987)
Carpentry and joinery	25, 139 (1981); Suppl. 7, 378 (1987)
Carrageenan	10, 181 (1976) (corr. 42, 255); 31, 79 (1983); Suppl. 7, 59 (1987)
Catechol	15, 155 (1977); Suppl. 7, 59 (1987)
CCNU (see 1-(2-Chloroethyl)-3-cyclohexyl-1-nitrosourea)	
Ceramic fibres (see Man-made mineral fibres)	
Chemotherapy, combined, including alkylating agents (see MOPP and other combined chemotherapy including alkylating agents)	
Chlorambucil	9, 125 (1975); 26, 115 (1981); Suppl. 7, 144 (1987)
Chloramphenicol	10, 85 (1976); Suppl. 7, 145 (1987); 50, 169 (1990)
Chlordane (see also Chlordane/Heptachlor)	20, 45 (1979) (corr. 42, 258)
Chlordane/Heptachlor	Suppl. 7, 146 (1987); 53, 115 (1991)
Chlordecone	20, 67 (1979); Suppl. 7, 59 (1987)
Chlordimeform	30, 61 (1983); Suppl. 7, 59 (1987)
Chlorendic acid	48, 45 (1990)
Chlorinated dibenzodioxins (other than TCDD)	15, 41 (1977); Suppl. 7, 59 (1987)
Chlorinated drinking-water	52, 45 (1991)
Chlorinated paraffins	48, 55 (1990)
α-Chlorinated toluenes	Suppl. 7, 148 (1987)
Chlormadinone acetate (see also Progestins; Combined oral contraceptives)	6, 149 (1974); 21, 365 (1979)
Chlornaphazine (see N,N-Bis(2-chloroethyl)-2-naphthylamine)	
Chloroacetonitrile (see Halogenated acetonitriles)	
para-Chloroaniline	57, 305 (1993)
Chlorobenzilate	5, 75 (1974); 30, 73 (1983); Suppl. 7, 60 (1987)
Chlorodibromomethane	52, 243 (1991)
Chlorodifluoromethane	41, 237 (1986) (corr. 51, 483); Suppl. 7, 149 (1987)
Chloroethane	52, 315 (1991)
1-(2-Chloroethyl)-3-cyclohexyl-1-nitrosourea (see also Chloroethyl nitrosoureas)	26, 137 (1981) (corr. 42, 260); Suppl. 7, 150 (1987)
1-(2-Chloroethyl)-3-(4-methylcyclohexyl)-1-nitrosourea (see also Chloroethyl nitrosoureas)	Suppl. 7, 150 (1987)
Chloroethyl nitrosoureas	Suppl. 7, 150 (1987)
Chlorofluoromethane	41, 229 (1986); Suppl. 7, 60 (1987)
Chloroform	1, 61 (1972); 20, 401 (1979); Suppl. 7, 152 (1987)
Chloromethyl methyl ether (technical-grade) (see also Bis(chloromethyl)ether)	4, 239 (1974); Suppl. 7, 131 (1987)
(4-Chloro-2-methylphenoxy)acetic acid (see MCPA)	
Chlorophenols	Suppl. 7, 154 (1987)
Chlorophenols (occupational exposures to)	41, 319 (1986)
Chlorophenoxy herbicides	Suppl. 7, 156 (1987)
Chlorophenoxy herbicides (occupational exposures to)	41, 357 (1986)
4-Chloro-ortho-phenylenediamine	27, 81 (1982); Suppl. 7, 60 (1987)
4-Chloro-meta-phenylenediamine	27, 82 (1982); Suppl. 7, 60 (1987)
Chloroprene	19, 131 (1979); Suppl. 7, 160 (1987)
Chloropropham	12, 55 (1976); Suppl. 7, 60 (1987)

Chloroquine	*13*, 47 (1977); *Suppl. 7*, 60 (1987)
Chlorothalonil	*30*, 319 (1983); *Suppl. 7*, 60 (1987)
para-Chloro-*ortho*-toluidine and its strong acid salts	*16*, 277 (1978); *30*, 65 (1983);
(*see also* Chlordimeform)	*Suppl. 7*, 60 (1987); *48*, 123 (1990)
Chlorotrianisene (*see also* Nonsteroidal oestrogens)	*21*, 139 (1979)
2-Chloro-1,1,1-trifluoroethane	*41*, 253 (1986); *Suppl. 7*, 60 (1987)
Chlorozotocin	*50*, 65 (1990)
Cholesterol	*10*, 99 (1976); *31*, 95 (1983); *Suppl. 7*, 161 (1987)
Chromic acetate (*see* Chromium and chromium compounds)	
Chromic chloride (*see* Chromium and chromium compounds)	
Chromic oxide (*see* Chromium and chromium compounds)	
Chromic phosphate (*see* Chromium and chromium compounds)	
Chromite ore (*see* Chromium and chromium compounds)	
Chromium and chromium compounds	*2*, 100 (1973); *23*, 205 (1980); *Suppl. 7*, 165 (1987); *49*, 49 (1990) (*corr. 51*, 483)
Chromium carbonyl (*see* Chromium and chromium compounds)	
Chromium potassium sulfate (*see* Chromium and chromium compounds)	
Chromium sulfate (*see* Chromium and chromium compounds)	
Chromium trioxide (*see* Chromium and chromium compounds)	
Chrysazin (*see* Dantron)	
Chrysene	*3*, 159 (1973); *32*, 247 (1983); *Suppl. 7*, 60 (1987)
Chrysoidine	*8*, 91 (1975); *Suppl. 7*, 169 (1987)
Chrysotile (*see* Asbestos)	
CI Acid Orange 3	*57*, 121 (1993)
CI Acid Red 114	*57*, 247 (1993)
CI Basic Red 9	*57*, 215 (1993)
Ciclosporin	*50*, 77 (1990)
CI Direct Blue 15	*57*, 235 (1993)
CI Disperse Yellow 3 (*see* Disperse Yellow 3)	
Cimetidine	*50*, 235 (1990)
Cinnamyl anthranilate	*16*, 287 (1978); *31*, 133 (1983); *Suppl. 7*, 60 (1987)
CI Pigment Red 3	*57*, 259 (1993)
CI Pigment Red 53:1 (*see* D&C Red No. 9)	
Cisplatin	*26*, 151 (1981); *Suppl. 7*, 170 (1987)
Citrinin	*40*, 67 (1986); *Suppl. 7*, 60 (1987)
Citrus Red No. 2	*8*, 101 (1975) (*corr. 42*, 254); *Suppl. 7*, 60 (1987)
Clofibrate	*24*, 39 (1980); *Suppl. 7*, 171 (1987)
Clomiphene citrate	*21*, 551 (1979); *Suppl. 7*, 172 (1987)
Coal gasification	*34*, 65 (1984); *Suppl. 7*, 173 (1987)
Coal-tar pitches (*see also* Coal-tars)	*35*, 83 (1985); *Suppl. 7*, 174 (1987)
Coal-tars	*35*, 83 (1985); *Suppl. 7*, 175 (1987)
Cobalt[III] acetate (*see* Cobalt and cobalt compounds)	
Cobalt–aluminium–chromium spinel (*see* Cobalt and cobalt compounds)	
Cobalt and cobalt compounds	*52*, 363 (1991)
Cobalt[II] chloride (*see* Cobalt and cobalt compounds)	

Cobalt–chromium alloy (see Chromium and chromium compounds)
Cobalt–chromium–molybdenum alloys (see Cobalt and cobalt compounds)
Cobalt metal powder (see Cobalt and cobalt compounds)
Cobalt naphthenate (see Cobalt and cobalt compounds)
Cobalt[II] oxide (see Cobalt and cobalt compounds)
Cobalt[II,III] oxide (see Cobalt and cobalt compounds)
Cobalt[II] sulfide (see Cobalt and cobalt compounds)

Coffee	51, 41 (1991) (corr. 52, 513)
Coke production	34, 101 (1984); Suppl. 7, 176 (1987)
Combined oral contraceptives (see also Oestrogens, progestins and combinations)	Suppl. 7, 297 (1987)
Conjugated oestrogens (see also Steroidal oestrogens)	21, 147 (1979)
Contraceptives, oral (see Combined oral contraceptives; Sequential oral contraceptives)	
Copper 8-hydroxyquinoline	15, 103 (1977); Suppl. 7, 61 (1987)
Coronene	32, 263 (1983); Suppl. 7, 61 (1987)
Coumarin	10, 113 (1976); Suppl. 7, 61 (1987)
Creosotes (see also Coal-tars)	35, 83 (1985); Suppl. 7, 177 (1987)
meta-Cresidine	27, 91 (1982); Suppl. 7, 61 (1987)
para-Cresidine	27, 92 (1982); Suppl. 7, 61 (1987)
Crocidolite (see Asbestos)	
Crude oil	45, 119 (1989)
Crystalline silica (see also Silica)	42, 39 (1987); Suppl. 7, 341 (1987)
Cycasin	1, 157 (1972) (corr. 42, 251); 10, 121 (1976); Suppl. 7, 61 (1987)
Cyclamates	22, 55 (1980); Suppl. 7, 178 (1987)
Cyclamic acid (see Cyclamates)	
Cyclochlorotine	10, 139 (1976); Suppl. 7, 61 (1987)
Cyclohexanone	47, 157 (1989)
Cyclohexylamine (see Cyclamates)	
Cyclopenta[cd]pyrene	32, 269 (1983); Suppl. 7, 61 (1987)
Cyclopropane (see Anaesthetics, volatile)	
Cyclophosphamide	9, 135 (1975); 26, 165 (1981); Suppl. 7, 182 (1987)

D

2,4-D (see also Chlorophenoxy herbicides; Chlorophenoxy herbicides, occupational exposures to)	15, 111 (1977)
Dacarbazine	26, 203 (1981); Suppl. 7, 184 (1987)
Dantron	50, 265 (1990) (corr. 59, 257)
D&C Red No. 9	8, 107 (1975); Suppl. 7, 61 (1987); 57, 203 (1993)
Dapsone	24, 59 (1980); Suppl. 7, 185 (1987)
Daunomycin	10, 145 (1976); Suppl. 7, 61 (1987)
DDD (see DDT)	
DDE (see DDT)	
DDT	5, 83 (1974) (corr. 42, 253); Suppl. 7, 186 (1987); 53, 179 (1991)
Decabromodiphenyl oxide	48, 73 (1990)
Deltamethrin	53, 251 (1991)

Deoxynivalenol (see Toxins derived from *Fusarium graminearum*,
  F. culmorum and *F. crookwellense*)
Diacetylaminoazotoluene — 8, 113 (1975); *Suppl. 7*, 61 (1987)
N,N'-Diacetylbenzidine — 16, 293 (1978); *Suppl. 7*, 61 (1987)
Diallate — 12, 69 (1976); 30, 235 (1983); *Suppl. 7*, 61 (1987)

2,4-Diaminoanisole — 16, 51 (1978); 27, 103 (1982); *Suppl. 7*, 61 (1987)

4,4'-Diaminodiphenyl ether — 16, 301 (1978); 29, 203 (1982); *Suppl. 7*, 61 (1987)

1,2-Diamino-4-nitrobenzene — 16, 63 (1978); *Suppl. 7*, 61 (1987)
1,4-Diamino-2-nitrobenzene — 16, 73 (1978); *Suppl. 7*, 61 (1987); 57, 185 (1993)

2,6-Diamino-3-(phenylazo)pyridine (see Phenazopyridine hydrochloride)
2,4-Diaminotoluene (see also Toluene diisocyanates) — 16, 83 (1978); *Suppl. 7*, 61 (1987)
2,5-Diaminotoluene (see also Toluene diisocyanates) — 16, 97 (1978); *Suppl. 7*, 61 (1987)
ortho-Dianisidine (see 3,3'-Dimethoxybenzidine)
Diazepam — 13, 57 (1977); *Suppl. 7*, 189 (1987)
Diazomethane — 7, 223 (1974); *Suppl. 7*, 61 (1987)
Dibenz[*a,h*]acridine — 3, 247 (1973); 32, 277 (1983); *Suppl. 7*, 61 (1987)

Dibenz[*a,j*]acridine — 3, 254 (1973); 32, 283 (1983); *Suppl. 7*, 61 (1987)

Dibenz[*a,c*]anthracene — 32, 289 (1983) (corr. 42, 262); *Suppl. 7*, 61 (1987)

Dibenz[*a,h*]anthracene — 3, 178 (1973) (corr. 43, 261); 32, 299 (1983); *Suppl. 7*, 61 (1987)

Dibenz[*a,j*]anthracene — 32, 309 (1983); *Suppl. 7*, 61 (1987)
7*H*-Dibenzo[*c,g*]carbazole — 3, 260 (1973); 32, 315 (1983); *Suppl. 7*, 61 (1987)

Dibenzodioxins, chlorinated (other than TCDD)
  [see Chlorinated dibenzodioxins (other than TCDD)]
Dibenzo[*a,e*]fluoranthene — 32, 321 (1983); *Suppl. 7*, 61 (1987)
Dibenzo[*h,rst*]pentaphene — 3, 197 (1973); *Suppl. 7*, 62 (1987)
Dibenzo[*a,e*]pyrene — 3, 201 (1973); 32, 327 (1983); *Suppl. 7*, 62 (1987)

Dibenzo[*a,h*]pyrene — 3, 207 (1973); 32, 331 (1983); *Suppl. 7*, 62 (1987)

Dibenzo[*a,i*]pyrene — 3, 215 (1973); 32, 337 (1983); *Suppl. 7*, 62 (1987)

Dibenzo[*a,l*]pyrene — 3, 224 (1973); 32, 343 (1983); *Suppl. 7*, 62 (1987)

Dibromoacetonitrile (see Halogenated acetonitriles)
1,2-Dibromo-3-chloropropane — 15, 139 (1977); 20, 83 (1979); *Suppl. 7*, 191 (1987)

Dichloroacetonitrile (see Halogenated acetonitriles)
Dichloroacetylene — 39, 369 (1986); *Suppl. 7*, 62 (1987)
ortho-Dichlorobenzene — 7, 231 (1974); 29, 213 (1982); *Suppl. 7*, 192 (1987)

para-Dichlorobenzene — 7, 231 (1974); 29, 215 (1982); *Suppl. 7*, 192 (1987)

3,3'-Dichlorobenzidine	4, 49 (1974); 29, 239 (1982); Suppl. 7, 193 (1987)
trans-1,4-Dichlorobutene	15, 149 (1977); Suppl. 7, 62 (1987)
3,3'-Dichloro-4,4'-diaminodiphenyl ether	16, 309 (1978); Suppl. 7, 62 (1987)
1,2-Dichloroethane	20, 429 (1979); Suppl. 7, 62 (1987)
Dichloromethane	20, 449 (1979); 41, 43 (1986); Suppl. 7, 194 (1987)
2,4-Dichlorophenol (see Chlorophenols; Chlorophenols, occupational exposures to)	
(2,4-Dichlorophenoxy)acetic acid (see 2,4-D)	
2,6-Dichloro-para-phenylenediamine	39, 325 (1986); Suppl. 7, 62 (1987)
1,2-Dichloropropane	41, 131 (1986); Suppl. 7, 62 (1987)
1,3-Dichloropropene (technical-grade)	41, 113 (1986); Suppl. 7, 195 (1987)
Dichlorvos	20, 97 (1979); Suppl. 7, 62 (1987); 53, 267 (1991)
Dicofol	30, 87 (1983); Suppl. 7, 62 (1987)
Dicyclohexylamine (see Cyclamates)	
Dieldrin	5, 125 (1974); Suppl. 7, 196 (1987)
Dienoestrol (see also Nonsteroidal oestrogens)	21, 161 (1979)
Diepoxybutane	11, 115 (1976) (corr. 42, 255); Suppl. 7, 62 (1987)
Diesel and gasoline engine exhausts	46, 41 (1989)
Diesel fuels	45, 219 (1989) (corr. 47, 505)
Diethyl ether (see Anaesthetics, volatile)	
Di(2-ethylhexyl)adipate	29, 257 (1982); Suppl. 7, 62 (1987)
Di(2-ethylhexyl)phthalate	29, 269 (1982) (corr. 42, 261); Suppl. 7, 62 (1987)
1,2-Diethylhydrazine	4, 153 (1974); Suppl. 7, 62 (1987)
Diethylstilboestrol	6, 55 (1974); 21, 173 (1979) (corr. 42, 259); Suppl. 7, 273 (1987)
Diethylstilboestrol dipropionate (see Diethylstilboestrol)	
Diethyl sulfate	4, 277 (1974); Suppl. 7, 198 (1987); 54, 213 (1992)
Diglycidyl resorcinol ether	11, 125 (1976); 36, 181 (1985); Suppl. 7, 62 (1987)
Dihydrosafrole	1, 170 (1972); 10, 233 (1976); Suppl. 7, 62 (1987)
1,8-Dihydroxyanthraquinone (see Dantron)	
Dihydroxybenzenes (see Catechol; Hydroquinone; Resorcinol)	
Dihydroxymethylfuratrizine	24, 77 (1980); Suppl. 7, 62 (1987)
Diisopropyl sulfate	54, 229 (1992)
Dimethisterone (see also Progestins; Sequential oral contraceptives)	6, 167 (1974); 21, 377 (1979)
Dimethoxane	15, 177 (1977); Suppl. 7, 62 (1987)
3,3'-Dimethoxybenzidine	4, 41 (1974); Suppl. 7, 198 (1987)
3,3'-Dimethoxybenzidine-4,4'-diisocyanate	39, 279 (1986); Suppl. 7, 62 (1987)
para-Dimethylaminoazobenzene	8, 125 (1975); Suppl. 7, 62 (1987)
para-Dimethylaminoazobenzenediazo sodium sulfonate	8, 147 (1975); Suppl. 7, 62 (1987)
trans-2-[(Dimethylamino)methylimino]-5-[2-(5-nitro-2-furyl)-vinyl]-1,3,4-oxadiazole	7, 147 (1974) (corr. 42, 253); Suppl. 7, 62 (1987)
4,4'-Dimethylangelicin plus ultraviolet radiation (see also Angelicin and some synthetic derivatives)	Suppl. 7, 57 (1987)

4,5'-Dimethylangelicin plus ultraviolet radiation (see also Angelicin and some synthetic derivatives)	Suppl. 7, 57 (1987)
2,6-Dimethylaniline	57, 323 (1993)
N,N-Dimethylaniline	57, 337 (1993)
Dimethylarsinic acid (see Arsenic and arsenic compounds)	
3,3'-Dimethylbenzidine	1, 87 (1972); Suppl. 7, 62 (1987)
Dimethylcarbamoyl chloride	12, 77 (1976); Suppl. 7, 199 (1987)
Dimethylformamide	47, 171 (1989)
1,1-Dimethylhydrazine	4, 137 (1974); Suppl. 7, 62 (1987)
1,2-Dimethylhydrazine	4, 145 (1974) (corr. 42, 253); Suppl. 7, 62 (1987)
Dimethyl hydrogen phosphite	48, 85 (1990)
1,4-Dimethylphenanthrene	32, 349 (1983); Suppl. 7, 62 (1987)
Dimethyl sulfate	4, 271 (1974); Suppl. 7, 200 (1987)
3,7-Dinitrofluoranthene	46, 189 (1989)
3,9-Dinitrofluoranthene	46, 195 (1989)
1,3-Dinitropyrene	46, 201 (1989)
1,6-Dinitropyrene	46, 215 (1989)
1,8-Dinitropyrene	33, 171 (1984); Suppl. 7, 63 (1987); 46, 231 (1989)
Dinitrosopentamethylenetetramine	11, 241 (1976); Suppl. 7, 63 (1987)
1,4-Dioxane	11, 247 (1976); Suppl. 7, 201 (1987)
2,4'-Diphenyldiamine	16, 313 (1978); Suppl. 7, 63 (1987)
Direct Black 38 (see also Benzidine-based dyes)	29, 295 (1982) (corr. 42, 261)
Direct Blue 6 (see also Benzidine-based dyes)	29, 311 (1982)
Direct Brown 95 (see also Benzidine-based dyes)	29, 321 (1982)
Disperse Blue 1	48, 139 (1990)
Disperse Yellow 3	8, 97 (1975); Suppl. 7, 60 (1987); 48, 149 (1990)
Disulfiram	12, 85 (1976); Suppl. 7, 63 (1987)
Dithranol	13, 75 (1977); Suppl. 7, 63 (1987)
Divinyl ether (see Anaesthetics, volatile)	
Dulcin	12, 97 (1976); Suppl. 7, 63 (1987)

E

Endrin	5, 157 (1974); Suppl. 7, 63 (1987)
Enflurane (see Anaesthetics, volatile)	
Eosin	15, 183 (1977); Suppl. 7, 63 (1987)
Epichlorohydrin	11, 131 (1976) (corr. 42, 256); Suppl. 7, 202 (1987)
1,2-Epoxybutane	47, 217 (1989)
1-Epoxyethyl-3,4-epoxycyclohexane	11, 141 (1976); Suppl. 7, 63 (1987)
3,4-Epoxy-6-methylcyclohexylmethyl-3,4-epoxy-6-methyl-cyclohexane carboxylate	11, 147 (1976); Suppl. 7, 63 (1987)
cis-9,10-Epoxystearic acid	11, 153 (1976); Suppl. 7, 63 (1987)
Erionite	42, 225 (1987); Suppl. 7, 203 (1987)
Ethinyloestradiol (see also Steroidal oestrogens)	6, 77 (1974); 21, 233 (1979)
Ethionamide	13, 83 (1977); Suppl. 7, 63 (1987)
Ethyl acrylate	19, 57 (1979); 39, 81 (1986); Suppl. 7, 63 (1987)
Ethylene	19, 157 (1979); Suppl. 7, 63 (1987)

Ethylene dibromide	15, 195 (1977); *Suppl. 7*, 204 (1987)
Ethylene oxide	11, 157 (1976); 36, 189 (1985) (*corr. 42*, 263); *Suppl. 7*, 205 (1987)
Ethylene sulfide	11, 257 (1976); *Suppl. 7*, 63 (1987)
Ethylene thiourea	7, 45 (1974); *Suppl. 7*, 207 (1987)
Ethyl methanesulfonate	7, 245 (1974); *Suppl. 7*, 63 (1987)
N-Ethyl-N-nitrosourea	1, 135 (1972); 17, 191 (1978); *Suppl. 7*, 63 (1987)
Ethyl selenac (*see also* Selenium and selenium compounds)	12, 107 (1976); *Suppl. 7*, 63 (1987)
Ethyl tellurac	12, 115 (1976); *Suppl. 7*, 63 (1987)
Ethynodiol diacetate (*see also* Progestins; Combined oral contraceptives)	6, 173 (1974); 21, 387 (1979)
Eugenol	36, 75 (1985); *Suppl. 7*, 63 (1987)
Evans blue	8, 151 (1975); *Suppl. 7*, 63 (1987)

F

Fast Green FCF	16, 187 (1978); *Suppl. 7*, 63 (1987)
Fenvalerate	53, 309 (1991)
Ferbam	12, 121 (1976) (*corr. 42*, 256); *Suppl. 7*, 63 (1987)
Ferric oxide	1, 29 (1972); *Suppl. 7*, 216 (1987)
Ferrochromium (*see* Chromium and chromium compounds)	
Fluometuron	30, 245 (1983); *Suppl. 7*, 63 (1987)
Fluoranthene	32, 355 (1983); *Suppl. 7*, 63 (1987)
Fluorene	32, 365 (1983); *Suppl. 7*, 63 (1987)
Fluorescent lighting (exposure to) (*see* Ultraviolet radiation)	
Fluorides (inorganic, used in drinking-water)	27, 237 (1982); *Suppl. 7*, 208 (1987)
5-Fluorouracil	26, 217 (1981); *Suppl. 7*, 210 (1987)
Fluorspar (*see* Fluorides)	
Fluosilicic acid (*see* Fluorides)	
Fluroxene (*see* Anaesthetics, volatile)	
Formaldehyde	29, 345 (1982); *Suppl. 7*, 211 (1987)
2-(2-Formylhydrazino)-4-(5-nitro-2-furyl)thiazole	7, 151 (1974) (*corr. 42*, 253); *Suppl. 7*, 63 (1987)
Frusemide (*see* Furosemide)	
Fuel oils (heating oils)	45, 239 (1989) (*corr. 47*, 505)
Fumonisin B$_1$ (*see* Toxins derived from *Fusarium moniliforme*)	
Fumonisin B$_2$ (*see* Toxins derived from *Fusarium moniliforme*)	
Furazolidone	31, 141 (1983); *Suppl. 7*, 63 (1987)
Furniture and cabinet-making	25, 99 (1981); *Suppl. 7*, 380 (1987)
Furosemide	50, 277 (1990)
2-(2-Furyl)-3-(5-nitro-2-furyl)acrylamide (*see* AF-2)	
Fusarenon-X (*see* Toxins derived from *Fusarium graminearum*, *F. culmorum* and *F. crookwellense*)	
Fusarenone-X (*see* Toxins derived from *Fusarium graminearum*, *F. culmorum* and *F. crookwellense*)	
Fusarin C (see Toxins derived from *Fusarium moniliforme*)	

G

Gasoline	45, 159 (1989) (*corr. 47*, 505)

Gasoline engine exhaust (see Diesel and gasoline engine exhausts)	
Glass fibres (see Man-made mineral fibres)	
Glass manufacturing industry, occupational exposures in	58, 347 (1993)
Glasswool (see Man-made mineral fibres)	
Glass filaments (see Man-made mineral fibres)	
Glu-P-1	40, 223 (1986); Suppl. 7, 64 (1987)
Glu-P-2	40, 235 (1986); Suppl. 7, 64 (1987)
L-Glutamic acid, 5-[2-(4-hydroxymethyl)phenylhydrazide] (see Agaritine)	
Glycidaldehyde	11, 175 (1976); Suppl. 7, 64 (1987)
Glycidyl ethers	47, 237 (1989)
Glycidyl oleate	11, 183 (1976); Suppl. 7, 64 (1987)
Glycidyl stearate	11, 187 (1976); Suppl. 7, 64 (1987)
Griseofulvin	10, 153 (1976); Suppl. 7, 391 (1987)
Guinea Green B	16, 199 (1978); Suppl. 7, 64 (1987)
Gyromitrin	31, 163 (1983); Suppl. 7, 391 (1987)

H

Haematite	1, 29 (1972); Suppl. 7, 216 (1987)
Haematite and ferric oxide	Suppl. 7, 216 (1987)
Haematite mining, underground, with exposure to radon	1, 29 (1972); Suppl. 7, 216 (1987)
Hairdressers and barbers (occupational exposure as)	57, 43 (1993)
Hair dyes, epidemiology of	16, 29 (1978); 27, 307 (1982);
Halogenated acetonitriles	52, 269 (1991)
Halothane (see Anaesthetics, volatile)	
HC Blue No. 1	57, 129 (1993)
HC Blue No. 2	57, 143 (1993)
α-HCH (see Hexachlorocyclohexanes)	
β-HCH (see Hexachlorocyclohexanes)	
γ-HCH (see Hexachlorocyclohexanes)	
HC Red No. 3	57, 153 (1993)
HC Yellow No. 4	57, 159 (1993)
Heating oils (see Fuel oils)	
Hepatitis B virus	59. 45 (1994)
Hepatitis C virus	59, 165 (1994)
Hepatitis D virus	59, 223 (1994)
Heptachlor (see also Chlordane/Heptachlor)	5, 173 (1974); 20, 129 (1979)
Hexachlorobenzene	20, 155 (1979); Suppl. 7, 219 (1987)
Hexachlorobutadiene	20, 179 (1979); Suppl. 7, 64 (1987)
Hexachlorocyclohexanes	5, 47 (1974); 20, 195 (1979) (corr. 42, 258); Suppl. 7, 220 (1987)
Hexachlorocyclohexane, technical-grade (see Hexachlorocyclohexanes)	
Hexachloroethane	20, 467 (1979); Suppl. 7, 64 (1987)
Hexachlorophene	20, 241 (1979); Suppl. 7, 64 (1987)
Hexamethylphosphoramide	15, 211 (1977); Suppl. 7, 64 (1987)
Hexoestrol (see Nonsteroidal oestrogens)	
Hycanthone mesylate	13, 91 (1977); Suppl. 7, 64 (1987)
Hydralazine	24, 85 (1980); Suppl. 7, 222 (1987)
Hydrazine	4, 127 (1974); Suppl. 7, 223 (1987)
Hydrochloric acid	54, 189 (1992)

Hydrochlorothiazide	50, 293 (1990)
Hydrogen peroxide	36, 285 (1985); Suppl. 7, 64 (1987)
Hydroquinone	15, 155 (1977); Suppl. 7, 64 (1987)
4-Hydroxyazobenzene	8, 157 (1975); Suppl. 7, 64 (1987)
17α-Hydroxyprogesterone caproate (see also Progestins)	21, 399 (1979) (corr. 42, 259)
8-Hydroxyquinoline	13, 101 (1977); Suppl. 7, 64 (1987)
8-Hydroxysenkirkine	10, 265 (1976); Suppl. 7, 64 (1987)
Hypochlorite salts	52, 159 (1991)

I

Indeno[1,2,3-cd]pyrene	3, 229 (1973); 32, 373 (1983); Suppl. 7, 64 (1987)
Inorganic acids (see Sulfuric acid and other strong inorganic acids, occupational exposures to mists and vapours from)	
Insecticides, occupational exposures in spraying and application of	53, 45 (1991)
IQ	40, 261 (1986); Suppl. 7, 64 (1987); 56, 165 (1993)
Iron and steel founding	34, 133 (1984); Suppl. 7, 224 (1987)
Iron-dextran complex	2, 161 (1973); Suppl. 7, 226 (1987)
Iron-dextrin complex	2, 161 (1973) (corr. 42, 252); Suppl. 7, 64 (1987)
Iron oxide (see Ferric oxide)	
Iron oxide, saccharated (see Saccharated iron oxide)	
Iron sorbitol–citric acid complex	2, 161 (1973); Suppl. 7, 64 (1987)
Isatidine	10, 269 (1976); Suppl. 7, 65 (1987)
Isoflurane (see Anaesthetics, volatile)	
Isoniazid (see Isonicotinic acid hydrazide)	
Isonicotinic acid hydrazide	4, 159 (1974); Suppl. 7, 227 (1987)
Isophosphamide	26, 237 (1981); Suppl. 7, 65 (1987)
Isopropanol	5, 223 (1977); Suppl. 7, 229 (1987)
Isopropanol manufacture (strong-acid process) (see also Isopropyl alcohol; Sulfuric acid and other strong inorganic acids, occupational exposures to mists and vapours from)	Suppl. 7, 229 (1987)
Isopropyl oils	15, 223 (1977); Suppl. 7, 229 (1987)
Isosafrole	1, 169 (1972); 10, 232 (1976); Suppl. 7, 65 (1987)

J

Jacobine	10, 275 (1976); Suppl. 7, 65 (1987)
Jet fuel	45, 203 (1989)
Joinery (see Carpentry and joinery)	

K

Kaempferol	31, 171 (1983); Suppl. 7, 65 (1987)
Kepone (see Chlordecone)	

L

Lasiocarpine	10, 281 (1976); Suppl. 7, 65 (1987)

Lauroyl peroxide	36, 315 (1985); Suppl. 7, 65 (1987)
Lead acetate (see Lead and lead compounds)	
Lead and lead compounds	1, 40 (1972) (corr. 42, 251); 2, 52, 150 (1973); 12, 131 (1976); 23, 40, 208, 209, 325 (1980); Suppl. 7, 230 (1987)
Lead arsenate (see Arsenic and arsenic compounds)	
Lead carbonate (see Lead and lead compounds)	
Lead chloride (see Lead and lead compounds)	
Lead chromate (see Chromium and chromium compounds)	
Lead chromate oxide (see Chromium and chromium compounds)	
Lead naphthenate (see Lead and lead compounds)	
Lead nitrate (see Lead and lead compounds)	
Lead oxide (see Lead and lead compounds)	
Lead phosphate (see Lead and lead compounds)	
Lead subacetate (see Lead and lead compounds)	
Lead tetroxide (see Lead and lead compounds)	
Leather goods manufacture	25, 279 (1981); Suppl. 7, 235 (1987)
Leather industries	25, 199 (1981); Suppl. 7, 232 (1987)
Leather tanning and processing	25, 201 (1981); Suppl. 7, 236 (1987)
Ledate (see also Lead and lead compounds)	12, 131 (1976)
Light Green SF	16, 209 (1978); Suppl. 7, 65 (1987)
d-Limonene	56, 135 (1993)
Lindane (see Hexachlorocyclohexanes)	
The lumber and sawmill industries (including logging)	25, 49 (1981); Suppl. 7, 383 (1987)
Luteoskyrin	10, 163 (1976); Suppl. 7, 65 (1987)
Lynoestrenol (see also Progestins; Combined oral contraceptives)	21, 407 (1979)

M

Magenta	4, 57 (1974) (corr. 42, 252); Suppl. 7, 238 (1987); 57, 215 (1993)
Magenta, manufacture of (see also Magenta)	Suppl. 7, 238 (1987)
Malathion	30, 103 (1983); Suppl. 7, 65 (1987)
Maleic hydrazide	4, 173 (1974) (corr. 42, 253); Suppl. 7, 65 (1987)
Malonaldehyde	36, 163 (1985); Suppl. 7, 65 (1987)
Maneb	12, 137 (1976); Suppl. 7, 65 (1987)
Man-made mineral fibres	43, 39 (1988)
Mannomustine	9, 157 (1975); Suppl. 7, 65 (1987)
Mate	51, 273 (1991)
MCPA (see also Chlorophenoxy herbicides; Chlorophenoxy herbicides, occupational exposures to)	30, 255 (1983)
MeA-α-C	40, 253 (1986); Suppl. 7, 65 (1987)
Medphalan	9, 168 (1975); Suppl. 7, 65 (1987)
Medroxyprogesterone acetate	6, 157 (1974); 21, 417 (1979) (corr. 42, 259); Suppl. 7, 289 (1987)
Megestrol acetate (see also Progestins; Combined oral contraceptives)	
MeIQ	40, 275 (1986); Suppl. 7, 65 (1987); 56, 197 (1993)

MeIQx   *40*, 283 (1986); *Suppl. 7*, 65 (1987); *56*, 211 (1993)

Melamine   *39*, 333 (1986); *Suppl. 7*, 65 (1987)
Melphalan   *9*, 167 (1975); *Suppl. 7*, 239 (1987)
6-Mercaptopurine   *26*, 249 (1981); *Suppl. 7*, 240 (1987)
Mercuric chloride (*see* Mercury and mercury compounds)
Mercury and mercury compounds   *58*, 239 (1993)
Merphalan   *9*, 169 (1975); *Suppl. 7*, 65 (1987)
Mestranol (*see also* Steroidal oestrogens)   *6*, 87 (1974); *21*, 257 (1979) (*corr. 42*, 259)

Metabisulfites (*see* Sulfur dioxide and some sulfites, bisulfites and metabisulfites)
Metallic mercury (*see* Mercury and mercury compounds)
Methanearsonic acid, disodium salt (*see* Arsenic and arsenic compounds)
Methanearsonic acid, monosodium salt (*see* Arsenic and arsenic compounds
Methotrexate   *26*, 267 (1981); *Suppl. 7*, 241 (1987)
Methoxsalen (*see* 8-Methoxypsoralen)
Methoxychlor   *5*, 193 (1974); *20*, 259 (1979); *Suppl. 7*, 66 (1987)

Methoxyflurane (*see* Anaesthetics, volatile)
5-Methoxypsoralen   *40*, 327 (1986); *Suppl. 7*, 242 (1987)
8-Methoxypsoralen (*see also* 8-Methoxypsoralen plus ultraviolet radiation)   *24*, 101 (1980)
8-Methoxypsoralen plus ultraviolet radiation   *Suppl. 7*, 243 (1987)
Methyl acrylate   *19*, 52 (1979); *39*, 99 (1986); *Suppl. 7*, 66 (1987)

5-Methylangelicin plus ultraviolet radiation (*see also* Angelicin and some synthetic derivatives)   *Suppl. 7*, 57 (1987)
2-Methylaziridine   *9*, 61 (1975); *Suppl. 7*, 66 (1987)
Methylazoxymethanol acetate   *1*, 164 (1972); *10*, 131 (1976); *Suppl. 7*, 66 (1987)
Methyl bromide   *41*, 187 (1986) (*corr. 45*, 283); *Suppl. 7*, 245 (1987)

Methyl carbamate   *12*, 151 (1976); *Suppl. 7*, 66 (1987)
Methyl-CCNU [*see* 1-(2-Chloroethyl)-3-(4-methylcyclohexyl)-1-nitrosourea]
Methyl chloride   *41*, 161 (1986); *Suppl. 7*, 246 (1987)
1-, 2-, 3-, 4-, 5- and 6-Methylchrysenes   *32*, 379 (1983); *Suppl. 7*, 66 (1987)
N-Methyl-*N*,4-dinitrosoaniline   *1*, 141 (1972); *Suppl. 7*, 66 (1987)
4,4'-Methylene bis(2-chloroaniline)   *4*, 65 (1974) (*corr. 42*, 252); *Suppl. 7*, 246 (1987); *57*, 271 (1993)

4,4'-Methylene bis(*N*,*N*-dimethyl)benzenamine   *27*, 119 (1982); *Suppl. 7*, 66 (1987)
4,4'-Methylene bis(2-methylaniline)   *4*, 73 (1974); *Suppl. 7*, 248 (1987)
4,4'-Methylenedianiline   *4*, 79 (1974) (*corr. 42*, 252); *39*, 347 (1986); *Suppl. 7*, 66 (1987)

4,4'-Methylenediphenyl diisocyanate   *19*, 314 (1979); *Suppl. 7*, 66 (1987)
2-Methylfluoranthene   *32*, 399 (1983); *Suppl. 7*, 66 (1987)
3-Methylfluoranthene   *32*, 399 (1983); *Suppl. 7*, 66 (1987)
Methylglyoxal   *51*, 443 (1991)

Methyl iodide	*15*, 245 (1977); *41*, 213 (1986); Suppl. 7, 66 (1987)
Methylmercury chloride (*see* Mercury and mercury compounds)	
Methylmercury compounds (*see* Mercury and mercury compounds)	
Methyl methacrylate	*19*, 187 (1979); Suppl. 7, 66 (1987)
Methyl methanesulfonate	*7*, 253 (1974); Suppl. 7, 66 (1987)
2-Methyl-1-nitroanthraquinone	*27*, 205 (1982); Suppl. 7, 66 (1987)
N-Methyl-*N*'-nitro-*N*-nitrosoguanidine	*4*, 183 (1974); Suppl. 7, 248 (1987)
3-Methylnitrosaminopropionaldehyde [*see* 3-(*N*-Nitrosomethylamino)-propionaldehyde]	
3-Methylnitrosaminopropionitrile [*see* 3-(*N*-Nitrosomethylamino)-propionitrile]	
4-(Methylnitrosamino)-4-(3-pyridyl)-1-butanal [*see* 4-(*N*-Nitrosomethylamino)-4-(3-pyridyl)-1-butanal]	
4-(Methylnitrosamino)-1-(3-pyridyl)-1-butanone [*see* 4-(*N*-Nitrosomethylamino)-1-(3-pyridyl)-1-butanone]	
N-Methyl-*N*-nitrosourea	*1*, 125 (1972); *17*, 227 (1978); Suppl. 7, 66 (1987)
N-Methyl-*N*-nitrosourethane	*4*, 211 (1974); Suppl. 7, 66 (1987)
Methyl parathion	*30*, 131 (1983); Suppl. 7, 392 (1987)
1-Methylphenanthrene	*32*, 405 (1983); Suppl. 7, 66 (1987)
7-Methylpyrido[3,4-*c*]psoralen	*40*, 349 (1986); Suppl. 7, 71 (1987)
Methyl red	*8*, 161 (1975); Suppl. 7, 66 (1987)
Methyl selenac (*see also* Selenium and selenium compounds)	*12*, 161 (1976); Suppl. 7, 66 (1987)
Methylthiouracil	*7*, 53 (1974); Suppl. 7, 66 (1987)
Metronidazole	*13*, 113 (1977); Suppl. 7, 250 (1987)
Mineral oils	*3*, 30 (1973); *33*, 87 (1984) (*corr. 42*, 262); Suppl. 7, 252 (1987)
Mirex	*5*, 203 (1974); *20*, 283 (1979) (*corr. 42*, 258); Suppl. 7, 66 (1987)
Mitomycin C	*10*, 171 (1976); Suppl. 7, 67 (1987)
MNNG [*see N*-Methyl-*N*'-nitro-*N*-nitrosoguanidine]	
MOCA [*see* 4,4'-Methylene bis(2-chloroaniline)]	
Modacrylic fibres	*19*, 86 (1979); Suppl. 7, 67 (1987)
Monocrotaline	*10*, 291 (1976); Suppl. 7, 67 (1987)
Monuron	*12*, 167 (1976); Suppl. 7, 67 (1987); *53*, 467 (1991)
MOPP and other combined chemotherapy including alkylating agents	Suppl. 7, 254 (1987)
Morpholine	*47*, 199 (1989)
5-(Morpholinomethyl)-3-[(5-nitrofurfurylidene)amino]-2-oxazolidinone	*7*, 161 (1974); Suppl. 7, 67 (1987)
Mustard gas	*9*, 181 (1975) (*corr. 42*, 254); Suppl. 7, 259 (1987)
Myleran (*see* 1,4-Butanediol dimethanesulfonate)	

N

Nafenopin	*24*, 125 (1980); Suppl. 7, 67 (1987)
1,5-Naphthalenediamine	*27*, 127 (1982); Suppl. 7, 67 (1987)
1,5-Naphthalene diisocyanate	*19*, 311 (1979); Suppl. 7, 67 (1987)

1-Naphthylamine　　　　　　　　　　　　　　　　　　4, 87 (1974) (corr. 42, 253);
　　　　　　　　　　　　　　　　　　　　　　　　　　Suppl. 7, 260 (1987)
2-Naphthylamine　　　　　　　　　　　　　　　　　　4, 97 (1974); Suppl. 7, 261 (1987)
1-Naphthylthiourea　　　　　　　　　　　　　　　　　30, 347 (1983); Suppl. 7, 263 (1987)
Nickel acetate (see Nickel and nickel compounds)
Nickel ammonium sulfate (see Nickel and nickel compounds)
Nickel and nickel compounds　　　　　　　　　　　　2, 126 (1973) (corr. 42, 252); 11, 75
　　　　　　　　　　　　　　　　　　　　　　　　　　(1976); Suppl. 7, 264 (1987)
　　　　　　　　　　　　　　　　　　　　　　　　　　(corr. 45, 283); 49, 257 (1990)
Nickel carbonate (see Nickel and nickel compounds)
Nickel carbonyl (see Nickel and nickel compounds)
Nickel chloride (see Nickel and nickel compounds)
Nickel-gallium alloy (see Nickel and nickel compounds)
Nickel hydroxide (see Nickel and nickel compounds)
Nickelocene (see Nickel and nickel compounds)
Nickel oxide (see Nickel and nickel compounds)
Nickel subsulfide (see Nickel and nickel compounds)
Nickel sulfate (see Nickel and nickel compounds)
Niridazole　　　　　　　　　　　　　　　　　　　　　13, 123 (1977); Suppl. 7, 67 (1987)
Nithiazide　　　　　　　　　　　　　　　　　　　　　31, 179 (1983); Suppl. 7, 67 (1987)
Nitrilotriacetic acid and its salts　　　　　　　　　　　48, 181 (1990)
5-Nitroacenaphthene　　　　　　　　　　　　　　　　16, 319 (1978); Suppl. 7, 67 (1987)
5-Nitro-ortho-anisidine　　　　　　　　　　　　　　　27, 133 (1982); Suppl. 7, 67 (1987)
9-Nitroanthracene　　　　　　　　　　　　　　　　　33, 179 (1984); Suppl. 7, 67 (1987)
7-Nitrobenz[a]anthracene　　　　　　　　　　　　　　46, 247 (1989)
6-Nitrobenzo[a]pyrene　　　　　　　　　　　　　　　33, 187 (1984); Suppl. 7, 67 (1987);
　　　　　　　　　　　　　　　　　　　　　　　　　　46, 255 (1989)
4-Nitrobiphenyl　　　　　　　　　　　　　　　　　　　4, 113 (1974); Suppl. 7, 67 (1987)
6-Nitrochrysene　　　　　　　　　　　　　　　　　　33, 195 (1984); Suppl. 7, 67 (1987);
　　　　　　　　　　　　　　　　　　　　　　　　　　46, 267 (1989)
Nitrofen (technical-grade)　　　　　　　　　　　　　　30, 271 (1983); Suppl. 7, 67 (1987)
3-Nitrofluoranthene　　　　　　　　　　　　　　　　　33, 201 (1984); Suppl. 7, 67 (1987)
2-Nitrofluorene　　　　　　　　　　　　　　　　　　　46, 277 (1989)
Nitrofural　　　　　　　　　　　　　　　　　　　　　7, 171 (1974); Suppl. 7, 67 (1987);
　　　　　　　　　　　　　　　　　　　　　　　　　　50, 195 (1990)
5-Nitro-2-furaldehyde semicarbazone (see Nitrofural)
Nitrofurantoin　　　　　　　　　　　　　　　　　　　50, 211 (1990)
Nitrofurazone (see Nitrofural)
1-[(5-Nitrofurfurylidene)amino]-2-imidazolidinone　　7, 181 (1974); Suppl. 7, 67 (1987)
N-[4-(5-Nitro-2-furyl)-2-thiazolyl]acetamide　　　　　1, 181 (1972); 7, 185 (1974);
　　　　　　　　　　　　　　　　　　　　　　　　　　Suppl. 7, 67 (1987)
Nitrogen mustard　　　　　　　　　　　　　　　　　　9, 193 (1975); Suppl. 7, 269 (1987)
Nitrogen mustard N-oxide　　　　　　　　　　　　　　9, 209 (1975); Suppl. 7, 67 (1987)
1-Nitronaphthalene　　　　　　　　　　　　　　　　　46, 291 (1989)
2-Nitronaphthalene　　　　　　　　　　　　　　　　　46, 303 (1989)
3-Nitroperylene　　　　　　　　　　　　　　　　　　　46, 313 (1989)
2-Nitro-para-phenylenediamine (see 1,4-Diamino-2-nitrobenzene)
2-Nitropropane　　　　　　　　　　　　　　　　　　　29, 331 (1982); Suppl. 7, 67 (1987)
1-Nitropyrene　　　　　　　　　　　　　　　　　　　　33, 209 (1984); Suppl. 7, 67 (1987);
　　　　　　　　　　　　　　　　　　　　　　　　　　46, 321 (1989)
2-Nitropyrene　　　　　　　　　　　　　　　　　　　　46, 359 (1989)
4-Nitropyrene　　　　　　　　　　　　　　　　　　　　46, 367 (1989)

N-Nitrosatable drugs	24, 297 (1980) (corr. 42, 260)
N-Nitrosatable pesticides	30, 359 (1983)
N'-Nitrosoanabasine	37, 225 (1985); Suppl. 7, 67 (1987)
N'-Nitrosoanatabine	37, 233 (1985); Suppl. 7, 67 (1987)
N-Nitrosodi-n-butylamine	4, 197 (1974); 17, 51 (1978); Suppl. 7, 67 (1987)
N-Nitrosodiethanolamine	17, 77 (1978); Suppl. 7, 67 (1987)
N-Nitrosodiethylamine	1, 107 (1972) (corr. 42, 251); 17, 83 (1978) (corr. 42, 257); Suppl. 7, 67 (1987)
N-Nitrosodimethylamine	1, 95 (1972); 17, 125 (1978) (corr. 42, 257); Suppl. 7, 67 (1987)
N-Nitrosodiphenylamine	27, 213 (1982); Suppl. 7, 67 (1987)
para-Nitrosodiphenylamine	27, 227 (1982) (corr. 42, 261); Suppl. 7, 68 (1987)
N-Nitrosodi-n-propylamine	17, 177 (1978); Suppl. 7, 68 (1987)
N-Nitroso-N-ethylurea (see N-Ethyl-N-nitrosourea)	
N-Nitrosofolic acid	17, 217 (1978); Suppl. 7, 68 (1987)
N-Nitrosoguvacine	37, 263 (1985); Suppl. 7, 68 (1987)
N-Nitrosoguvacoline	37, 263 (1985); Suppl. 7, 68 (1987)
N-Nitrosohydroxyproline	17, 304 (1978); Suppl. 7, 68 (1987)
3-(N-Nitrosomethylamino)propionaldehyde	37, 263 (1985); Suppl. 7, 68 (1987)
3-(N-Nitrosomethylamino)propionitrile	37, 263 (1985); Suppl. 7, 68 (1987)
4-(N-Nitrosomethylamino)-4-(3-pyridyl)-1-butanal	37, 205 (1985); Suppl. 7, 68 (1987)
4-(N-Nitrosomethylamino)-1-(3-pyridyl)-1-butanone	37, 209 (1985); Suppl. 7, 68 (1987)
N-Nitrosomethylethylamine	17, 221 (1978); Suppl. 7, 68 (1987)
N-Nitroso-N-methylurea (see N-Methyl-N-nitrosourea)	
N-Nitroso-N-methylurethane (see N-Methyl-N-nitrosourethane)	
N-Nitrosomethylvinylamine	17, 257 (1978); Suppl. 7, 68 (1987)
N-Nitrosomorpholine	17, 263 (1978); Suppl. 7, 68 (1987)
N'-Nitrosonornicotine	17, 281 (1978); 37, 241 (1985); Suppl. 7, 68 (1987)
N-Nitrosopiperidine	17, 287 (1978); Suppl. 7, 68 (1987)
N-Nitrosoproline	17, 303 (1978); Suppl. 7, 68 (1987)
N-Nitrosopyrrolidine	17, 313 (1978); Suppl. 7, 68 (1987)
N-Nitrososarcosine	17, 327 (1978); Suppl. 7, 68 (1987)
Nitrosoureas, chloroethyl (see Chloroethyl nitrosoureas)	
5-Nitro-ortho-toluidine	48, 169 (1990)
Nitrous oxide (see Anaesthetics, volatile)	
Nitrovin	31, 185 (1983); Suppl. 7, 68 (1987)
Nivalenol (see Toxins derived from Fusarium graminearum, F. culmorum and F. crookwellense)	
NNA [see 4-(N-Nitrosomethylamino)-4-(3-pyridyl)-1-butanal]	
NNK [see 4-(N-Nitrosomethylamino)-1-(3-pyridyl)-1-butanone]	
Nonsteroidal oestrogens (see also Oestrogens, progestins and combinations)	Suppl. 7, 272 (1987)
Norethisterone (see also Progestins; Combined oral contraceptives)	6, 179 (1974); 21, 461 (1979)
Norethynodrel (see also Progestins; Combined oral contraceptives	6, 191 (1974); 21, 461 (1979) (corr. 42, 259)
Norgestrel (see also Progestins, Combined oral contraceptives)	6, 201 (1974); 21, 479 (1979)
Nylon 6	19, 120 (1979); Suppl. 7, 68 (1987)

O

Ochratoxin A	10, 191 (1976); 31, 191 (1983) (corr. 42, 262); Suppl. 7, 271 (1987); 56, 489 (1993)
Oestradiol-17β (see also Steroidal oestrogens)	6, 99 (1974); 21, 279 (1979)
Oestradiol 3-benzoate (see Oestradiol-17β)	
Oestradiol dipropionate (see Oestradiol-17β)	
Oestradiol mustard	9, 217 (1975)
Oestradiol-17β-valerate (see Oestradiol-17β)	
Oestriol (see also Steroidal oestrogens)	6, 117 (1974); 21, 327 (1979)
Oestrogen–progestin combinations (see Oestrogens, progestins and combinations)	
Oestrogen–progestin replacement therapy (see also Oestrogens, progestins and combinations)	Suppl. 7, 308 (1987)
Oestrogen replacement therapy (see also Oestrogens, progestins and combinations)	Suppl. 7, 280 (1987)
Oestrogens (see Oestrogens, progestins and combinations)	
Oestrogens, conjugated (see Conjugated oestrogens)	
Oestrogens, nonsteroidal (see Nonsteroidal oestrogens)	
Oestrogens, progestins and combinations	6 (1974); 21 (1979); Suppl. 7, 272 (1987)
Oestrogens, steroidal (see Steroidal oestrogens)	
Oestrone (see also Steroidal oestrogens)	6, 123 (1974); 21, 343 (1979) (corr. 42, 259)
Oestrone benzoate (see Oestrone)	
Oil Orange SS	8, 165 (1975); Suppl. 7, 69 (1987)
Oral contraceptives, combined (see Combined oral contraceptives)	
Oral contraceptives, investigational (see Combined oral contraceptives)	
Oral contraceptives, sequential (see Sequential oral contraceptives)	
Orange I	8, 173 (1975); Suppl. 7, 69 (1987)
Orange G	8, 181 (1975); Suppl. 7, 69 (1987)
Organolead compounds (see also Lead and lead compounds)	Suppl. 7, 230 (1987)
Oxazepam	13, 58 (1977); Suppl. 7, 69 (1987)
Oxymetholone [see also Androgenic (anabolic) steroids]	13, 131 (1977)
Oxyphenbutazone	13, 185 (1977); Suppl. 7, 69 (1987)

P

Paint manufacture and painting (occupational exposures in)	47, 329 (1989)
Panfuran S (see also Dihydroxymethylfuratrizine)	24, 77 (1980); Suppl. 7, 69 (1987)
Paper manufacture (see Pulp and paper manufacture)	
Paracetamol	50, 307 (1990)
Parasorbic acid	10, 199 (1976) (corr. 42, 255); Suppl. 7, 69 (1987)
Parathion	30, 153 (1983); Suppl. 7, 69 (1987)
Patulin	10, 205 (1976); 40, 83 (1986); Suppl. 7, 69 (1987)
Penicillic acid	10, 211 (1976); Suppl. 7, 69 (1987)
Pentachloroethane	41, 99 (1986); Suppl. 7, 69 (1987)
Pentachloronitrobenzene (see Quintozene)	

Pentachlorophenol (see also Chlorophenols; Chlorophenols, occupational exposures to)	20, 303 (1979); 53, 371 (1991)
Permethrin	53, 329 (1991)
Perylene	32, 411 (1983); Suppl. 7, 69 (1987)
Petasitenine	31, 207 (1983); Suppl. 7, 69 (1987)
Petasites japonicus (see Pyrrolizidine alkaloids)	
Petroleum refining (occupational exposures in)	45, 39 (1989)
Some petroleum solvents	47, 43 (1989)
Phenacetin	13, 141 (1977); 24, 135 (1980); Suppl. 7, 310 (1987)
Phenanthrene	32, 419 (1983); Suppl. 7, 69 (1987)
Phenazopyridine hydrochloride	8, 117 (1975); 24, 163 (1980) (corr. 42, 260); Suppl. 7, 312 (1987)
Phenelzine sulfate	24, 175 (1980); Suppl. 7, 312 (1987)
Phenicarbazide	12, 177 (1976); Suppl. 7, 70 (1987)
Phenobarbital	13, 157 (1977); Suppl. 7, 313 (1987)
Phenol	47, 263 (1989) (corr. 50, 385)
Phenoxyacetic acid herbicides (see Chlorophenoxy herbicides)	
Phenoxybenzamine hydrochloride	9, 223 (1975); 24, 185 (1980); Suppl. 7, 70 (1987)
Phenylbutazone	13, 183 (1977); Suppl. 7, 316 (1987)
meta-Phenylenediamine	16, 111 (1978); Suppl. 7, 70 (1987)
para-Phenylenediamine	16, 125 (1978); Suppl. 7, 70 (1987)
Phenyl glycidyl ether (see Glycidyl ethers)	
N-Phenyl-2-naphthylamine	16, 325 (1978) (corr. 42, 257); Suppl. 7, 318 (1987)
ortho-Phenylphenol	30, 329 (1983); Suppl. 7, 70 (1987)
Phenytoin	13, 201 (1977); Suppl. 7, 319 (1987)
PhIP	56, 229 (1993)
Pickled vegetables	56, 83 (1993)
Picloram	53, 481 (1991)
Piperazine oestrone sulfate (see Conjugated oestrogens)	
Piperonyl butoxide	30, 183 (1983); Suppl. 7, 70 (1987)
Pitches, coal-tar (see Coal-tar pitches)	
Polyacrylic acid	19, 62 (1979); Suppl. 7, 70 (1987)
Polybrominated biphenyls	18, 107 (1978); 41, 261 (1986); Suppl. 7, 321 (1987)
Polychlorinated biphenyls	7, 261 (1974); 18, 43 (1978) (corr. 42, 258); Suppl. 7, 322 (1987)
Polychlorinated camphenes (see Toxaphene)	
Polychloroprene	19, 141 (1979); Suppl. 7, 70 (1987)
Polyethylene	19, 164 (1979); Suppl. 7, 70 (1987)
Polymethylene polyphenyl isocyanate	19, 314 (1979); Suppl. 7, 70 (1987)
Polymethyl methacrylate	19, 195 (1979); Suppl. 7, 70 (1987)
Polyoestradiol phosphate (see Oestradiol-17β)	
Polypropylene	19, 218 (1979); Suppl. 7, 70 (1987)
Polystyrene	19, 245 (1979); Suppl. 7, 70 (1987)
Polytetrafluoroethylene	19, 288 (1979); Suppl. 7, 70 (1987)
Polyurethane foams	19, 320 (1979); Suppl. 7, 70 (1987)
Polyvinyl acetate	19, 346 (1979); Suppl. 7, 70 (1987)
Polyvinyl alcohol	19, 351 (1979); Suppl. 7, 70 (1987)

Polyvinyl chloride	7, 306 (1974); 19, 402 (1979); Suppl. 7, 70 (1987)
Polyvinyl pyrrolidone	19, 463 (1979); Suppl. 7, 70 (1987)
Ponceau MX	8, 189 (1975); Suppl. 7, 70 (1987)
Ponceau 3R	8, 199 (1975); Suppl. 7, 70 (1987)
Ponceau SX	8, 207 (1975); Suppl. 7, 70 (1987)
Potassium arsenate (see Arsenic and arsenic compounds)	
Potassium arsenite (see Arsenic and arsenic compounds)	
Potassium bis(2-hydroxyethyl)dithiocarbamate	12, 183 (1976); Suppl. 7, 70 (1987)
Potassium bromate	40, 207 (1986); Suppl. 7, 70 (1987)
Potassium chromate (see Chromium and chromium compounds)	
Potassium dichromate (see Chromium and chromium compounds)	
Prednimustine	50, 115 (1990)
Prednisone	26, 293 (1981); Suppl. 7, 326 (1987)
Procarbazine hydrochloride	26, 311 (1981); Suppl. 7, 327 (1987)
Proflavine salts	24, 195 (1980); Suppl. 7, 70 (1987)
Progesterone (see also Progestins; Combined oral contraceptives)	6, 135 (1974); 21, 491 (1979) (corr. 42, 259)
Progestins (see also Oestrogens, progestins and combinations)	Suppl. 7, 289 (1987)
Pronetalol hydrochloride	13, 227 (1977) (corr. 42, 256); Suppl. 7, 70 (1987)
1,3-Propane sultone	4, 253 (1974) (corr. 42, 253); Suppl. 7, 70 (1987)
Propham	12, 189 (1976); Suppl. 7, 70 (1987)
β-Propiolactone	4, 259 (1974) (corr. 42, 253); Suppl. 7, 70 (1987)
n-Propyl carbamate	12, 201 (1976); Suppl. 7, 70 (1987)
Propylene	19, 213 (1979); Suppl. 7, 71 (1987)
Propylene oxide	11, 191 (1976); 36, 227 (1985) (corr. 42, 263); Suppl. 7, 328 (1987)
Propylthiouracil	7, 67 (1974); Suppl. 7, 329 (1987)
Ptaquiloside (see also Bracken fern)	40, 55 (1986); Suppl. 7, 71 (1987)
Pulp and paper manufacture	25, 157 (1981); Suppl. 7, 385 (1987)
Pyrene	32, 431 (1983); Suppl. 7, 71 (1987)
Pyrido[3,4-c]psoralen	40, 349 (1986); Suppl. 7, 71 (1987)
Pyrimethamine	13, 233 (1977); Suppl. 7, 71 (1987)
Pyrrolizidine alkaloids (see Hydroxysenkirkine; Isatidine; Jacobine; Lasiocarpine; Monocrotaline; Retrorsine; Riddelliine; Seneciphylline; Senkirkine)	

Q

Quercetin (see also Bracken fern)	31, 213 (1983); Suppl. 7, 71 (1987)
para-Quinone	15, 255 (1977); Suppl. 7, 71 (1987)
Quintozene	5, 211 (1974); Suppl. 7, 71 (1987)

R

Radon	43, 173 (1988) (corr. 45, 283)
Reserpine	10, 217 (1976); 24, 211 (1980) (corr. 42, 260); Suppl. 7, 330 (1987)
Resorcinol	15, 155 (1977); Suppl. 7, 71 (1987)

Retrorsine	*10*, 303 (1976); *Suppl. 7*, 71 (1987)
Rhodamine B	*16*, 221 (1978); *Suppl. 7*, 71 (1987)
Rhodamine 6G	*16*, 233 (1978); *Suppl. 7*, 71 (1987)
Riddelliine	*10*, 313 (1976); *Suppl. 7*, 71 (1987)
Rifampicin	*24*, 243 (1980); *Suppl. 7*, 71 (1987)
Rockwool (*see* Man-made mineral fibres)	
The rubber industry	*28* (1982) (*corr. 42*, 261); *Suppl. 7*, 332 (1987)
Rugulosin	*40*, 99 (1986); *Suppl. 7*, 71 (1987)

S

Saccharated iron oxide	*2*, 161 (1973); *Suppl. 7*, 71 (1987)
Saccharin	*22*, 111 (1980) (*corr. 42*, 259); *Suppl. 7*, 334 (1987)
Safrole	*1*, 169 (1972); *10*, 231 (1976); *Suppl. 7*, 71 (1987)
Salted fish	*56*, 41 (1993)
The sawmill industry (including logging) [*see* The lumber and sawmill industry (including logging)]	
Scarlet Red	*8*, 217 (1975); *Suppl. 7*, 71 (1987)
Selenium and selenium compounds	*9*, 245 (1975) (*corr. 42*, 255); *Suppl. 7*, 71 (1987)
Selenium dioxide (*see* Selenium and selenium compounds)	
Selenium oxide (*see* Selenium and selenium compounds)	
Semicarbazide hydrochloride	*12*, 209 (1976) (*corr. 42*, 256); *Suppl. 7*, 71 (1987)
Senecio jacobaea L. (*see* Pyrrolizidine alkaloids)	
Senecio longilobus (*see* Pyrrolizidine alkaloids)	
Seneciphylline	*10*, 319, 335 (1976); *Suppl. 7*, 71 (1987)
Senkirkine	*10*, 327 (1976); *31*, 231 (1983); *Suppl. 7*, 71 (1987)
Sepiolite	*42*, 175 (1987); *Suppl. 7*, 71 (1987)
Sequential oral contraceptives (*see also* Oestrogens, progestins and combinations)	*Suppl. 7*, 296 (1987)
Shale-oils	*35*, 161 (1985); *Suppl. 7*, 339 (1987)
Shikimic acid (*see also* Bracken fern)	*40*, 55 (1986); *Suppl. 7*, 71 (1987)
Shoe manufacture and repair (*see* Boot and shoe manufacture and repair)	
Silica (*see also* Amorphous silica; Crystalline silica)	*42*, 39 (1987)
Simazine	*53*, 495 (1991)
Slagwool (*see* Man-made mineral fibres)	
Sodium arsenate (*see* Arsenic and arsenic compounds)	
Sodium arsenite (*see* Arsenic and arsenic compounds)	
Sodium cacodylate (*see* Arsenic and arsenic compounds)	
Sodium chlorite	*52*, 145 (1991)
Sodium chromate (*see* Chromium and chromium compounds)	
Sodium cyclamate (*see* Cyclamates)	
Sodium dichromate (*see* Chromium and chromium compounds)	
Sodium diethyldithiocarbamate	*12*, 217 (1976); *Suppl. 7*, 71 (1987)
Sodium equilin sulfate (*see* Conjugated oestrogens)	

Sodium fluoride (see Fluorides)
Sodium monofluorophosphate (see Fluorides)
Sodium oestrone sulfate (see Conjugated oestrogens)
Sodium ortho-phenylphenate (see also ortho-Phenylphenol)   30, 329 (1983); Suppl. 7, 392 (1987)
Sodium saccharin (see Saccharin)
Sodium selenate (see Selenium and selenium compounds)
Sodium selenite (see Selenium and selenium compounds)
Sodium silicofluoride (see Fluorides)
Solar radiation   55 (1992)
Soots   3, 22 (1973); 35, 219 (1985); Suppl. 7, 343 (1987)

Spironolactone   24, 259 (1980); Suppl. 7, 344 (1987)
Stannous fluoride (see Fluorides)
Steel founding (see Iron and steel founding)
Sterigmatocystin   1, 175 (1972); 10, 245 (1976); Suppl. 7, 72 (1987)

Steroidal oestrogens (see also Oestrogens, progestins and   Suppl. 7, 280 (1987)
   combinations)
Streptozotocin   4, 221 (1974); 17, 337 (1978); Suppl. 7, 72 (1987)

Strobane® (see Terpene polychlorinates)
Strontium chromate (see Chromium and chromium compounds)
Styrene   19, 231 (1979) (corr. 42, 258); Suppl. 7, 345 (1987)

Styrene-acrylonitrile copolymers   19, 97 (1979); Suppl. 7, 72 (1987)
Styrene-butadiene copolymers   19, 252 (1979); Suppl. 7, 72 (1987)
Styrene oxide   11, 201 (1976); 19, 275 (1979); 36, 245 (1985); Suppl. 7, 72 (1987)

Succinic anhydride   15, 265 (1977); Suppl. 7, 72 (1987)
Sudan I   8, 225 (1975); Suppl. 7, 72 (1987)
Sudan II   8, 233 (1975); Suppl. 7, 72 (1987)
Sudan III   8, 241 (1975); Suppl. 7, 72 (1987)
Sudan Brown RR   8, 249 (1975); Suppl. 7, 72 (1987)
Sudan Red 7B   8, 253 (1975); Suppl. 7, 72 (1987)
Sulfafurazole   24, 275 (1980); Suppl. 7, 347 (1987)
Sulfallate   30, 283 (1983); Suppl. 7, 72 (1987)
Sulfamethoxazole   24, 285 (1980); Suppl. 7, 348 (1987)
Sulfites (see Sulfur dioxide and some sulfites, bisulfites and metabisulfites)
Sulfur dioxide and some sulfites, bisulfites and metabisulfites   54, 131 (1992)
Sulfur mustard (see Mustard gas)
Sulfuric acid and other strong inorganic acids, occupational exposures 54, 41 (1992)
   to mists and vapours from
Sulfur trioxide   54, 121 (1992)
Sulphisoxazole (see Sulfafurazole)
Sunset Yellow FCF   8, 257 (1975); Suppl. 7, 72 (1987)
Symphytine   31, 239 (1983); Suppl. 7, 72 (1987)

T

2,4,5-T (see also Chlorophenoxy herbicides; Chlorophenoxy   15, 273 (1977)
   herbicides, occupational exposures to)
Talc   42, 185 (1987); Suppl. 7, 349 (1987)

Tannic acid	10, 253 (1976) (corr. 42, 255); Suppl. 7, 72 (1987)
Tannins (see also Tannic acid)	10, 254 (1976); Suppl. 7, 72 (1987)
TCDD (see 2,3,7,8-Tetrachlorodibenzo-*para*-dioxin)	
TDE (see DDT)	
Tea	51, 207 (1991)
Terpene polychlorinates	5, 219 (1974); Suppl. 7, 72 (1987)
Testosterone (see also Androgenic (anabolic) steroids)	6, 209 (1974); 21, 519 (1979)
Testosterone oenanthate (see Testosterone)	
Testosterone propionate (see Testosterone)	
2,2′,5,5′-Tetrachlorobenzidine	27, 141 (1982); Suppl. 7, 72 (1987)
2,3,7,8-Tetrachlorodibenzo-*para*-dioxin	15, 41 (1977); Suppl. 7, 350 (1987)
1,1,1,2-Tetrachloroethane	41, 87 (1986); Suppl. 7, 72 (1987)
1,1,2,2-Tetrachloroethane	20, 477 (1979); Suppl. 7, 354 (1987)
Tetrachloroethylene	20, 491 (1979); Suppl. 7, 355 (1987)
2,3,4,6-Tetrachlorophenol (see Chlorophenols; Chlorophenols, occupational exposures to)	
Tetrachlorvinphos	30, 197 (1983); Suppl. 7, 72 (1987)
Tetraethyllead (see Lead and lead compounds)	
Tetrafluoroethylene	19, 285 (1979); Suppl. 7, 72 (1987)
Tetrakis(hydroxymethyl) phosphonium salts	48, 95 (1990)
Tetramethyllead (see Lead and lead compounds)	
Textile manufacturing industry, exposures in	48, 215 (1990) (corr. 51, 483)
Theobromine	51, 421 (1991)
Theophylline	51, 391 (1991)
Thioacetamide	7, 77 (1974); Suppl. 7, 72 (1987)
4,4′-Thiodianiline	16, 343 (1978); 27, 147 (1982); Suppl. 7, 72 (1987)
Thiotepa	9, 85 (1975); Suppl. 7, 368 (1987); 50, 123 (1990)
Thiouracil	7, 85 (1974); Suppl. 7, 72 (1987)
Thiourea	7, 95 (1974); Suppl. 7, 72 (1987)
Thiram	12, 225 (1976); Suppl. 7, 72 (1987); 53, 403 (1991)
Titanium dioxide	47, 307 (1989)
Tobacco habits other than smoking (see Tobacco products, smokeless)	
Tobacco products, smokeless	37 (1985) (corr. 42, 263; 52, 513); Suppl. 7, 357 (1987)
Tobacco smoke	38 (1986) (corr. 42, 263); Suppl. 7, 357 (1987)
Tobacco smoking (see Tobacco smoke)	
ortho-Tolidine (see 3,3′-Dimethylbenzidine)	
2,4-Toluene diisocyanate (see also Toluene diisocyanates)	19, 303 (1979); 39, 287 (1986)
2,6-Toluene diisocyanate (see also Toluene diisocyanates)	19, 303 (1979); 39, 289 (1986)
Toluene	47, 79 (1989)
Toluene diisocyanates	39, 287 (1986) (corr. 42, 264); Suppl. 7, 72 (1987)
Toluenes, α-chlorinated (see α-Chlorinated toluenes)	
ortho-Toluenesulfonamide (see Saccharin)	
ortho-Toluidine	16, 349 (1978); 27, 155 (1982); Suppl. 7, 362 (1987)

Toxaphene 20, 327 (1979); *Suppl. 7*, 72 (1987)
T-2 Toxin (*see* Toxins derived from *Fusarium sporotrichioides*)
Toxins derived from *Fusarium graminearum*, *F. culmorum* and 11, 169 (1976); 31, 153, 279 (1983);
  F. crookwellense *Suppl. 7*, 64, 74 (1987); 56, 397 (1993)
Toxins derived from *Fusarium moniliforme* 56, 445 (1993)
Toxins derived from *Fusarium sporotrichioides* 31, 265 (1983); *Suppl. 7*, 73 (1987);
  56, 467 (1993)

Tremolite (*see* Asbestos)
Treosulfan 26, 341 (1981); *Suppl. 7*, 363 (1987)
Triaziquone [*see* Tris(aziridinyl)-*para*-benzoquinone]
Trichlorfon 30, 207 (1983); *Suppl. 7*, 73 (1987)
Trichlormethine 9, 229 (1975); *Suppl. 7*, 73 (1987);
  50, 143 (1990)

Trichloroacetonitrile (*see* Halogenated acetonitriles)
1,1,1-Trichloroethane 20, 515 (1979); *Suppl. 7*, 73 (1987)
1,1,2-Trichloroethane 20, 533 (1979); *Suppl. 7*, 73 (1987);
  52, 337 (1991)
Trichloroethylene 11, 263 (1976); 20, 545 (1979);
  Suppl. 7, 364 (1987)
2,4,5-Trichlorophenol (*see also* Chlorophenols; Chlorophenols 20, 349 (1979)
  occupational exposures to)
2,4,6-Trichlorophenol (*see also* Chlorophenols; Chlorophenols, 20, 349 (1979)
  occupational exposures to)
(2,4,5-Trichlorophenoxy)acetic acid (*see* 2,4,5-T)
Trichlorotriethylamine hydrochloride (*see* Trichlormethine)
T₂-Trichothecene (*see* Toxins derived from *Fusarium sporotrichioides*)
Triethylene glycol diglycidyl ether 11, 209 (1976); *Suppl. 7*, 73 (1987)
Trifluralin 53, 515 (1991)
4,4',6-Trimethylangelicin plus ultraviolet radiation (*see also* *Suppl. 7*, 57 (1987)
  Angelicin and some synthetic derivatives)
2,4,5-Trimethylaniline 27, 177 (1982); *Suppl. 7*, 73 (1987)
2,4,6-Trimethylaniline 27, 178 (1982); *Suppl. 7*, 73 (1987)
4,5',8-Trimethylpsoralen 40, 357 (1986); *Suppl. 7*, 366 (1987)
Trimustine hydrochloride (*see* Trichlormethine)
Triphenylene 32, 447 (1983); *Suppl. 7*, 73 (1987)
Tris(aziridinyl)-*para*-benzoquinone 9, 67 (1975); *Suppl. 7*, 367 (1987)
Tris(1-aziridinyl)phosphine oxide 9, 75 (1975); *Suppl. 7*, 73 (1987)
Tris(1-aziridinyl)phosphine sulphide (*see* Thiotepa)
2,4,6-Tris(1-aziridinyl)-*s*-triazine 9, 95 (1975); *Suppl. 7*, 73 (1987)
Tris(2-chloroethyl) phosphate 48, 109 (1990)
1,2,3-Tris(chloromethoxy)propane 15, 301 (1977); *Suppl. 7*, 73 (1987)
Tris(2,3-dibromopropyl)phosphate 20, 575 (1979); *Suppl. 7*, 369 (1987)
Tris(2-methyl-1-aziridinyl)phosphine oxide 9, 107 (1975); *Suppl. 7*, 73 (1987)
Trp-P-1 31, 247 (1983); *Suppl. 7*, 73 (1987)
Trp-P-2 31, 255 (1983); *Suppl. 7*, 73 (1987)
Trypan blue 8, 267 (1975); *Suppl. 7*, 73 (1987)
Tussilago farfara L. (*see* Pyrrolizidine alkaloids)

U

Ultraviolet radiation 40, 379 (1986); 55 (1992)
Underground haematite mining with exposure to radon 1, 29 (1972); *Suppl. 7*, 216 (1987)

Uracil mustard	9, 235 (1975); *Suppl. 7*, 370 (1987)
Urethane	7, 111 (1974); *Suppl. 7*, 73 (1987)

V

Vat Yellow 4	*48*, 161 (1990)
Vinblastine sulfate	*26*, 349 (1981) (*corr. 42*, 261); *Suppl. 7*, 371 (1987)
Vincristine sulfate	*26*, 365 (1981); *Suppl. 7*, 372 (1987)
Vinyl acetate	*19*, 341 (1979); *39*, 113 (1986); *Suppl. 7*, 73 (1987)
Vinyl bromide	*19*, 367 (1979); *39*, 133 (1986); *Suppl. 7*, 73 (1987)
Vinyl chloride	7, 291 (1974); *19*, 377 (1979) (*corr. 42*, 258); *Suppl. 7*, 373 (1987)
Vinyl chloride–vinyl acetate copolymers	7, 311 (1976); *19*, 412 (1979) (*corr. 42*, 258); *Suppl. 7*, 73 (1987)
4-Vinylcyclohexene	*11*, 277 (1976); *39*, 181 (1986); *Suppl. 7*, 73 (1987)
Vinyl fluoride	*39*, 147 (1986); *Suppl. 7*, 73 (1987)
Vinylidene chloride	*19*, 439 (1979); *39*, 195 (1986); *Suppl. 7*, 376 (1987)
Vinylidene chloride–vinyl chloride copolymers	*19*, 448 (1979) (*corr. 42*, 258); *Suppl. 7*, 73 (1987)
Vinylidene fluoride	*39*, 227 (1986); *Suppl. 7*, 73 (1987)
N-Vinyl-2-pyrrolidone	*19*, 461 (1979); *Suppl. 7*, 73 (1987)

W

Welding	*49*, 447 (1990) (*corr. 52*, 513)
Wollastonite	*42*, 145 (1987); *Suppl. 7*, 377 (1987)
Wood industries	*25* (1981); *Suppl. 7*, 378 (1987)

X

Xylene	*47*, 125 (1989)
2,4-Xylidine	*16*, 367 (1978); *Suppl. 7*, 74 (1987)
2,5-Xylidine	*16*, 377 (1978); *Suppl. 7*, 74 (1987)
2,6-Xylidine (*see* 2,6-Dimethylaniline)	

Y

Yellow AB	*8*, 279 (1975); *Suppl. 7*, 74 (1987)
Yellow OB	*8*, 287 (1975); *Suppl. 7*, 74 (1987)

Z

Zearalenone (*see* Toxins derived from *Fusarium graminearum*, *F. culmorum* and *F. crookwellense*)

Zectran	*12*, 237 (1976); *Suppl. 7*, 74 (1987)
Zinc beryllium silicate (*see* Beryllium and beryllium compounds)	

Zinc chromate (*see* Chromium and chromium compounds)
Zinc chromate hydroxide (*see* Chromium and chromium compounds)
Zinc potassium chromate (*see* Chromium and chromium compounds)
Zinc yellow (*see* Chromium and chromium compounds)
Zineb *12*, 245 (1976); *Suppl. 7*, 74 (1987)
Ziram *12*, 259 (1976); *Suppl. 7*, 74 (1987); *53*, 423 (1991)

PUBLICATIONS OF THE INTERNATIONAL AGENCY FOR RESEARCH ON CANCER

Scientific Publications Series

(Available from Oxford University Press through local bookshops)

No. 1 **Liver Cancer**
1971; 176 pages (*out of print*)

No. 2 **Oncogenesis and Herpesviruses**
Edited by P.M. Biggs, G. de-Thé and L.N. Payne
1972; 515 pages (*out of print*)

No. 3 ***N*-Nitroso Compounds: Analysis and Formation**
Edited by P. Bogovski, R. Preussman and E.A. Walker
1972; 140 pages (*out of print*)

No. 4 **Transplacental Carcinogenesis**
Edited by L. Tomatis and U. Mohr
1973; 181 pages (*out of print*)

No. 5/6 **Pathology of Tumours in Laboratory Animals, Volume 1, Tumours of the Rat**
Edited by V.S. Turusov
1973/1976; 533 pages (*out of print*)

No. 7 **Host Environment Interactions in the Etiology of Cancer in Man**
Edited by R. Doll and I. Vodopija
1973; 464 pages (*out of print*)

No. 8 **Biological Effects of Asbestos**
Edited by P. Bogovski, J.C. Gilson, V. Timbrell and J.C. Wagner
1973; 346 pages (*out of print*)

No. 9 ***N*-Nitroso Compounds in the Environment**
Edited by P. Bogovski and E.A. Walker
1974; 243 pages (*out of print*)

No. 10 **Chemical Carcinogenesis Essays**
Edited by R. Montesano and L. Tomatis
1974; 230 pages (*out of print*)

No. 11 **Oncogenesis and Herpesviruses II**
Edited by G. de-Thé, M.A. Epstein and H. zur Hausen
1975; Part I: 511 pages
Part II: 403 pages (*out of print*)

No. 12 **Screening Tests in Chemical Carcinogenesis**
Edited by R. Montesano, H. Bartsch and L. Tomatis
1976; 666 pages (*out of print*)

No. 13 **Environmental Pollution and Carcinogenic Risks**
Edited by C. Rosenfeld and W. Davis
1975; 441 pages (*out of print*)

No. 14 **Environmental *N*-Nitroso Compounds. Analysis and Formation**
Edited by E.A. Walker, P. Bogovski and L. Griciute
1976; 512 pages (*out of print*)

No. 15 **Cancer Incidence in Five Continents, Volume III**
Edited by J.A.H. Waterhouse, C. Muir, P. Correa and J. Powell
1976; 584 pages (*out of print*)

No. 16 **Air Pollution and Cancer in Man**
Edited by U. Mohr, D. Schmähl and L. Tomatis
1977; 328 pages (*out of print*)

No. 17 **Directory of On-going Research in Cancer Epidemiology 1977**
Edited by C.S. Muir and G. Wagner
1977; 599 pages (*out of print*)

No. 18 **Environmental Carcinogens. Selected Methods of Analysis. Volume 1: Analysis of Volatile Nitrosamines in Food**
Editor-in-Chief: H. Egan
1978; 212 pages (*out of print*)

No. 19 **Environmental Aspects of *N*-Nitroso Compounds**
Edited by E.A. Walker, M. Castegnaro, L. Griciute and R.E. Lyle
1978; 561 pages (*out of print*)

No. 20 **Nasopharyngeal Carcinoma: Etiology and Control**
Edited by G. de-Thé and Y. Ito
1978; 606 pages (*out of print*)

No. 21 **Cancer Registration and its Techniques**
Edited by R. MacLennan, C. Muir, R. Steinitz and A. Winkler
1978; 235 pages (*out of print*)

No. 22 **Environmental Carcinogens. Selected Methods of Analysis. Volume 2: Methods for the Measurement of Vinyl Chloride in Poly(vinyl chloride), Air, Water and Foodstuffs**
Editor-in-Chief: H. Egan
1978; 142 pages (*out of print*)

No. 23 **Pathology of Tumours in Laboratory Animals. Volume II: Tumours of the Mouse**
Editor-in-Chief: V.S. Turusov
1979; 669 pages (*out of print*)

No. 24 **Oncogenesis and Herpesviruses III**
Edited by G. de-Thé, W. Henle and F. Rapp
1978; Part I: 580 pages, Part II: 512 pages (*out of print*)

Prices, valid for February 1994 are subject to change without notice

List of IARC Publications

No. 25 Carcinogenic Risk. Strategies for Intervention
Edited by W. Davis and C. Rosenfeld
1979; 280 pages (*out of print*)

No. 26 Directory of On-going Research in Cancer Epidemiology 1978
Edited by C.S. Muir and G. Wagner
1978; 550 pages (*out of print*)

No. 27 Molecular and Cellular Aspects of Carcinogen Screening Tests
Edited by R. Montesano, H. Bartsch and L. Tomatis
1980; 372 pages £30.00

No. 28 Directory of On-going Research in Cancer Epidemiology 1979
Edited by C.S. Muir and G. Wagner
1979; 672 pages (*out of print*)

No. 29 Environmental Carcinogens. Selected Methods of Analysis. Volume 3: Analysis of Polycyclic Aromatic Hydrocarbons in Environmental Samples
Editor-in-Chief: H. Egan
1979; 240 pages (*out of print*)

No. 30 Biological Effects of Mineral Fibres
Editor-in-Chief: J.C. Wagner
1980; **Volume 1:** 494 pages **Volume 2:** 513 pages (*out of print*)

No. 31 N-Nitroso Compounds: Analysis, Formation and Occurrence
Edited by E.A. Walker, L. Griciute, M. Castegnaro and M. Börzsönyi
1980; 835 pages (*out of print*)

No. 32 Statistical Methods in Cancer Research. Volume 1. The Analysis of Case-control Studies
By N.E. Breslow and N.E. Day
1980; 338 pages £18.00

No. 33 Handling Chemical Carcinogens in the Laboratory
Edited by R. Montesano *et al.*
1979; 32 pages (*out of print*)

No. 34 Pathology of Tumours in Laboratory Animals. Volume III. Tumours of the Hamster
Editor-in-Chief: V.S. Turusov
1982; 461 pages (*out of print*)

No. 35 Directory of On-going Research in Cancer Epidemiology 1980
Edited by C.S. Muir and G. Wagner
1980; 660 pages (*out of print*)

No. 36 Cancer Mortality by Occupation and Social Class 1851-1971
Edited by W.P.D. Logan
1982; 253 pages (*out of print*)

No. 37 Laboratory Decontamination and Destruction of Aflatoxins B_1, B_2, G_1, G_2 in Laboratory Wastes
Edited by M. Castegnaro *et al.*
1980; 56 pages (*out of print*)

No. 38 Directory of On-going Research in Cancer Epidemiology 1981
Edited by C.S. Muir and G. Wagner
1981; 696 pages (*out of print*)

No. 39 Host Factors in Human Carcinogenesis
Edited by H. Bartsch and B. Armstrong
1982; 583 pages (*out of print*)

No. 40 Environmental Carcinogens. Selected Methods of Analysis. Volume 4: Some Aromatic Amines and Azo Dyes in the General and Industrial Environment
Edited by L. Fishbein, M. Castegnaro, I.K. O'Neill and H. Bartsch
1981; 347 pages (*out of print*)

No. 41 N-Nitroso Compounds: Occurrence and Biological Effects
Edited by H. Bartsch, I.K. O'Neill, M. Castegnaro and M. Okada
1982; 755 pages £50.00

No. 42 Cancer Incidence in Five Continents, Volume IV
Edited by J. Waterhouse, C. Muir, K. Shanmugaratnam and J. Powell
1982; 811 pages (*out of print*)

No. 43 Laboratory Decontamination and Destruction of Carcinogens in Laboratory Wastes: Some N-Nitrosamines
Edited by M. Castegnaro *et al.*
1982; 73 pages £7.50

No. 44 Environmental Carcinogens. Selected Methods of Analysis. Volume 5: Some Mycotoxins
Edited by L. Stoloff, M. Castegnaro, P. Scott, I.K. O'Neill and H. Bartsch
1983; 455 pages £32.50

No. 45 Environmental Carcinogens. Selected Methods of Analysis. Volume 6: N-Nitroso Compounds
Edited by R. Preussmann, I.K. O'Neill, G. Eisenbrand, B. Spiegelhalder and H. Bartsch
1983; 508 pages £32.50

No. 46 Directory of On-going Research in Cancer Epidemiology 1982
Edited by C.S. Muir and G. Wagner
1982; 722 pages (*out of print*)

No. 47 Cancer Incidence in Singapore 1968–1977
Edited by K. Shanmugaratnam, H.P. Lee and N.E. Day
1983; 171 pages (*out of print*)

No. 48 Cancer Incidence in the USSR (2nd Revised Edition)
Edited by N.P. Napalkov, G.F. Tserkovny, V.M. Merabishvili, D.M. Parkin, M. Smans and C.S. Muir
1983; 75 pages (*out of print*)

No. 49 Laboratory Decontamination and Destruction of Carcinogens in Laboratory Wastes: Some Polycyclic Aromatic Hydrocarbons
Edited by M. Castegnaro *et al.*
1983; 87 pages (*out of print*)

No. 50 Directory of On-going Research in Cancer Epidemiology 1983
Edited by C.S. Muir and G. Wagner
1983; 731 pages (*out of print*)

No. 51 Modulators of Experimental Carcinogenesis
Edited by V. Turusov and R. Montesano
1983; 307 pages (*out of print*)

List of IARC Publications

No. 52 Second Cancers in Relation to Radiation Treatment for Cervical Cancer: Results of a Cancer Registry Collaboration
Edited by N.E. Day and J.C. Boice, Jr
1984; 207 pages (*out of print*)

No. 53 Nickel in the Human Environment
Editor-in-Chief: F.W. Sunderman, Jr
1984; 529 pages (*out of print*)

No. 54 Laboratory Decontamination and Destruction of Carcinogens in Laboratory Wastes: Some Hydrazines
Edited by M. Castegnaro et al.
1983; 87 pages (*out of print*)

No. 55 Laboratory Decontamination and Destruction of Carcinogens in Laboratory Wastes: Some N-Nitrosamides
Edited by M. Castegnaro et al.
1984; 66 pages (*out of print*)

No. 56 Models, Mechanisms and Etiology of Tumour Promotion
Edited by M. Börzsönyi, N.E. Day, K. Lapis and H. Yamasaki
1984; 532 pages (*out of print*)

No. 57 N-Nitroso Compounds: Occurrence, Biological Effects and Relevance to Human Cancer
Edited by I.K. O'Neill, R.C. von Borstel, C.T. Miller, J. Long and H. Bartsch
1984; 1013 pages (*out of print*)

No. 58 Age-related Factors in Carcinogenesis
Edited by A. Likhachev, V. Anisimov and R. Montesano
1985; 288 pages (*out of print*)

No. 59 Monitoring Human Exposure to Carcinogenic and Mutagenic Agents
Edited by A. Berlin, M. Draper, K. Hemminki and H. Vainio
1984; 457 pages (*out of print*)

No. 60 Burkitt's Lymphoma: A Human Cancer Model
Edited by G. Lenoir, G. O'Conor and C.L.M. Olweny
1985; 484 pages (*out of print*)

No. 61 Laboratory Decontamination and Destruction of Carcinogens in Laboratory Wastes: Some Haloethers
Edited by M. Castegnaro et al.
1985; 55 pages (*out of print*)

No. 62 Directory of On-going Research in Cancer Epidemiology 1984
Edited by C.S. Muir and G. Wagner
1984; 717 pages (*out of print*)

No. 63 Virus-associated Cancers in Africa
Edited by A.O. Williams, G.T. O'Conor, G.B. de-Thé and C.A. Johnson
1984; 773 pages (*out of print*)

No. 64 Laboratory Decontamination and Destruction of Carcinogens in Laboratory Wastes: Some Aromatic Amines and 4-Nitrobiphenyl
Edited by M. Castegnaro et al.
1985; 84 pages (*out of print*)

No. 65 Interpretation of Negative Epidemiological Evidence for Carcinogenicity
Edited by N.J. Wald and R. Doll
1985; 232 pages (*out of print*)

No. 66 The Role of the Registry in Cancer Control
Edited by D.M. Parkin, G. Wagner and C.S. Muir
1985; 152 pages £10.00

No. 67 Transformation Assay of Established Cell Lines: Mechanisms and Application
Edited by T. Kakunaga and H. Yamasaki
1985; 225 pages (*out of print*)

No. 68 Environmental Carcinogens. Selected Methods of Analysis. Volume 7. Some Volatile Halogenated Hydrocarbons
Edited by L. Fishbein and I.K. O'Neill
1985; 479 pages (*out of print*)

No. 69 Directory of On-going Research in Cancer Epidemiology 1985
Edited by C.S. Muir and G. Wagner
1985; 745 pages (*out of print*)

No. 70 The Role of Cyclic Nucleic Acid Adducts in Carcinogenesis and Mutagenesis
Edited by B. Singer and H. Bartsch
1986; 467 pages (*out of print*)

No. 71 Environmental Carcinogens. Selected Methods of Analysis. Volume 8: Some Metals: As, Be, Cd, Cr, Ni, Pb, Se, Zn
Edited by I.K. O'Neill, P. Schuller and L. Fishbein
1986; 485 pages (*out of print*)

No. 72 Atlas of Cancer in Scotland, 1975–1980. Incidence and Epidemiological Perspective
Edited by I. Kemp, P. Boyle, M. Smans and C.S. Muir
1985; 285 pages (*out of print*)

No. 73 Laboratory Decontamination and Destruction of Carcinogens in Laboratory Wastes: Some Antineoplastic Agents
Edited by M. Castegnaro et al.
1985; 163 pages £12.50

No. 74 Tobacco: A Major International Health Hazard
Edited by D. Zaridze and R. Peto
1986; 324 pages £22.50

No. 75 Cancer Occurrence in Developing Countries
Edited by D.M. Parkin
1986; 339 pages £22.50

No. 76 Screening for Cancer of the Uterine Cervix
Edited by M. Hakama, A.B. Miller and N.E. Day
1986; 315 pages £30.00

No. 77 Hexachlorobenzene: Proceedings of an International Symposium
Edited by C.R. Morris and J.R.P. Cabral
1986; 668 pages (*out of print*)

No. 78 Carcinogenicity of Alkylating Cytostatic Drugs
Edited by D. Schmähl and J.M. Kaldor
1986; 337 pages (*out of print*)

No. 79 Statistical Methods in Cancer Research. Volume III: The Design and Analysis of Long-term Animal Experiments
By J.J. Gart, D. Krewski, P.N. Lee, R.E. Tarone and J. Wahrendorf
1986; 213 pages £22.00

List of IARC Publications

No. 80 Directory of On-going Research in Cancer Epidemiology 1986
Edited by C.S. Muir and G. Wagner
1986; 805 pages (*out of print*)

No. 81 Environmental Carcinogens: Methods of Analysis and Exposure Measurement. Volume 9: Passive Smoking
Edited by I.K. O'Neill, K.D. Brunnemann, B. Dodet and D. Hoffmann
1987; 383 pages £35.00

No. 82 Statistical Methods in Cancer Research. Volume II: The Design and Analysis of Cohort Studies
By N.E. Breslow and N.E. Day
1987; 404 pages £25.00

No. 83 Long-term and Short-term Assays for Carcinogens: A Critical Appraisal
Edited by R. Montesano, H. Bartsch, H. Vainio, J. Wilbourn and H. Yamasaki
1986; 575 pages £35.00

No. 84 The Relevance of *N*-Nitroso Compounds to Human Cancer: Exposure and Mechanisms
Edited by H. Bartsch, I.K. O'Neill and R. Schulte-Hermann
1987; 671 pages (*out of print*)

No. 85 Environmental Carcinogens: Methods of Analysis and Exposure Measurement. Volume 10: Benzene and Alkylated Benzenes
Edited by L. Fishbein and I.K. O'Neill
1988; 327 pages £40.00

No. 86 Directory of On-going Research in Cancer Epidemiology 1987
Edited by D.M. Parkin and J. Wahrendorf
1987; 676 pages (*out of print*)

No. 87 International Incidence of Childhood Cancer
Edited by D.M. Parkin, C.A. Stiller, C.A. Bieber, G.J. Draper, B. Terracini and J.L. Young
1988; 401 pages £35.00

No. 88 Cancer Incidence in Five Continents Volume V
Edited by C. Muir, J. Waterhouse, T. Mack, J. Powell and S. Whelan
1987; 1004 pages £55.00

No. 89 Method for Detecting DNA Damaging Agents in Humans: Applications in Cancer Epidemiology and Prevention
Edited by H. Bartsch, K. Hemminki and I.K. O'Neill
1988; 518 pages £50.00

No. 90 Non-occupational Exposure to Mineral Fibres
Edited by J. Bignon, J. Peto and R. Saracci
1989; 500 pages £50.00

No. 91 Trends in Cancer Incidence in Singapore 1968–1982
Edited by H.P. Lee, N.E. Day and K. Shanmugaratnam
1988; 160 pages (*out of print*)

No. 92 Cell Differentiation, Genes and Cancer
Edited by T. Kakunaga, T. Sugimura, L. Tomatis and H. Yamasaki
1988; 204 pages £27.50

No. 93 Directory of On-going Research in Cancer Epidemiology 1988
Edited by M. Coleman and J. Wahrendorf
1988; 662 pages (*out of print*)

No. 94 Human Papillomavirus and Cervical Cancer
Edited by N. Muñoz, F.X. Bosch and O.M. Jensen
1989; 154 pages £22.50

No. 95 Cancer Registration: Principles and Methods
Edited by O.M. Jensen, D.M. Parkin, R. MacLennan, C.S. Muir and R. Skeet
1991; 288 pages £28.00

No. 96 Perinatal and Multigeneration Carcinogenesis
Edited by N.P. Napalkov, J.M. Rice, L. Tomatis and H. Yamasaki
1989; 436 pages £50.00

No. 97 Occupational Exposure to Silica and Cancer Risk
Edited by L. Simonato, A.C. Fletcher, R. Saracci and T. Thomas
1990; 124 pages £22.50

No. 98 Cancer Incidence in Jewish Migrants to Israel, 1961–1981
Edited by R. Steinitz, D.M. Parkin, J.L. Young, C.A. Bieber and L. Katz
1989; 320 pages £35.00

No. 99 Pathology of Tumours in Laboratory Animals, Second Edition, Volume 1, Tumours of the Rat
Edited by V.S. Turusov and U. Mohr
740 pages £85.00

No. 100 Cancer: Causes, Occurrence and Control
Editor-in-Chief L. Tomatis
1990; 352 pages £24.00

No. 101 Directory of On-going Research in Cancer Epidemiology 1989/90
Edited by M. Coleman and J. Wahrendorf
1989; 818 pages £40.00

No. 102 Patterns of Cancer in Five Continents
Edited by S.L. Whelan, D.M. Parkin & E. Masuyer
1990; 162 pages £25.00

No. 103 Evaluating Effectiveness of Primary Prevention of Cancer
Edited by M. Hakama, V. Beral, J.W. Cullen and D.M. Parkin
1990; 250 pages £32.00

No. 104 Complex Mixtures and Cancer Risk
Edited by H. Vainio, M. Sorsa and A.J. McMichael
1990; 442 pages £38.00

No. 105 Relevance to Human Cancer of *N*-Nitroso Compounds, Tobacco Smoke and Mycotoxins
Edited by I.K. O'Neill, J. Chen and H. Bartsch
1991; 614 pages £70.00

No. 106 Atlas of Cancer Incidence in the Former German Democratic Republic
Edited by W.H. Mehnert, M. Smans, C.S. Muir, M. Möhner & D. Schön
1992; 384 pages £55.00

List of IARC Publications

No. 107 **Atlas of Cancer Mortality in the European Economic Community**
Edited by M. Smans, C.S. Muir and P. Boyle
1992; 280 pages £35.00

No. 108 **Environmental Carcinogens: Methods of Analysis and Exposure Measurement. Volume 11: Polychlorinated Dioxins and Dibenzofurans**
Edited by C. Rappe, H.R. Buser, B. Dodet and I.K. O'Neill
1991; 426 pages £45.00

No. 109 **Environmental Carcinogens: Methods of Analysis and Exposure Measurement. Volume 12: Indoor Air Contaminants**
Edited by B. Seifert, H. van de Wiel, B. Dodet and I.K. O'Neill
1993; 384 pages £45.00

No. 110 **Directory of On-going Research in Cancer Epidemiology 1991**
Edited by M. Coleman and J. Wahrendorf
1991; 753 pages £38.00

No. 111 **Pathology of Tumours in Laboratory Animals, Second Edition, Volume 2, Tumours of the Mouse**
Edited by V.S. Turusov and U. Mohr
1993; 776 pages; £90.00

No. 112 **Autopsy in Epidemiology and Medical Research**
Edited by E. Riboli and M. Delendi
1991; 288 pages £25.00

No. 113 **Laboratory Decontamination and Destruction of Carcinogens in Laboratory Wastes: Some Mycotoxins**
Edited by M. Castegnaro, J. Barek, J.–M. Frémy, M. Lafontaine, M. Miraglia, E.B. Sansone and G.M. Telling
1991; 64 pages £11.00

No. 114 **Laboratory Decontamination and Destruction of Carcinogens in Laboratory Wastes: Some Polycyclic Heterocyclic Hydrocarbons**
Edited by M. Castegnaro, J. Barek J. Jacob, U. Kirso, M. Lafontaine, E.B. Sansone, G.M. Telling and T. Vu Duc
1991; 50 pages £8.00

No. 115 **Mycotoxins, Endemic Nephropathy and Urinary Tract Tumours**
Edited by M. Castegnaro, R. Plestina, G. Dirheimer, I.N. Chernozemsky and H Bartsch
1991; 340 pages £45.00

No. 116 **Mechanisms of Carcinogenesis in Risk Identification**
Edited by H. Vainio, P.N. Magee, D.B. McGregor & A.J. McMichael
1992; 616 pages £65.00

No. 117 **Directory of On-going Research in Cancer Epidemiology 1992**
Edited by M. Coleman, J. Wahrendorf & E. Démaret
1992; 773 pages £42.00

No. 118 **Cadmium in the Human Environment: Toxicity and Carcinogenicity**
Edited by G.F. Nordberg, R.F.M. Herber & L. Alessio
1992; 470 pages £60.00

No. 119 **The Epidemiology of Cervical Cancer and Human Papillomavirus**
Edited by N. Muñoz, F.X. Bosch, K.V. Shah & A. Meheus
1992; 288 pages £28.00

No. 120 **Cancer Incidence in Five Continents, Volume VI**
Edited by D.M. Parkin, C.S. Muir, S.L. Whelan, Y.T. Gao, J. Ferlay & J.Powell
1992; 1080 pages £120.00

No. 121 **Trends in Cancer Incidence and Mortality**
M.P. Coleman, J. Estève, P. Damiecki, A. Arslan and H. Renard
1993; 806 pages, £120.00

No. 122 **International Classification of Rodent Tumours. Part 1. The Rat**
Editor-in-Chief: U. Mohr
1992/93; 10 fascicles of 60–100 pages, £120.00

No. 123 **Cancer in Italian Migrant Populations**
Edited by M. Geddes, D.M. Parkin, M. Khlat, D. Balzi and E. Buiatti
1993; 292 pages, £40.00

No. 124 **Postlabelling Methods for Detection of DNA Adducts**
Edited by D.H. Phillips, M. Castegnaro and H. Bartsch
1993; 392 pages; £46.00

No. 125 **DNA Adducts: Identification and Biological Significance**
Edited by K. Hemminki, A. Dipple, D. Shuker, F.F. Kadlubar, D. Segerbäck and H. Bartsch
1994; 480 pages; £52.00

No. 127 **Butadiene and Styrene: Assessment of Health Hazards.**
Edited by M. Sorsa, K. Peltonen, H. Vainio and K. Hemminki
1993; 412 pages; £54.00

No. 130 **Directory of On-going Research in Cancer Epidemiology 1994**
Edited by R. Sankaranarayanan, J. Wahrendorf and E. Démaret
1994; 792 pages, £46.00

List of IARC Publications

IARC MONOGRAPHS ON THE EVALUATION OF CARCINOGENIC RISKS TO HUMANS

(Available from booksellers through the network of WHO Sales Agents)

Volume 1 **Some Inorganic Substances, Chlorinated Hydrocarbons, Aromatic Amines, N-Nitroso Compounds, and Natural Products**
1972; 184 pages (*out of print*)

Volume 2 **Some Inorganic and Organometallic Compounds**
1973; 181 pages (*out of print*)

Volume 3 **Certain Polycyclic Aromatic Hydrocarbons and Heterocyclic Compounds**
1973; 271 pages (*out of print*)

Volume 4 **Some Aromatic Amines, Hydrazine and Related Substances, N-Nitroso Compounds and Miscellaneous Alkylating Agents**
1974; 286 pages Sw. fr. 18.–

Volume 5 **Some Organochlorine Pesticides**
1974; 241 pages (*out of print*)

Volume 6 **Sex Hormones**
1974; 243 pages (*out of print*)

Volume 7 **Some Anti-Thyroid and Related Substances, Nitrofurans and Industrial Chemicals**
1974; 326 pages (*out of print*)

Volume 8 **Some Aromatic Azo Compounds**
1975; 357 pages Sw. fr. 44.–

Volume 9 **Some Aziridines, N-, S- and O-Mustards and Selenium**
1975; 268 pages Sw.fr. 33.–

Volume 10 **Some Naturally Occurring Substances**
1976; 353 pages (*out of print*)

Volume 11 **Cadmium, Nickel, Some Epoxides, Miscellaneous Industrial Chemicals and General Considerations on Volatile Anaesthetics**
1976; 306 pages (*out of print*)

Volume 12 **Some Carbamates, Thiocarbamates and Carbazides**
1976; 282 pages Sw. fr. 41.-

Volume 13 **Some Miscellaneous Pharmaceutical Substances**
1977; 255 pages Sw. fr. 36.–

Volume 14 **Asbestos**
1977; 106 pages (*out of print*)

Volume 15 **Some Fumigants, The Herbicides 2,4-D and 2,4,5-T, Chlorinated Dibenzodioxins and Miscellaneous Industrial Chemicals**
1977; 354 pages (*out of print*)

Volume 16 **Some Aromatic Amines and Related Nitro Compounds - Hair Dyes, Colouring Agents and Miscellaneous Industrial Chemicals**
1978; 400 pages Sw. fr. 60.–

Volume 17 **Some N-Nitroso Compounds**
1978; 365 pages Sw. fr. 60.–

Volume 18 **Polychlorinated Biphenyls and Polybrominated Biphenyls**
1978; 140 pages Sw. fr. 24.–

Volume 19 **Some Monomers, Plastics and Synthetic Elastomers, and Acrolein**
1979; 513 pages (*out of print*)

Volume 20 **Some Halogenated Hydrocarbons**
1979; 609 pages (*out of print*)

Volume 21 **Sex Hormones (II)**
1979; 583 pages Sw. fr. 72.–

Volume 22 **Some Non-Nutritive Sweetening Agents**
1980; 208 pages Sw. fr. 30.–

Volume 23 **Some Metals and Metallic Compounds**
1980; 438 pages (*out of print*)

Volume 24 **Some Pharmaceutical Drugs**
1980; 337 pages Sw. fr. 48.–

Volume 25 **Wood, Leather and Some Associated Industries**
1981; 412 pages Sw. fr. 72.–

Volume 26 **Some Antineoplastic and Immunosuppressive Agents**
1981; 411 pages Sw. fr. 75.–

Volume 27 **Some Aromatic Amines, Anthraquinones and Nitroso Compounds, and Inorganic Fluorides Used in Drinking Water and Dental Preparations**
1982; 341 pages Sw. fr. 48.–

Volume 28 **The Rubber Industry**
1982; 486 pages Sw. fr. 84.–

Volume 29 **Some Industrial Chemicals and Dyestuffs**
1982; 416 pages Sw. fr. 72.–

Volume 30 **Miscellaneous Pesticides**
1983; 424 pages Sw. fr. 72.–

Volume 31 **Some Food Additives, Feed Additives and Naturally Occurring Substances**
1983; 314 pages Sw. fr. 66.–

Volume 32 **Polynuclear Aromatic Compounds, Part 1: Chemical, Environmental and Experimental Data**
1983; 477 pages Sw. fr. 88.–

Volume 33 **Polynuclear Aromatic Compounds, Part 2: Carbon Blacks, Mineral Oils and Some Nitroarenes**
1984; 245 pages (*out of print*)

Volume 34 **Polynuclear Aromatic Compounds, Part 3: Industrial Exposures in Aluminium Production, Coal Gasification, Coke Production, and Iron and Steel Founding**
1984; 219 pages Sw. fr. 53.–

Volume 35 **Polynuclear Aromatic Compounds, Part 4: Bitumens, Coal-tars and Derived Products, Shale-oils and Soots**
1985; 271 pages Sw. fr. 77.–

List of IARC Publications

Volume 36 **Allyl Compounds, Aldehydes, Epoxides and Peroxides**
1985; 369 pages Sw. fr. 77.–

Volume 37 **Tobacco Habits Other than Smoking: Betel-quid and Areca-nut Chewing; and some Related Nitrosamines**
1985; 291 pages Sw. fr. 77.–

Volume 38 **Tobacco Smoking**
1986; 421 pages Sw. fr. 83.–

Volume 39 **Some Chemicals Used in Plastics and Elastomers**
1986; 403 pages Sw. fr. 83.–

Volume 40 **Some Naturally Occurring and Synthetic Food Components, Furocoumarins and Ultraviolet Radiation**
1986; 444 pages Sw. fr. 83.–

Volume 41 **Some Halogenated Hydrocarbons and Pesticide Exposures**
1986; 434 pages Sw. fr. 83.–

Volume 42 **Silica and Some Silicates**
1987; 289 pages Sw. fr. 72.

Volume 43 **Man-Made Mineral Fibres and Radon**
1988; 300 pages Sw. fr. 72.–

Volume 44 **Alcohol Drinking**
1988; 416 pages Sw. fr. 83.

Volume 45 **Occupational Exposures in Petroleum Refining; Crude Oil and Major Petroleum Fuels**
1989; 322 pages Sw. fr. 72.–

Volume 46 **Diesel and Gasoline Engine Exhausts and Some Nitroarenes**
1989; 458 pages Sw. fr. 83.–

Volume 47 **Some Organic Solvents, Resin Monomers and Related Compounds, Pigments and Occupational Exposures in Paint Manufacture and Painting**
1989; 535 pages Sw. fr. 94.–

Volume 48 **Some Flame Retardants and Textile Chemicals, and Exposures in the Textile Manufacturing Industry**
1990; 345 pages Sw. fr. 72.–

Volume 49 **Chromium, Nickel and Welding**
1990; 677 pages Sw. fr. 105.–

Volume 50 **Pharmaceutical Drugs**
1990; 415 pages Sw. fr. 93.–

Volume 51 **Coffee, Tea, Mate, Methylxanthines and Methylglyoxal**
1991; 513 pages Sw. fr. 88.–

Volume 52 **Chlorinated Drinking-water; Chlorination By-products; Some Other Halogenated Compounds; Cobalt and Cobalt Compounds**
1991; 544 pages Sw. fr. 88.–

Volume 53 **Occupational Exposures in Insecticide Application and some Pesticides**
1991; 612 pages Sw. fr. 105.–

Volume 54 **Occupational Exposures to Mists and Vapours from Strong Inorganic Acids; and Other Industrial Chemicals**
1992; 336 pages Sw. fr. 72.–

Volume 55 **Solar and Ultraviolet Radiation**
1992; 316 pages Sw. fr. 65.–

Volume 56 **Some Naturally Occurring Substances: Food Items and Constituents, Heterocyclic Aromatic Amines and Mycotoxins**
1993; 600 pages Sw. fr. 95.–

Volume 57 **Occupational Exposures of Hairdressers and Barbers and Personal Use of Hair Colourants; Some Hair Dyes, Cosmetic Colourants, Industrial Dyestuffs and Aromatic Amines**
1993; 428 pages Sw. fr. 75.–

Volume 58 **Beryllium, Cadmium, Mercury and Exposures in the Glass Manufacturing Industry**
1993; 426 pages Sw. fr. 75.–

Volume 59 **Hepatitis Viruses**
1994; 286 pages Sw. fr. 65.–

Supplement No. 1
Chemicals and Industrial Processes Associated with Cancer in Humans (IARC Monographs, Volumes 1 to 20)
1979; 71 pages (*out of print*)

Supplement No. 2
Long-term and Short-term Screening Assays for Carcinogens: A Critical Appraisal
1980; 426 pages Sw. fr. 40.–

Supplement No. 3
Cross Index of Synonyms and Trade Names in Volumes 1 to 26
1982; 199 pages (*out of print*)

Supplement No. 4
Chemicals, Industrial Processes and Industries Associated with Cancer in Humans (IARC Monographs, Volumes 1 to 29)
1982; 292 pages (*out of print*)

Supplement No. 5
Cross Index of Synonyms and Trade Names in Volumes 1 to 36
1985; 259 pages (*out of print*)

Supplement No. 6
Genetic and Related Effects: An Updating of Selected IARC Monographs from Volumes 1 to 42
1987; 729 pages Sw. fr. 80.–

Supplement No. 7
Overall Evaluations of Carcinogenicity: An Updating of IARC Monographs Volumes 1-42
1987; 440 pages Sw. fr. 65.–

Supplement No. 8
Cross Index of Synonyms and Trade Names in Volumes 1 to 46
1990; 346 pages Sw. fr. 60.–

List of IARC Publications

IARC TECHNICAL REPORTS*

No. 1 **Cancer in Costa Rica**
Edited by R. Sierra,
R. Barrantes, G. Muñoz Leiva, D.M. Parkin, C.A. Bieber and
N. Muñoz Calero
1988; 124 pages Sw. fr. 30.-

No. 2 **SEARCH: A Computer Package to Assist the Statistical Analysis of Case-control Studies**
Edited by G.J. Macfarlane,
P. Boyle and P. Maisonneuve
1991; 80 pages (*out of print*)

No. 3 **Cancer Registration in the European Economic Community**
Edited by M.P. Coleman and
E. Démaret
1988; 188 pages Sw. fr. 30.-

No. 4 **Diet, Hormones and Cancer: Methodological Issues for Prospective Studies**
Edited by E. Riboli and
R. Saracci
1988; 156 pages Sw. fr. 30.-

No. 5 **Cancer in the Philippines**
Edited by A.V. Laudico,
D. Esteban and D.M. Parkin
1989; 186 pages Sw. fr. 30.-

No. 6 **La genèse du Centre International de Recherche sur le Cancer**
Par R. Sohier et A.G.B. Sutherland
1990; 104 pages Sw. fr. 30.-

No. 7 **Epidémiologie du cancer dans les pays de langue latine**
1990; 310 pages Sw. fr. 30.-

No. 8 **Comparative Study of Antismoking Legislation in Countries of the European Economic Community**
Edited by A. Sasco, P. Dalla Vorgia and P. Van der Elst
1992; 82 pages Sw. fr. 30.-

No. 9 **Epidemiologie du cancer dans les pays de langue latine**
1991 346 pages Sw. fr. 30.-

No. 11 **Nitroso Compounds: Biological Mechanisms, Exposures and Cancer Etiology**
Edited by I.K. O'Neill & H. Bartsch
1992; 149 pages Sw. fr. 30.-

No. 12 **Epidémiologie du cancer dans les pays de langue latine**
1992; 375 pages Sw. fr. 30.-

No. 13 **Health, Solar UV Radiation and Environmental Change**
By A. Kricker, B.K. Armstrong, M.E. Jones and R.C. Burton
1993; 216 pages Sw.fr. 30.—

No. 14 **Epidémiologie du cancer dans les pays de langue latine**
1993; 385 pages Sw. fr. 30.-

No. 15 **Cancer in the African Population of Bulawayo, Zimbabwe, 1963–1977: Incidence, Time Trends and Risk Factors**
By M.E.G. Skinner, D.M. Parkin, A.P. Vizcaino and A. Ndhlovu
1993; 123 pages Sw. fr. 30.-

No. 16 **Cancer in Thailand, 1988–1991**
By V. Vatanasapt, N. Martin, H. Sriplung, K. Vindavijak, S. Sontipong, S. Sriamporn, D.M. Parkin and J. Ferlay
1993; 164 pages Sw. fr. 30.-

DIRECTORY OF AGENTS BEING TESTED FOR CARCINOGENICITY (Until Vol. 13 Information Bulletin on the Survey of Chemicals Being Tested for Carcinogenicity)*

No. 8 Edited by M.-J. Ghess,
H. Bartsch and L. Tomatis
1979; 604 pages Sw. fr. 40.-

No. 9 Edited by M.-J. Ghess,
J.D. Wilbourn, H. Bartsch and
L. Tomatis
1981; 294 pages Sw. fr. 41.-

No. 10 Edited by M.-J. Ghess,
J.D. Wilbourn and H. Bartsch
1982; 362 pages Sw. fr. 42.-

No. 11 Edited by M.-J. Ghess,
J.D. Wilbourn, H. Vainio and
H. Bartsch
1984; 362 pages Sw. fr. 50.-

No. 12 Edited by M.-J. Ghess,
J.D. Wilbourn, A. Tossavainen and H. Vainio
1986; 385 pages Sw. fr. 50.-

No. 13 Edited by M.-J. Ghess,
J.D. Wilbourn and A. Aitio 1988; 404 pages Sw. fr. 43.-

No. 14 Edited by M.-J. Ghess,
J.D. Wilbourn and H. Vainio
1990; 370 pages Sw. fr. 45.-

No. 15 Edited by M.-J. Ghess, J.D. Wilbourn and H. Vainio
1992; 318 pages Sw. fr. 45.-

NON-SERIAL PUBLICATIONS

Alcool et Cancer†
By A. Tuyns (in French only)
1978; 42 pages Fr. fr. 35.-

Cancer Morbidity and Causes of Death Among Danish Brewery Workers†
By O.M. Jensen
1980; 143 pages Fr. fr. 75.-

Directory of Computer Systems Used in Cancer Registries†
By H.R. Menck and D.M. Parkin
1986; 236 pages Fr. fr. 50.-

Facts and Figures of Cancer in the European Community*
Edited by J. Estève, A. Kricker, J. Ferlay and D.M. Parkin
1993; 52 pages Sw. fr. 10.-

---

* Available from booksellers through the network of WHO Sales agents.

† Available directly from IARC

IARC Monographs are distributed
by the
World Health Organization,
Distribution and Sales Service,
1211 Geneva 27, Switzerland
and are available from booksellers
through the network of WHO Sales Agents.

A list of these Agents may be obtained
by writing to the above address.